# Exploring New Vistas in Health Care

# Exploring New Vistas in Health Care

*Edited by*

## JOHN M. VIRGO

*Atlantic Economic Society*
*International Health Economics and Management Institute*
*Southern Illinois University at Edwardsville*


*Foreword by*

## C. EVERETT KOOP
*Surgeon General, United States Public Health Services*


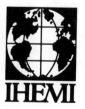

*International Health Economics and Management Institute*
*Box 101, Southern Illinois University at Edwardsville*
*Edwardsville, Illinois 62026*

Published by the International Health Economics and Management Institute, which assumes no responsibility for statements expressed by authors.

ISBN   0-914943-01-4
Library of Congress Catalog Card Number: 85-080123

*Printed in the United States of America*

# Contents

# PART SIX MANAGEMENT SYSTEMS

# PART SEVEN FRAUD AND THIRD PARTY REIMBURSEMENT

# PART EIGHT MARKETING HEALTH SERVICES

# PART NINE CASE STUDIES AND ANALYSES

# Foreword

## C. EVERETT KOOP

Surgeon General, United States Public Health Service

The preamble of the World Health Organization's constitution states, "The enjoyment of the highest attainable standard of health is one of the fundamental rights of every human being." This volume represents the initial collection of essays from the first official conference of the International Health Economics and Management Institute (IHEMI). It represents an important first step toward fostering improved international health among the nations of the world.

Health care offers probably the best and most fruitful opportunity to change the basic quality of life for all the people of the world. To the extent that the international health issue does not suffer political pressures and is free from parochial interests, providing adequate health care enjoys virtually universal support. To a large extent this commitment can be traced to the long history of battles against such fearful diseases as smallpox, malaria, yellow fever, and various diarrheal diseases, some of which still afflict much of the developing world. Although for some nations it might be said that a pure self-interest motivates their concern about the health of other nations, this concern stems primarily,from long-standing cultural traditions of broad humanitarianism. For an effective commitment to international health, what is required is a willingness among nations, and the best minds within these nations, to develop a world-wide agenda to cope with the problems posed by poor health care.

Today health care is being given a higher and higher priority by heads of state than it has received in the past. This enhanced recognition is no doubt due in part to the recognition of the impact that a nation's health can have upon its own economic and social development.

The papers contained in this volume are another vehicle for the transfer of information concerning the explosion of ever escalating health care technology and knowledge among the nations of the world. Only by an international sharing of information and a bringing together of the best minds dealing with all facets of health care throughout the world can progress in this crucial area be accelerated. This volume hopefully will provide a foundation upon which subsequent conferences can build. The range of subjects covered is broad and diverse and the range of applicability extensive. Although still in its infancy, the International Health Economics and Management Institute fills a very real void and can complement greatly existing efforts in understanding and bringing about change in the field of economics of international health. The continued growth and expansion of the International Health Economics and Management Institute is looked forward to with high expectation.

# Introduction

## JOHN M. VIRGO, Editor

Fundamental changes are occurring today in health care systems throughout the world. In past decades, the health care environment remained relatively stable, highly isolated from governmental controls. Physicians and hospitals enjoyed a relative monopoly in the marketplace. This tranquility erupted when, in the past 20 years, governments infused massive amounts of money to bring high-quality care to all of society. Economic repercussions were pushed into the background because society felt a price tag could not be placed upon the right of the individual to receive needed health services.

By 1980, however, significant erosion of this philosophical construct started to occur. Increasing consumer demand, especially by a growing elderly population; esoteric technologies; new types of delivery systems; rising consumer expectations; and spiraling inflation forced a reevaluation of the impact economics has on the health sector. Today, many no longer view health services as distinct from other sectors of the economy. Conventional economic forces impact health care, just as they affect other industries in the private sector. In the pursuit of equal access to quality health care and improved quality of life for society, two fundamental problems have developed: increasing costs and the inability of governments to cover these costs.

Faced with financial insolvency in health programs, governments have now started to search for ways to allocate the limited health care resources. In many industrialized countries, this has led to a restructuring of health care delivery systems and financial institutions. The economic realities of rational and cost-effective use of a nation's limited resources are being applied in a revolutionary fashion to health care. The revolution, however, must not cause one to lose sight of the fundamental objective: providing citizens with their basic health care needs.

It is within this revolution that the International Health Economics and Management Institute was founded. The primary goal of the Institute is to improve and expand knowledge in health care economics and management systems. Fundamental health care issues are assessed by the Institute from an interdisciplinary, comparative viewpoint. Specialists in economics, management, finance, data processing, and marketing join forces to discuss and analyze the future of health care around the world. Industrialized countries, despite historical, cultural, political, and social diversity, share many common perspectives on health care problems. Much can be learned through open discussion of fundamental health issues and the ways in which various governments are responding to the challenge.

The International Health Economics and Management Institute addresses the needs of hospital administrators, educators, government officials, and business leaders interested in keeping up-to-date in the health care field by discussing innovative ideas and alternatives with top-level policymakers from around the world.

An initial meeting of world health leaders was held in Paris in 1983 to provide an open forum for assessing fundamental health care issues among industrialized countries. The success and interest stimulated by these meetings led to the formalization of the new International Health Economics and Management Institute. The Institute's inaugural conference was held in March 1984 in San Juan, Puerto Rico. Puerto Rico was an ideal setting for the charter meeting since that island state has undergone dramatic changes in health policy in recent years. Furthermore, Puerto Rico serves as a focal point for other Caribbean nations and is establishing itself as a world leader in innovative health care systems.

At the charter meeting in San Juan, the Institute brought together leading health care specialists from around the world. They addressed a wide range of current topics in over 40 seminars, dealing with all major aspects of the health care field. Recommendations were made about future governmental policies and programs needed to address the overriding issues of manageability of programs, cost-effectiveness, inefficiency, and the future viability of health care in a dynamically changing national and international environment.

The Institute holds one such international conference each year in order to provide an opportunity for health practitioners, educators, and business leaders to meet with high-level policymakers. Every odd-numbered year the conference is held in Europe and every even-numbered year it is held in the Caribbean. Selected papers from each conference are published in order to disseminate and initiate further discussion of pressing health issues.

This book represents the major areas of discussion of the 1984 Puerto Rican conference. The contributors to this book collectively represent a broad spectrum of views and ideas about present health care systems in a variety of countries. Ideas exchanged at the conference, through formal seminars and informal discussion meetings, were then incorporated into the authors' original manuscripts.

The book is not designed to answer all questions about health care policy but, rather, is designed to stimulate discussion and critical thinking. For the hospital administrator, certain chapters should prove helpful in obtaining greater understanding of how management systems are changing and of how new strategic management, financing, and marketing techniques can aid in meeting the changing internal and external environments. Business leaders will gain a better understanding of the changing dynamics of health policy, along with new and innovative ways that business can take advantage of new approaches to health care delivery. Policymakers will gain greater insight into the impact their decisions have on the industry and on society. The book should provide an indispensable aid to policymakers in their quest to overcome internal and external challenges to the health care environments.

Graduate-level students will find a wealth of state-of-the-art topics, ranging from governmental impact on the health care structure, to proactive management responses, to horizon scanning of future health sector developments. A unique array of the latest innovative management and governmental responses to today's health care revolution will provide the student with a firmer grasp of the economic, social, ethical, and political challenges faced by health care leaders in the mid-1980's.

In any work of this magnitude, no one person can be singled out for his or her efforts. The book has been the result of a truly group effort over the past two years. At the planning level for the conference in San Juan that set the stage for the book, special mention should be made of Enrique Baquero from San Juan and William Toby, Regional Director of the U.S. Health Care Financing Administration. Both freely gave endless hours of their time in helping to create a program that was professionally stimulating, educational, and demanding. Governor of Puerto Rico, Carlos Romero-Barceló, Secretary of Health for Puerto Rico, Jaime Rivera Dueno, Cooperativa de Seguros de Vida de Puerto Rico, Seguros de Servicio de Salud de Puerto Rico, Inc., the Tourism Company of Puerto Rico, and Blue Cross of Puerto Rico provided an open and receptive environment, a deeper appreciation for Caribbean health problems, and an unsurpassed hospitality.

The extraordinary support of Sol Seltzer, President of MCAUTO Systems Group, Inc., has made this book possible. Harry M. Neer, President of Presbyterian Hospital in Oklahoma City, has been a guiding and dedicated leader whose vision, search for excellence, and belief in the goals of the Institute provided the impetus to carry it forward during the formative years since 1983.

The editor would like to thank Kathy S. Virgo, Executive Administrator of the Institute, for her unwavering dedication, enormous enthusiasm, and total unselfishness in devoting endless hours to the creation of the new Institute. She willingly gave up vacations, holidays, and weekends to work on the enormous task of solidifying the contents of this book, working and reworking it for consistency, and rewriting the editor's scrambled notes. Her willingness to be a sounding board for the editor's unravelling thoughts has provided a constant source of tranquility and understanding.

Jonalyn S. Atherton, Assistant Coordinator of the Institute, performed the unenviable task of trying to keep the editor on schedule, communicating with authors, and typing the manuscripts. Her attention to detail and consistency has added to quality and readability throughout. Often working overtime, she injected an element of enthusiasm and excitement into an often laborious task.

Finally, endless hours of writing and rewriting by the authors, their commitment to improving the health care delivery system, and a willingness to share their knowledge and ideas with others have established the quality of their respective chapters. All of them deserve a special note of thanks for their hard work and devotion to health care.

# Part One

The Issues

# Chapter One

## Restructuring of the Health Care System

JOHN M. VIRGO

### Introduction

Criticism has rapidly grown in developing countries over the efficacy and adequacy of current health care delivery systems. Health care systems have come under close scrutiny because of spiraling costs; inequities in access to health care; conflicts among providers, patients, and third party payors; disparity of care; and moral and ethical dilemmas. Health care, as a right or a privilege for society, is being questioned. Conflicts are arising between traditional ideals of the sanctity of life and the quality of life. How should a society's scarce resources for health care be explicitly and implicitly rationed?

Two basic approaches to these issues are described throughout this chapter. Most countries, including the United States, have developed systems on a needs-based approach, providing health services to society regardless of the expected return on resource investment. Until recently, such an approach was considered socially responsible. Today, the needs-based approach is being questioned because of the inability of governments to contain rapidly rising costs in health care.

Becoming increasingly popular is the cost-benefit or utilitarian approach. This approach measures the cost of resources and the rate of return on investment. Policy is being altered to emphasize maximum net benefits to society, rather than the needs of the individual.

Whichever approach, or combination of approaches, is taken, fundamental economic, philosophical, and ethical issues must be considered. The question of who should receive health care must pass the close examination of people in a democratic society.

Major policy issues in Canada, the United States, and the Caribbean are described in this chapter. Significant reforms in the U.S. Medicare program are then evaluated, followed by an analysis of the impact those changes have had on the strategic management process in hospitals. Evolving management systems in the U.S., Canada, and Germany are described. Problems with fraud, abuse, and waste in health insurance programs are reviewed, followed by a study of new marketing techniques in a changing competitive environment. The final section describes case studies in a variety of health care settings.

1

## Health Care Policy

Health care policy is an integral part of the political, economic, legal, and social environment of any country. In democratic countries there exists a pluralistic arena in which semiautonomous and autonomous groups compete for influence in the decision making process.

As more and more groups enter this pluralistic arena, policymaking becomes more complex. When governments increase their spheres of influence to meet the competing demands of different pluralistic groups, hospital administrators find themselves faced with less autonomy and greater governmental regulation. In addition, attempts by governments to lower costs by interjecting more competition into the health sector has, ironically, increased regulation and lessened freedom of choice by management. It can be argued that the private market mechanism has given way to market control by governmental administrative agencies.

Recently, the rising cost of health care and the commensurate drain on the economy has led to an increased outcry in many countries to convert the health care industry into a more competitive, free-market environment. Consumer sovereignty and market freedom for health care providers, it has been argued, will bring about economic equilibrium on both the demand and supply sides of the health care market.

Movement toward market competition can bring about increased efficiency, increased use of limited resources, better management techniques, and a greater appreciation by the consumer of the cost of health care. The critical question is, will the consumer of health care services be punished for this increased competitive structure through diminution of quality and services, while paying a higher price?

These issues are addressed in the following three chapters. National health policy is critically analyzed in Chapter 2. Recent recommendations by the National Citizens' Board of Inquiry on American health care have suggested that the Canadian system should be used as a model in the United States. Malcolm G. Taylor compares the politics and historical development of the Canadian system with some of the main features found in the U.S. system.

Unlike the U.S. system, regulation of health care in Canada falls within the jurisdiction of the provinces rather than within the jurisdiction of federal government. However, as in the U.S., the federal government of Canada can exert pressure over the provinces by establishing eligibility requirements for provinces before they can receive federal grant monies. With total health expenditures rising to about 8 percent of Canadian GNP, strong incentives are being implemented by the federal government to restrict the rise in health care costs. Such incentives may well lead to a conflict situation among the provinces, special interest groups, and the federal government.

The Canadian experience demonstrates one of several reasonable alternatives U.S. policymakers should explore. If these alternative systems will work given the culture and political environment of the United States, these alternatives should be carefully analyzed. Critics of the Canadian system argue that it would not provide the necessary degree of market competition and is, therefore, not a viable solution. These critics see consumer and provider sovereignty in the market place as the only rational approach to cost containment in health care.

However, there are numerous pitfalls in the argument that laissez-faire competition will improve current health care problems. Free competition in the health sector is unrealistic, given the governmental and private institutional constraints that have developed over the years. Certainly, some of this institutionalization can be privitized and some movement can be made toward increased competition, even though one could realistically only expect such movement to be marginal at best.

An analysis of the underlying assumptions of the competitive marketplace, of health sector institutional constraints, and of the positive and negative implications of increased health sector competition are found in Chapter 3. Roger M. Battistella feels that the advantages of increased competition must be balanced against ethical and social considerations for the consumer. The philosophy of increased competition must not free the policymaker from moral responsibility for care of the sick. Consumer integrity and sovereignty must be preserved. Equity in the accessibility and quality of care must not give way to the pursuit of self-interest in a free-enterprise setting for the sake of cost containment. To do so, would be to circumvent the underlying ideals of the Medicare system.

To achieve a balance between the need for cost containment and the need for equity and quality of health care is the challenge facing today's policymakers. Disincentives toward cost containment were built into the Medicare system which must now be eliminated. Established hospital and physician practices must be reevaluated by both the private and governmental sectors. If the private sector does not respond in a positive manner, governmental agencies will be forced to step in to fill the void.

The private and public approaches to cost containment are now being heavily debated throughout the United States. If the public sector increases regulation through changing payment mechanisms, hospital administrators, physicians, and other groups will find increased restraints placed upon their decision making perogatives.

The current policy, according to Gloria R. Smith and Pamela Paul-Shaheen (Chapter 4), is simply a short-term attempt to shift costs and hold back spending by reducing benefit eligibility. True cost containment, in the long run, requires not only a reform of the existing delivery system, but also a shift of resources from a sickness to a wellness system. A number of policy approaches are suggested in Chapter 4 that will constrain expenditures, develop new delivery strategies for wellness and prevention, and encourage creation of additional revenues for new program development.

**Health Care Policy in the Caribbean**

The Caribbean islands have undergone dramatic change in recent decades. These islands are moving from the depths of poverty and disease to economic development, growth, and improved living standards. Most of the islands are moving forward through participatory democracy and are starting to overcome the problems of overpopulation, lack of mineral resources, an agrarian-based economy, geographic isolation, and years of colonialism. In the past 10 years, Caribbean Basin exports have increased 700 percent to over $700 million.

The Caribbean island of Puerto Rico provides an excellent example of how one such island state has propelled itself into a technologically sophisticated, industrialized society. Carlos Romero-Barceló, Governor of Puerto Rico, describes in Chapter 5 the remarkable success of the island over recent years. Much of Puerto Rico's economic growth has been in the service and high-tech industries. Assembling heart pacemakers; manufacturing of pharmaceuticals and computer components; communications; banking; data processing; and a variety of other industries have transformed the island into a competitive leader in the Caribbean.

Through the application of an aggressive health care policy, Puerto Rico has increased the life expectancy of its inhabitants from 46 years of age in the late 1930's to 74 years in 1984. Puerto Rico has emphasized the need for preventive medicine and democratized medical services. High-quality health care is guaranteed to all citizens. Cost containment has been accomplished through economies of scale.

Equity of care has been established in Puerto Rico by a unique system designed to eliminate the distinction between private and public hospitals. In the past six years, the government has constructed and equipped public hospitals. Private companies are then contracted to administer and staff the public hospitals. The result has been high-quality health care for all while decreasing the rate of expenditure increases.

Jaime Rivera Dueno, Puerto Rico's Secretary of Health, was instrumental in developing and implementing this new and unique health policy. In Chapter 6, he describes how democratization of health care has impacted on the quality of life of the Puerto Rican people. Responsibility for providing health care is divided by regions to increase efficiency, decrease costs, and increase availability of high quality care to all people. Preventive care is provided at the local level; curative care at a secondary level in area hospitals; and highly specialized care at a tertiary level in medical centers.

This three-tiered health system, combined with government-built hospitals contracting out to private management firms, has established a more efficient and equitable use of health care resources. Quality and access of health care has improved, while costs have decreased.

The Puerto Rican system is, however, not without its critics. Some argue that the democratization policy will, over time, lead to socialized medicine and an eroding of the private market system. Reinaldo A. Ferrer (Chapter 7) analyzes the new Puerto Rican system and evaluates its strengths and weaknesses.

Further complicating health care in Puerto Rico is the close relationship and dependency it has on the changing U.S. economy. For example, capital formation, technological change, employment, industrialization, and economic growth are all inexplicably linked to the ebbs and flows of changing policy in Washington. Jesus M. Rodriguez (Chapter 8) reviews the implications of these interrelationships on the health care sector in Puerto Rico. He concludes that strong leadership in Puerto Rico's health care sector is needed if Puerto Rico is to adjust to the complexities of an ever changing political and economic environment.

## Medicare

Health care policy today, for all countries, must address the issue of controlling spiraling costs while maintaining equity, access, and quality of care. In 1965, Medicare was introduced in the United States to provide basic protection for the elderly and disabled. By 1980, it became apparent that if Medicare was to avoid bankruptcy, prompt and decisive policies needed to be enacted.

In the political arena, and throughout the entire country, questions regarding the fundamental objectives of Medicare, its financial drain on society, and in what form it should survive became hotly debated. These debates have resulted in the initiation of a landmark period in health care reform by the Reagan Administration. A new and controversial prospective payment system has been applied to hospitals and will be extended to physicians in the near future.

John M. Virgo (Chapter 9) considers the historical circumstances leading to the development of the new prospective payment system and the economic, political, and social environments of its implementation. Several areas have been impacted by prospective payment, including manpower, cost-shifting, and strategic management. Virgo also evaluates the future of Medicare and presents a number of alternative strategies to improve the present system.

Since the prospective payment system has not yet been fully phased in, it is difficult to accurately assess its long-term impact. In the short run, however, several positive economic externalities can be pointed out. Hospital administrators are starting to apply economic techniques, such as cost-benefit analysis, to their decision making. Medical record keeping in hospitals is being converted to a product line accounting system, composed of direct and indirect patient care expenditures. The federal government now pays for specific types of care at specific payment levels, based upon the types of care provided.

Carolyne K. Davis (Chapter 10), who is responsible for implementation of the new system, evaluates its various components, including outpatient payments, payments for rehabilitative and psychiatric services, and payments for physicians' services. Medical educational expenses and capital expenses are being considered for possible inclusion within the output-related payment system. Based upon the latest available data, Davis sees a clear pattern emerging: hospitals are concentrating on those types of care with high volume and high quality, which will promote greater overall specialization within the industry.

Professional Review Organizations (PRO's) have been established to evaluate any adverse reaction to the new prospective payment system. PRO's are responsible for ensuring that the quality of care is maintained. Any unnecessary utilization patterns by hospitals and physicians will be closely examined by the PRO's. The overall intent of PRO's, according to Davis, is to stimulate competition among hospitals in admissions and to promote the highest quality care at the lowest possible price.

Other initiatives have also been enacted which are designed to increase competition in health care. Health Maintenance Organizations (HMO's) and Competitive Medical Programs (CMP's) are two such initiatives. These developments are creating a revolution in the structure of the health care system. The entire industry is realigning itself, with new hybrid organizations being formed. Government policymakers and industry specialists are closely evaluating these changes and analyzing the future impact.

One such evaluation started in 1982 when the Advisory Council on Social Security was appointed to review the Medicare system. After 15 months of investigation, the Council made 26 sweeping recommendations to make Medicare financially viable. The chairman of the Council, former Governor of Indiana, Otis R. Bowen (Chapter 11); and two of its members, Richard W. Rahn (Chapter 12) and Thomas R. Burke (Chapter 13) discuss the findings of the Council and suggest alternatives for restructuring the Medicare system.

Six general areas are covered by the Council's recommendations: financing, eligibility, benefit structure, reimbursement, general issues, and future concerns. If implemented, these recommendations will provide solvency for the Medicare trust fund by 1995, according to Bowen. The Reagan Administration initiated some of those recommendations within a few months after they were presented to Congress. More controversial suggestions are now openly being debated and will take longer to become operational.

Health care policy, according to Rahn, should be changed so that health care is no longer a free economic good for the elderly. Since free goods are over-utilized, the introduction of prices will provide an incentive to switch to lower cost alternatives, such as home health care and nursing homes. To introduce the pricing mechanism into the system, however, requires providing the elderly with a means by which they can increase their savings for health care over their working years.

Establishment of a "health credit account" and a tax deductible health bank Individual Retirement Account would according to Rahn, provide a working person with a tax incentive to save now for health care expenditures upon retirement. Such a system would avoid tax increases, increase private market incentives, increase individual control and choice over medical coverage, and reduce health expenditures by the federal government.

An extension of this proposal is given by Burke. He recommends extending coverage to include catastrophic coverage, with Medicare continuing to cover basic health care needs. Part A and Part B would be combined and financed by a payroll tax. A new coinsurance program under Medicare would cover all medical expenses during a 12-month period, up to a catastrophic cap. Medicare costs would decrease, individual cost-consciousness would increase, and cost of catastrophic care would shift from Medicare to the individual's IMA. Freedom of choice by the individual is increased, since he can decide how his health care savings are to be spent.

**Strategic Planning**

The new prospective payment system, introduced in 1983, represented a major policy change in the way hospitals (and eventually physicians) were to be paid for services to Medicare patients. A rush of anxiety swept through the hospitals upon its introduction. Management called in consultants, bought systems to track costs, reduced staffs, and implemented new strategic planning techniques.

Management also closely reevaluated its quantitative and qualitative strategic planning techniques to discover the manner in which to adjust to the new policy directives. New ways had to be found for quantifying and evaluating data which had not previously been needed. More sophisticated use of computers, merging of clinical and financial information, and analyses of external environmental factors gave added emphasis to the need for strategic planning.

Lyndsey Stone (Chapter 14) sees the need for strategic planning increasing because of the complex internal and external environments in which the hospitals of today must operate. The new medical-industrial complex, dominated by for-profit corporations, uses strategic planning to remain at the forefront of these changing environments. Computerized management information systems provide an opportunity for system-wide strategic planning. Eight major obstacles are noted by Stone which must be overcome if strategic planning is to be successful in the hospital setting.

Movement to the new prospective payment system has also created strong incentives for administrators to shift costs to non-regulated payors. This may create higher costs for patients who are not covered by Medicare. Hospitals successful at cost-shifting will have less incentive to initiate cost-containment programs.

A model of hospital cost-shifting is developed by Michael D. Rosko in Chapter 15. The model is based upon the New Jersey Standard Hospital Accounting and Rate Evaluation program and illustrates how cost-shifting incentives may be created under prospective payment mechanisms. The implications of cost-shifting incentives are analyzed for inner-city hospitals as well as for hospitals located in other areas.

Strategic planning is essential for management control and survival. Integrative strategic management requires the application of policy, planning, and resources to the long-term goals and objectives of the hospital. In Chapter 16, Richard C. McKibbin views this new emphasis on strategic planning as it affects health professionals, non-professional health workers, and the structure of the delivery system. Traditional roles and relationships among all health care employees will be significantly altered. Hospital administrators are now working more closely with representatives from medical staffs, accounting, medical records, and nursing.

Conflict will surely increase between administrators, physicians, and nurses as professional and staffing relationships are reevaluated and changed. Physician autonomy will decrease as administrators emphasize limiting length of stay, reducing testing, and eliminating unnecessary procedures—all of which reduce the physician's income.

With drastic changes in strategic management, the budgeting, financing, accounting, costing, pricing, and marketing strategies have come under intensive scrutiny. Charles T. Wood (Chapter 17) analyzes new techniques of cost control, productivity, and resource usage in and among hospitals. He emphasizes the need to establish a networking system of two or more hospitals through the development of six management systems. Such a technique will lead to better cost identification, better productivity measurements, and increase resource utilization control.

## Management Systems

Response to environmental change causes all organizations to reevaluate their goals and objectives. Organizational change takes place internally and through external relationships, often leading to new management systems. Such systems can be behavioral or holistic in nature, can use input-output approaches, or can use a combination of these techniques. By taking a systems approach, unstructured environmental changes, which impact directly or indirectly on the organization, can be logically organized and delineated.

The system concept is applied to the health care field by Ronald E. Beller in Chapter 18. A model is developed for analyzing health care delivery systems through zones of interest, goals of the system and subsystems, system variables, and the environment. The model is applied to a specific example of a maternal and infant care program.

One of the problems of instituting new systems is the built-in resistance to change by many of those affected. The organization must attempt to modify this resistance by careful planning and communication throughout the hospital. R. Kenneth McGeorge (Chapter 19) considers the Canadian health care program and the response by one hospital to implement organizational change through a case mix management system.

Helmut Jung (Chapter 20) gives an example of a Berlin hospital that also anticipated negative reaction to organizational change and implemented a hospital information system. He analyzes why information systems are not typically used in German hospitals and suggests ways to implement organizational change and development.

Concern over behavior modification and changing delivery systems is at the heart of the present prospective payment system in the United States. Organizational change has started to take place as a result of a rapidly changing economic environment, the growth of for-profit multihospital corporations, reduced hospital revenues, and the government's incursion into the physician reward system.

Behavior modification, as assessed by Martha S. Albert in Chapter 21, leads to increased use of HMO's, self-improvement, and corporate health improvement plans. For individual health behavior to be modified, strategies need to be introduced to decrease resistance by those asked to accept more responsibility for their own health care. Wellness rather than illness must be emphasized. Health care delivery systems should be modified to include more physical fitness programs, carefully-devised motivational techniques, convenience of participation, and strong peer support. The responsibility for wellness should be shared by all groups: individuals; families; employers; and local, state, and federal governments.

Hospitals have reacted in a variety of ways to the new prospective payment delivery system. Resistance to the system has been vocal and hotly debated. Edward P. Robinson (Chapter 22) reviews these reactions and repercussions from the viewpoint of the hospital administrator who must adapt and implement these new systems. He feels that behavior modification and the creation of HMO's and PPO's may well increase the competitive health care environment. However, he warns that if hospitals are not compensated fairly and equitably, reactions will be triggered that might lead to a lower quality of care, refusal of care to indigent patients, and reduced services. Suggested alternatives are developed and analyzed.

### Fraud and Third Party Reimbursement

One area of recent concern over rising health care costs involves fraud, abuse, and waste in health insurance programs. Prices for new medical technology are not established in a competitive market setting, rather, they are heavily affected by governmental regulations and through negotiations with third party payors. Once prices are established, they become inflexible in a downward direction due to institutional constraints.

To test this hypothesis, Lewis Freiberg (Chapter 23) develops a model to describe the price-setting mechanism between providers and third parties, under conditions of high uncertainty. He concludes that the potential for significant overpayment by society for new technology exists because of the failure of the political and institutional processes. In addition, third party approval of high prices can lead to significant overpayment.

In Chapter 24, Frank W. Fournier agrees, in principle, with Freiberg but suggests that it is also necessary to look at three additional issues. The type of intervention, the instruments for intervention, and the mechanisms for intervention must be agreed upon to control fraud, abuse, and waste. Fournier describes a program taking place in Puerto Rico designed to implement incentives to reduce inefficient use of health resources. The key to reduction of fraud and abuse is prevention. Strong penalties are needed, coupled with mass media publicity to communicate to the public how these new mechanisms will control abuse, fraud, and waste.

## Marketing

Hospitals are becoming increasingly aware of the degree of competitiveness in the arena in which they compete. Modern marketing techniques, similar to those used by business in the private sector, are being implemented in many hospitals. Unfortunately, a larger number of hospitals do not recognize the nature and role of the marketing function. They instead use marketing activities in a random and haphazard manner.

Research by William J. Winston (Chapter 25) indicates that only recently have administrators targeted their potential markets with any degree of sophistication and planning. Psychographic and life-style analysis can be used in segmenting and targeting. From refined segments and targets, individualized marketing strategies can then be created and implemented to maximize the marketing effort. Using advanced statistical tools, the relationship between consumer's life-style and health service utilization can be constantly monitored and updated, leading to increased sensitivity in marketing health services.

For survival in today's rapidly changing environment, hospitals must develop a marketing campaign that would have been considered unprofessional as little as three years ago. As hospitals increase their services to the community, hospital structure and shape frequently change. Paul F. Detrick (Chapter 26) analyzes the impact this movement has had on hospitals and the stimulation of the entrepreneurial spirit within administration. Several examples are cited that typify dramatic changes occurring in marketing, finance, and entrepreneurship. Hospitals are venturing into for-profit, private enterprises that are often quite diversified from the hospital setting.

The life of the free-standing hospital will quickly end, according to Detrick. Remaining will be those hospitals whose administrators have broken out of the traditional, narrow image and have openly accepted the realities of the business world and the free market mechanism.

## Case Studies and Analyses

Patient scheduling can be an expensive part of clinical operations. Fixed and variable costs, if not properly contained, can lead to substantial losses if a clinic does not operate near full capacity. In Chapter 27, Voeller, Clegg, Wilcox, Straub, and Elevich develop a model for cost effective patient scheduling, using multiple variable techniques. Their model has widespread application to clinics, in general. The chapter explains how an appropriate level of overbooking can be determined in order to minimize the costs of under- and overbooking.

P. Donald Muhlenthaler (Chapter 28) analyzes labor productivity in a rural hospital setting. With fluctuating levels of admissions, a management system was implemented to control payroll and productivity. An incentive system for each hospital department was established, and every hospital employee was eligible to receive financial benefits if target rates were met or exceeded. The result was an increase in productivity, lower payroll costs, and a feeling by employees that they were partners with management in working for the hospital's success.

Increased public assistance to the elderly is reviewed by John P. Kemph in Chapter 29. Feelings of social responsibility to the aged and increased voting power by this cohort group have provided motivation for continued expenditures for their health benefits. Kemph evaluates legislation by the State of Ohio which required each of the state's medical schools to establish a division of geriatrics. He uses one specific medical school as an example of how the program was implemented and the positive impact it had on elderly patient care.

A study of a primary care delivery system for pregnant adolescents in New Jersey was conducted by Silverberg, Tama, Wallner, and Braitman (Chapter 30). The authors evaluated the short-term effectiveness of primary nursing care between pregnant adolescents in an experimental group and a control group. Results of the study surprisingly found that no significant differences existed in the short run between the two groups. The authors recommend that further long run factors need to be analyzed to see if a primary care delivery system is beneficial to pregnant adolescents.

Transforming a deficit hospital dental service into a self-supporting program is described in Chapter 31 by Stephen M. Patz. The dental profession, like other groups in health care, has been faced with increasing costs and a decreasing client population. Higher dental insurance deductibles and co-payments have exacerbated the problem. In a depressed urban environment, the local hospital often becomes the focal point for the poor and indigent seeking dental care. Development of an outpatient dental facility in a major urban setting is described by Patz, with special emphasis on cost control and hospital structure. He concludes that a strong dental service can have definite financial benefits, as well as other benefits for the hospital, while providing much needed dental care.

# Part Two

Evolving Health Care Policy

# Chapter Two

## The Politics of Canadian Health Policy

MALCOLM G. TAYLOR

"The friend of humanity cannot recognize a distinction between what is political and what is not.
"There is nothing that is not political. Everything is politics."

Thomas Mann,
*The Magic Mountain*

"Politics is but medicine writ large."

Rudolph Virchow

## Introduction

If one accepts the wisdom of these two statements, then it is appropriate to be discussing "politics" or "political economics" at this International Health Economics and Management Conference. And, of course, in the context of the title of this paper that means that the author shall confine himself primarily to Canadian politics. However, as in many countries, even that is not a consistent element for, as one wag has classified the Canadian political scene:

"In the Atlantic provinces, politics is a disease; in Quebec, politics is religion; in Ontario, politics is business; in the Western prairies, politics is protest; and in British Columbia, politics is entertainment."

It is regrettable that in democratic societies, the word "politics" has come to have an increasingly pejorative connotation. Public opinion polls show that confidence in the political system has declined along with that in other institutions. Whether they be corporations, unions, the universities, or even the churches. But the author feels that in their innermost being people know that politics—or in more precise terms, the political process—is the means by which a democratic society of free people governs itself, seeks to make progress, guarantees its civil liberties, protects its territory, and struggles to resolve peacefully its inevitable conflicts. One certainly knows, in Canada, that it is the political process that created the federation, built its railways, extended its territory from sea to sea, created its educational systems, assisted its commerce, mobilized for two World Wars, provided family allowances and social security, and, certainly not least, created one of the most comprehensive and equitably financed health care treatment systems in the world. It is in this positive sense that the author shall deal with the politics of Canadian health policy.

15

## The Political Process in Canada

The political process in Canada is unusually complex, with several layers, similar to an onion. The main reason for its complexity is, of course, that, like the American States in 1787, the framers of Canada's constitution adopted the *Federal System*. Unlike the American statesmen, however, they were determined that the central government should be the dominant partner in the relationship. But, interestingly, the vagaries of history, court decisions, and the fact that those growth industries of the twentieth century—health, welfare, and education—fall within the jurisdiction of the provinces, have frustrated that original intention. The federal government's power reached its apogee during World War II but since then the pendulum has swung inexorably to the provinces, with the result that negotiating with provincial governments became, in Professor Smiley's words, "Akin to those of effective international diplomacy."

The second major characteristic of the Canadian constitution is that it adopted the British *Cabinet System* rather than the U.S. separation of powers between executive and legislature. That is, all cabinet ministers must be members of Parliament and the government remains in office only as long as it can command a majority in the House of Commons. The majority is normally composed of one party, but since World War II three minority governments have been kept in office for as long as two years by the votes of one or another of the opposition parties.

The essential point here is what the author's political science professors at Berkeley used to emphasize: if public opinion in favor of a policy is strong, if the government has a majority, if the party caucus and cabinet are in agreement, then legislation will pass substantially as it was drafted. When the conditions are right, therefore, the British model provides for very strong and responsible government. Normally, there can be no buck–passing; one party, and one alone, is responsible.

All this, of course, depends on the third layer: the *political parties*. Here the picture is more confusing than in the United States. The traditional Canadian parties are the Liberals and Conservatives. But, since the Depression there have been four, the two new ones being the New Democratic Party and Social Credit. Moreover, each of the parties in Parliament controlled one or more provincial governments. The presence of third and fourth parties can be very disruptive, leading to minority governments or unstable coalitions. On the other hand, they can provide (as the era of the Lafollette Progressives attests) leadership for progressive legislation and leverage to get it passed. The New Democratic Party (NDP) did both, for it was the Saskatchewan New Democratic Government that first introduced universal hospital insurance and medical care insurance at the provincial level, and it was the NDP support in the House of Commons in Ottawa that enabled (and some would say, indirectly forced) the minority government of Lester Pearson to pass the Medical Care Act of 1966.

The fourth layer of this particular onion is the political role of the *organized medical profession*. Because health is a provincial responsibility, there are in each province two medical bodies: (1) the licensing authority, known as the College of Physicians and Surgeons; and (2) the political arm of the profession, the provincial Medical Association. The ten of these are linked in a federated system as divisions of the Canadian Medical Association (CMA). Each provincial division has a Committee on Economics and their ten chairmen form the CMA Council on Economics.

## Health Care and the Government

The beginning of the involvement of the profession with government in the payment for medical services for the general population dates back to 1914 when the first Municipal Doctor Plan was introduced in Saskatchewan. That story was well-documented by Dr. C. Rufus Rorem in the monograph he wrote for the Committee on the Costs of Medical Care in 1931. Rural municipalities entered into a contract with a doctor to provide general practitioner services to all the property tax payers and their dependants, usually without a user fee. The idea quickly spread in Saskatchewan and there were also a number of such plans in Alberta and Manitoba.

As with practically every other sector of Canadian society, the Depression fell with devastating impact on the medical profession. It is no wonder, then, that the CMA's Committee on Economics devoted two years in the preparation of a 50,000 word, *Report on Medical Economics*, which was presented at the CMA 1934 Annual Meeting. Its major contribution was to propose 19 principles to guide the development of any health insurance program: the foremost principle being that any government program should be administered by a representative, independent, non-political commission.

The first encounter between the profession and a provincial government occurred in 1935. In that year, the government of British Columbia (B.C.) passed a health insurance bill. However, because it did not provide for those on welfare and the medically indigent, and would have imposed a new tax on employers, the plan was aborted by the opposition of the B.C. Medical Association and the B.C. Manufacturers' Association.

The next significant event in the politics of health was the outbreak of World War II. Three factors occurred. First, the rejection rates of the armed forces for preventable or remediable conditions focused public attention on the inadequacy of health care services and the ability of people to afford them.

Second, the sacrifices of war, piled on top of the deprivations of the depression, created new aspirations for a better world that were encapsulated in the ringing words of Roosevelt's four freedoms and Churchill's and Roosevelt's Atlantic Charter.

Third, no government could ignore the ground swell of public opinion casting off the pessimism of depression or the evidence in the extraordinary war effort of a maturing nation becoming aware of undreamed-of strengths and daily growing in resolve that not only *must* there be, there *could* be a higher quality of life.

A politician has been described as a man who channelizes an existing stream—in a land where there is no water he digs in vain. Here were vast rivers of discontent and of hope, just waiting for someone to direct the forces.

He came by accident, through that part of the Canadian political process known as the "cabinet shuffle." And it happened this way.

When war was declared at the beginning of September 1939, the Canadian Minister of Defense was a gifted parliamentarian by the name of Ian Mackenzie, M.P. from Vancouver, who was fully informed about British Columbia's health insurance proposals in the mid-1930's. But it was clear at the first cabinet meeting following the declaration that he was not the man to direct the Defense Department in war time. On September 19, several ministers were moved, and Mackenzie found himself as minister of a very small Health Department. Mackenzie was disappointed, but he was not dismayed; there were other campaigns to be fought, greener fields to conquer, new terrain to be occupied.

As a result, there occurred that catalytic reaction when an able, committed, and idealistic politician is joined with a dedicated, and knowledgeable civil servant, as Mackenzie, the new Minister of Health, met Dr. J. J. Heagerty, Director of Public Health Services.

Within four months, Mackenzie wrote to the Prime Minister urging unemployment insurance and health insurance as immediate and positive wartime goals for the Canadian people. The cabinet turned it down.

Mackenzie then invited 14 health and consumer interest groups—medical, hospital, farm, labor, and others—to appoint advisory committees to an interdepartmental committee or task force which produced a 500 page report in 1942. The importance to the medical profession of such collaboration was extraordinary, for practically all of the 19 principles they had enunciated in 1934 were embodied in the two draft bills, one for the Canadian Parliament and the other a model bill for the provinces.

Still the cabinet would not act, and so a series of public hearings was held by a Parliamentary committee in 1943 and 1944. The format of the hearings was similar to those held by the U.S. Congress in 1945, but the spirit was different. The Canadian Hospital Association endorsed the proposals; the insurance industry endorsed them; the Canadian Medical Association endorsed them, and ended its submission with these ringing words:

> "The CMA desires to assure the committee that our entire organization stretching from sea to sea, stands ready to render any assistance in its power towards the solution of one of the country's most important problems, namely, the safeguarding of the health of our people."

It was Canadian organized medicine's finest hour, but it was not to be, even though a 1944 Gallup Poll revealed 80 percent of the Canadian voters desiring and willing to pay for a national program.

The reason was that health insurance ceased to be a single proposal but became enmeshed in a series of social security and reconstruction measures that the federal government felt would be imperative to forestall any return of the 1930's depression, and these huge expenditures would require transfer to Ottawa from the provinces of major tax fields, mainly personal and corporation income taxes.

At the 1945–46 Federal–Provincial Conference on Reconstruction the whole package was rejected, owing to the opposition of the wealthier provinces.

The great federal post–war design for Canada was now in disarray, as was the financial position of most of the provinces. So Canada began to pick up the pieces: (1) a massive re–establishment program for returning members of the armed forces; (2) tax agreements with seven of the nine provinces; and (3) the introduction of universal hospital insurance plans by the three western provincial governments.

But an equally important development was the rapid expansion of the voluntary prepayment plans sponsored by the hospital and medical associations and the insurance industry as they rushed in to fill the vacuum left by the failure of the provinces to accept the 1945 federal offer. By 1949, there were 10 physician–sponsored plans, and six Blue Cross Plans selling insurance in all provinces except British Columbia and Saskatchewan, where there had never been a Blue Cross Plan.

With this degree of success, as well as increased sales by commercial insurance, in 1949 all three associations reversed their 1943 policy of endorsing a governmental program, and favored the extension of the voluntary and commercial insurance plans with governments paying in whole or in part the premiums on behalf of those who could not pay for themselves.

At the same time, a 1949 Gallup Poll continued to show 80 percent of the Canadian population in favor of a national government program.

## Development of a National Health Program

One now needs to shift to the politics of the political parties and the federal and provincial governments in the period of the early 1950's. Several things had changed.

1. The battle over taxes that had aborted the 1945 reconstruction proposals had been settled. Block Grants (equalization payments) from the federal government to the provinces had brought the fiscal capacity of all the provinces to the average of the two highest revenue–producing provinces.

2. Four provinces now had government hospital insurance programs in place.

3. Voluntary prepayment plans and commercial insurance had increased dramatically but had been able to insure no more than 40 percent of the total population for hospital coverage, nor more than 27 percent for medical coverage. Moreover, except in provinces having universal hospital insurance, hospitals were continuing to incur substantial deficits.

4. The main political difference, however, was that the new Liberal Prime Minister of Canada, the Hon. Louis St. Laurent, was totally opposed to health insurance of any kind. But he was trapped in the long–term commitment of the Liberal Party. In the 1953 election he came up with a brilliant escape hatch: the Liberals were still in favor of health insurance but the federal government would not act until a majority of the provinces, representing a majority of the population, had programs in operation. That meant two more provinces, and one would have to be either Quebec or Ontario, and everyone knew Quebec would not act. That left Ontario, and everyone knew if Ontario acted, a sixth province would not be difficult to find. That meant that the Conservative Premier of Ontario, Mr. Leslie Frost, and his large majority in the legislature would make the decision. He, too, was not enthusiastic, but equally determined that he would not bear the onus for saying "No."

Accordingly, at the next regular Federal–Provincial Conference, in 1955, Mr. Frost proposed a federal–provincial program, in effect, saying to the Liberals, "Put up or shut up." Mr. St. Laurent continued to oppose, but when his Minister of Health, the Hon. Paul Martin (Mackenzie had become Minister of Veterans' Affairs), threatened to resign he agreed to propose a national insurance program, administered by the provinces, in which the federal government would pay 50 percent of the national costs. By 1961, all provinces were in the system and virtually the total population of Canada was insured for unlimited days of care at the standard ward level. Millions were also insured for semi–private and extended benefits.

Once again the politics of political parties enters, the New Democratic Party of Saskatchewan (named, at that time, the Cooperative Commonwealth Federation) had been elected in 1944 with a commitment to a full range of health services but had been able to afford only hospital insurance introduced in 1947. But now 50 percent of the costs of that program would be contributed by the federal government. Here were windfall revenues that clearly belonged to the health sector, and with a 1960 election approaching, the decision to go forward with medical care was announced.

The party was returned to office and appointed a citizens' advisory committee, including three physicians representing the College of Physicians and Surgeons, opposed to a government administered program.

These actions by the Saskatchewan government triggered yet another response by the Canadian Medical Association. Fearful that medical care insurance would become a political football, both in other provinces and at the federal level, in 1960 the CMA asked the Conservative Prime Minister, Mr. Diefenbaker, who had succeeded Mr. St. Laurent, to appoint a Royal Commission which could give "dispassionate and objective consideration of the future pattern of health care in this country."

Mr. Diefenbaker agreed. The Royal Commission of seven members, chaired by Chief Justice Hall of Saskatchewan, and including two medical doctors, was appointed in 1961 and reported in 1964. To the dismay of the CMA, it unanimously recommended a comprehensive range of health services to be administered by the provincial governments, and subsidized, like hospital insurance, through federal grants–in–aid.

The early 1960's thus presented the volatility and turbulence of a kaleidoscope. Here was a ringing endorsement of health insurance by a Royal Commission appointed by a conservative government which had been defeated in 1963. The three wealthiest provinces immediately introduced province–wide programs modelled on the CMA and insurance industry recommendations, whose anti–government publicity and lobbying were stepped up. Farmer, labor, women's, and church groups formed a Health Coalition. But in the author's judgement, the most significant event that was to determine the outcome was that with the election of Lester Pearson's government in 1963, he appointed as Minister of Finance the only man ever to hold that position who genuinely believed in health insurance—Mr. Walter Gordon. Although Pearson's was a minority government, on this issue he could count on the votes of the New Democratic Party, to achieve an over–all majority on the vote.

So, at a Federal–Provincial Conference in July 1965, the offer was made. In 1966, the legislation was passed by a vote of 177–to–2, almost rivalling the unanimous vote on hospital insurance a decade earlier. In July 1968, the program went into effect, over strong external opposition. By January 1971, all provinces were in the system. Such is—or was—the power of the federal government under its blanket power to spend.

### Financial Issues

Since the inauguration of the programs, the "politics of health policy" has focused mainly on financial issues.

As stated, these were federal–provincial, conditional grant–in–aid, or "shared–cost" programs. There were two flaws in the original arrangements:

1. From the point of view of the provinces, an imbalance was created in provincial health programs by the fact that only treatment services costs were shared; and

2. From the federal point of view, the problem was that its costs were determined by provincial medical and hospital expenditures.

By 1977, it was agreed that the Basic Financial Arrangements Act, the federal government transferred 50 percent of its former contribution by reducing its personal income tax by 12.5 percent and its corporations income tax by 1.0 percent, permitting the provinces to occupy this tax room. Secondly, it continues to make cash payments equivalent to the other half of its former payments in the base year, 1975–1976, increased each year by the percentage increase in Gross National Product (GNP).

There have been several results of the new formula:

1. Since the federal contribution is linked to Gross National Product rather than to provincial expenditures, the federal government has now gained control, or at least predictability, over its health budget.

2. Under the new formula, the federal contribution to medical and hospital care has increased, as planned, from 50.3 percent, under the old formula, to about 57 percent in 1979–1980, and 51.3 percent in 1984.

3. The provinces are now free to allocate their resources, including the federal contribution, to whatever health program they wish; the federal formula no longer has any steering effect on their decisions.

4. Since the provinces are solely responsible for the full amount by which the percentage increase in health expenditures exceeds the percentage increase in the GNP, their incentives for cost–containment are much higher and their efforts, indeed, much greater.

## Hospital Payments

The second major political area is the payment of hospitals. With inflation, reduced revenues, and more militant unions, the adequacy of hospital funding has become a primary issue in public debate. In administering the hospital services programs and the new imperatives of cost–containment, provincial governments have some advantages over their U.S. counterparts. One agency, the Ministry of Health, is responsible for the three major functions:

1. It is the central planning agency, responsible for approving what are called (in the United States) "certificates of need" for beds, programs, and high technology.

2. It is the rate–setting agency, responsible for negotiating annual "prospective" budgets.

3. It is the paying agency for all basic services, although other bodies, such as Blue Cross, may pay for supplementary benefits such as semi–private care.

## Physician Payments

The third major political area is the payment of physicians. Here, again, there is a basic difference with the United States in that the medical profession in Canada never adopted the "customary, prevailing, and reasonable" methodology, for, in the operation of their own "Blue Shield" prepayment plans, the provincial Medical Associations adopted a standardized, province–wide fee schedule that, typically, paid specialists (who must be certificated by the Royal College of Physicians and Surgeons) at a rate 50 percent higher than general practitioners. Governments simply adopted the same system, and negotiate one or two year contracts with the Medical Association.

Even under the Blue Shield plans, however, there were always some physicians who were non–members or "opted out" and who billed their patients for their self–determined fee, with the patient obtaining reimbursement of the standard fee. The results are mixed. There is no extra–billing in Quebec or British Columbia. In Ontario, the percentage of doctors billing some patients is about 15 percent. In the Atlantic provinces, with the exception of Nova Scotia, the numbers of doctors extra–billing is negligible. In the prairie provinces, it is high only in Alberta. It has been estimated that extra–billing adds about 2 percent to the total expenditures on the government medical care programs.

In 1979–80, in the *Report of a National Review* of the system, Commissioner Hall said:

> "If extra–billing is permitted as a right and practiced by physicians in their sole discretion, it will, over the years, destroy the program, creating in that downward path the two–tier system incompatible with the societal level which Canadians have attained."

## Current Issues

As indicated, the field of health falls within the constitutional jurisdiction of the provinces, so the federal government cannot legislate in that area. What it can and does do, however, is attach conditions to its grants. The five conditions attached to the medical care insurance programs were: the programs must be universal, comprehensive, and administered by public authority; the benefits must be portable and no user fee or physicians' extra–billing should deny reasonable access.

The issue of user fees and extra–billing has now become the hottest political issue in Canada. To curb what is called the "erosion" of the program's principles, the federal government has just introduced a new Canada Health Act which incorporates the two separate Hospital and Medical Care Insurance Acts, and, further, penalizes provinces which authorize user fees and permit extra–billing by deducting from federal cash payments an amount equal to whatever amount hospitals and doctors charge patients.

If the provinces act within three years to abolish extra–billing, the penalty deductions will be repaid.

Aware of overwhelming public opinion supporting this proposal, the Liberal Party, facing an election in the next year (and down in the public opinion polls), clearly believed it had a major election issue. To its consternation—and to the dismay of the medical profession and several provincial governments—the Conservative Opposition party also endorsed the measure, so of course it would pass. The provincial governments must now decide whether to accept the penalties (about $50 million in Ontario, for example) or do battle with the medical profession which considers the right to set its fees fundamental to professional autonomy. It will be fascinating to observe the battles ahead.

Almost every key actor in the health care system can be said, as the current expression goes, to find him or herself between a rock and a hard place. The hospital administrator faces, on the one hand, a combination of medical demands, militant unions, and inflating prices, and on the other, a health ministry committed to cost-containment. The Minister of Health and his senior officials confront, on the one hand, the hospital and nurses' unions and the medical profession whose members have established the 1970 incomes, inflated by the introduction of Medicare, as their baseline, and, on the other, the Minister of Finance. The Finance officials, of course, face not only the Health Department, already accounting for from 25 to 30 percent of provincial budgets but a host of other ministers responsible for equally important activities. At the same time, they and the government face an electorate whose tolerance for (and capacity to pay) taxes has declined as their utilization of government services has risen.

### Conclusion

What this paper has been describing is, of course, not new. The essence of the political process has always been: "Who gets what and when?" But what *is* new, at least for most of this generation, is that the country is in a period of recession, with all governments encountering declining revenues and mostly, increasing deficits.

During the 1970's, total expenditures on all health services accounted for about 7 percent of GNP but this year, because of the decline in real GNP, it may reach as high as 8 percent.

There have been complaints by medical and hospital spokespersons that the system is being underfunded, but an all-party Parliamentary Committee that held public hearings across the nation last year concluded that it would not be in the public interest to expand the treatment system further.

There have been, and there are, problems in the health care programs— conflicts between the federal and provincial governments over cost-sharing and political credit; conflicts between health professions, union, and governments over payment levels; conflicts with hospitals over bed-closings, high technology purchases, and operating budgets. But given that health services programs are the most complex of the social insurances to administer, it is perhaps remarkable that there have been as few problems and foul-ups as experienced. Clearly, there has been a remarkable degree of responsibility exercised by all participants in the enterprise, and the programs retain the highest degree of citizen approval of any programs administered by government. Few, if any, would turn back the clock, although there are many advocating, and working for, their improvement. But they, too, must rely on "politics" to achieve their goals.

# Chapter Three

## National Health Policy: Role of Market Competition

### ROGER M. BATTISTELLA

## Introduction

Rhetoric espousing competition as the answer to the many problems convulsing the health sector is not to be taken literally. The possibility that the untrammelled infusion of commercial values and free market transactions will culminate in an optimal use of costly resources, devoid of troublesome social inequities, is wildly fanciful.[1] Fulfillment of this and corollary visions of total consumer and provider sovereignty, free of public controls, compels suspension of practical experience for consummate faith in the power of theory untested outside the realm of abstract logic [Ginzberg, 1980, pp. 1112-15].

This essay has two purposes: first, to lay bare the underlying assumptions impairing the relevance of competitive panaceas; and second, to identify some of the practical reasons why appeals to competitive values nevertheless persist as expedients for accelerating cumbersome, large-scale changes in the organization and financing of health services. Compelling imperatives for pragmatism are assessed in terms of efficiency-equity trade-offs and implications for public regulation.

## Perfect Competition

Put into historical perspective, the dogma of perfect competition is a derivative of eighteenth century political and economic beliefs apotheosizing the beneficence of the self-regulating market. Long discredited for having a highly tenuous relationship to reality, the ideals depicted nevertheless acquired from the start a catechistic influence in the minds of political-economic reformers distrustful of human nature and goverment power. The appeal of competitive dogma is enhanced by the elegance of its logic and the simplicity of its guidelines for salvation, unencumbered

---

[1] Proclamations of the superiority of private markets are a hallmark of the Reagan Administration's policy espousing: deregulation, competition consumer choice, free entry and exit of capital and labor, economic discipline through the assumption of financial risks and rewards among providers and consumers, and reclassification of health care from a social good to an economic good. The thrust of the competitive strategy has been conveniently summarized by the director of the politically powerful Office of Management and Budget. See [Stockman, 1981, pp. 5-19; Meyer, 1983].

by practical considerations of the opportunity costs of change. In practice, however, redemption demands strict observance of carefully specified but arduous rules of conduct [Galbraith, 1977, pp. 11-9].

*Necessary Conditions*

As described in introductory textbooks on the subject, equality of economic power among buyers and sellers is fundamental to unstructured competition [Leftwich, 1976]. The elaborate self-regulatory machinery featured in pristine theory requires that individuals and groups be powerless to influence the price of what is bought and sold. Second, prices must be allowed to move freely in response to changes in supply and demand. Third, restrictions over market entry and exit are strictly prohibited so that market prices may set the best use of scarce resources. Fourth, complete knowledge of market vacillations and the value of goods and services is mandatory among all participants. Laxity in pursuit of information is discouraged by fear of the consequences foretold in the underlying dictum, "let the buyer beware."

There are, moreover, a number of important secondary assumptions. The first of these centers on self-interest. Altruism and public service is suspect in competitive market doctrine because of the penchant for acquisitiveness attributed to human nature. This is conveyed in the archetype of "economically rational man," in which individuals are admonished against undertaking actions for themselves whereby others obtain an unintended free benefit. Exclusive consumption of benefits is a cardinal principle of self-interest. All of these conditions are predicated, furthermore, on a steadfast conviction in competition as a dynamic for continuous economic and social progress, including the eventual perfectability of man.[2]

If, as mentioned earlier, the key assumptions for perfect competition have seldom, if ever, been encountered in actuality, there are few instances where the mismatch is generally acknowledged to be greater than in the health sector, where service values have been important for centuries [Culyer, 1981, pp. 25-55].

## Health-Sector Market Constraints

Price and income rationing have never been totally excluded from the health sector, but from ancient times onward society has intervened to restrain the full power of commercial values and unchecked self-interest. Considerations of community welfare and social cohesion underlie the many ethical constraints traditionally imposed on physicians and other health professions. These constraints arise from the understanding that emotional fears of disability and death constitute an invitation to exploita-

---

[2] A discussion of the secondary assumptions essential to an understanding of perfect competition may be found in Bell and Kristal [1971].

tion detrimental to community economic and social welfare.[3]

*Service Ethic Origins*

In return for a commitment to strive within human limitations to place the well-being of patients ahead of self-interest, the medical profession has been granted monopoly powers over diagnosis and treatment. Social status, high material rewards, and freedom to govern itself are the rewards for adherence to a special social trust in which members of the profession promise to uphold the sanctity of life and to provide a uniformly high standard of care, regardless of ability to pay and other differences among individuals.

Privilege and responsibility is what differentiates a profession from other occupations. The extraordinarily high status enjoyed by medicine originates out of practical necessity, rather than weakness and misguided idealism as often alleged by critics of the service ethic. At the core of this special relationship is the understanding that gaps in technical knowledge, in association with emotional stress, hamper the ability of individuals to ascertain the medical significance of symptoms and the most appropriate course of treatment. Formidable complexities of definition and measurement, regarding cause and effect relationships between health-services product mix and health outcomes, additionally limit consumers' ability to assess either the quality of treatment or accuracy of diagnosis [Pauly, 1982, pp. 3-24]. There is, therefore, an inescapable asymmetry in the doctor-patient relationship that curtails the exercise of consumer sovereignty and impels physicians to make important decisions on behalf of the sick. It is within this framework of expectations that physicians initiate diagnostic and treatment decisions which today account for about 70 percent of the money spent on personal health services in the U.S. [Gibson, 1979, p. 6; *Congressional Quarterly,* 1980(a), p. 37].

Admittedly imperfect, this arrangement nevertheless gives consumers a larger degree of protection than conceivable in the anarchistic world of perfect competition. Monitoring and accountability for quality is intrinsically easier in structured than unstructured situations. Monopolization of medical practice also benefits the overall community in important ways. Economic and social chaos would ensue if individuals were free to determine independently whether they were too sick to report to work or undertake their usual family and community obligations, given the fact that responsibility frequently entails hardship and self-denial.

Both for utilitarian and humanitarian reasons, society has conferred special privileges on the ill and disabled; notably, compassion and absolution from personal responsibility for illness, together with relief from one's

---

[3] Perhaps the most erudite and widely cited explanation of the social considerations underlying the service ethic and the special status granted the medical profession is provided by Parsons [1951, pp. 428-79].

normal duties. In modern economies, the privileges extended to sick persons include legal entitlements to treatment and cash allowances to offset illness-related wage losses. In return for these privileges, the sick are expected to seek technically competent medical assistance and to cooperate fully with physicians for a speedy recovery. Temptations to feign sickness as a way of avoiding unpleasant responsibility or to profit from monetary entitlements no doubt would be multiplied if there were no restrictions on who could practice medicine, and self-proclaimed practitioners were allowed to aggressively market for clientele. The negative consequences for public health and economic growth are disturbing to contemplate.

*Additional Sources of Market Failure*

That the service ethic has persevered in this and other countries with strong free-market beliefs is no mere happenstance. Its resiliency speaks to the many important ways in which health and health services differ from economic goods and services in general.[4] In addition to emotional vulnerability to commercial exploitation, consumer rationality is limited by the intangibility of health and health services. Despite the progress made in medical science, considerable doubt persists about what consumers get when they purchase medical care. Unlike a pair of shoes or a new car, individuals are buying, at best, a significant but unknown reduction in the risks of illness and a postponement of disability and death. In the end, all medicine fails.

Health itself is highly subjective, a problem compounded by contemporary liberalization of the definition to include a state of total mental and emotional well-being, as well as freedom from illness and disability [Fox, 1977, pp. 9-22]. Uncertainty prevails, even in the case of less ambiguous illness treatment and preventive services. Guarantees that compliance with medical advice precludes disease or the progression of disability are few. Other dilemmas stem from the uneven and unpredictable occurrence of illness. In contemporary medicine, the most accurate predictions are statistical. Reliability of findings is directly correlated with group size.

At the individual level, persons most in need of health services can least afford to pay for them because of the inverse relationship between sickness and severity of sickness with income and social class. Except for the very rich, the cost of health care is beyond the reach of out-of-pocket payment. Contemporary advances in medical technology have exacerbated this problem in so far as the cost of treatment has become more expensive.

---

[4] The definitive discussion of the special features of health services underlying the shortcomings of efforts to obtain optimal resource allocation through the market is provided by Arrow [1963, pp. 941-69]. For the perspective of a respected health economist see [Klarman, 1965, pp. 1-19].

*Limitations of Experience Rating*

Were it not for the development of prepayment health insurance, it is doubtful whether even middle class families could escape dependence on public assistance for their health care. The predictability of large numbers, pooling of risks, and economies of group enrollment enable voluntary health insurance to provide a measure of protection against economic insecurity. Approximately four-fifths of all Americans with some form of private health insurance are enrolled in groups, mainly as the result of employment-related fringe benefits [Dicker, 1983].

The scope and adequacy of private insurance coverage would be higher were it not for the dysfunctionality of competition for profits. Aggressive marketing of experience rating and appeals to individual gain over values of mutual aid undermine the ability of nonprofit insurers to extend the benefits of prepayment to low-income groups through community-rating principles whereby the young and healthy subsidize the premiums of elderly and sick subscribers.

Since stockholders seek competitive rates of return on their money, investor-owned insurance firms understandably seek to avoid high-risk subscribers. Profit margins depend upon an ability, through experience rating, to offer lower premiums to persons least in need of insurance protection. Therefore, competition based on experience rating culminates in the exclusion of low income persons. The elderly also are disadvantaged by a system granting preference to young healthy persons. Retirement from the labor force multiplies the plight of the aged, since most voluntary health insurance is provided as a condition of employment in which employers usually pay from two-thirds to four-fifths of the premium.

More so than anything else, the dysfunctionalities of experience rating created the political pressures behind government's intervention in the mid-1960's to protect the poor, the medically indigent, and retired persons through the Medicaid and Medicare programs [Davis and Schoen, 1978]. The groundwork is being laid for still more government intervention in the future. Because of recession induced profit declines, private business and industry are beginning to shift from community-rated to experience-rated health plans in order to save money. Others find it financially advantageous in the short run to self-insure. In recent years, self-insurance has grown to account for nearly 20 percent of the health insurance market, in comparison with only 5 percent in 1975 [Samors and Sullivan, 1983, pp. 144-59].

Anticipation of having to assume a larger financial role, combined with difficulties of managing already existing public commitments is, of course, a root cause of unremitting nonpartisan federal and state efforts to obtain efficiencies in health services following passage of Medicare and Medicaid. The aim is to contain not only unit costs but total spending in both public and private sectors. Health care costs exercise an inflationary effect on the economy as a whole, as well as adding to the problems government faces in bringing public sector borrowing requirements under control. Growth in the size and political strength of the aged population imposes unavoidable responsibilities in the decades ahead.

*Supply Generated Demand*

Fundamental to ongoing restructuring efforts is the assumption that, due to the special properties characteristic of health services delivery, ordinary laws of supply and demand do not function; instead, supply creates its own demand. Concurrently, it is generally accepted among policymakers at all levels that an oversupply of hospitals and physicians aggrevates the practical political difficulties of bringing health costs under control [Abel-Smith, 1974, pp. 17-28]. This conclusion is evident in the relationship between regional variations in surgical rates and the number of surgeons in an area [Wennberg and Gittelsohn, 1973, pp. 1102-08]. There are many ways whereby physicians are able to generate their own demand, including: flexibility of diagnostic labeling in cases of ambiguous symptomology and multiple causation (a situation typical of chronic disease); command over referrals; latitude in scheduling the number and location of follow-up visits; number of diagnostic tests ordered; mix of treatment services provided; and authority to alter the mix of services in pursuit of quality [Battistella and Chester, 1978(b), pp. 219-52].

Few policymakers doubt any longer that adding more money to the health sector will prove anything but wasteful, without changes in incentives for economy and a greater division of labor conducive to economies of scale for monitoring and evaluating the quality and cost effectiveness of services. In matters of health policy, reversal of orthodox economic laws of supply and demand is the rule and not the exception.

The fiscal leverage possessed by insurance companies and government are realities having little in common with textbook descriptions of pure competition, in which equilibrium of supply and demand is unsullied by the power of market participants to influence events. Ideologues' entreaties to give the theory a try are oblivious to the opportunity costs of foregoing the benefits of collective safeguards that have evolved from a process of trial and error.

**Positive Spillovers of Health Spending**

In addition to the protections given to consumers, voluntary insurance and government programs help to secure the financial stability of the health sector, which has grown to become one of the two largest components of the modern economy in terms of size of employment and magnitude of economic activity. Five percent of the labor force and 10 percent of the gross national product cannot be destabilized without potentially enormous harm, direct and indirect, to the economy as a whole. That the health economy has acquired such strategic importance in all highly developed countries indicates the rising public expectations for quality of life and growth in the role of social services in improving living standards [Battistella, 1978(a), pp. 23-51].

The significance of public financing parallels the quantum improvements in the ability of clinical services to alter the natural course of disease since scientific medicine reached the takeoff stage shortly before World War II. In company with earlier advances in public health technology for disease prevention, improvement in the efficaciousness of clinical medicine has solidified the perception that government spending can be targeted to raise the quality and productivity of the labor force. Priorities for economic growth inevitably encompass investments in labor force quality, producing a relaxation of ideological beliefs confining government authority in free market economies to control of contagious disease and other serious environmental threats to community health and safety.

Possibly more important from the standpoint of practical politics, the widely held view in public opinion that health services ought to be made available on the basis of need rather than the ability to pay, because of their perceived significance for quality of life, makes it academic whether health care meets the test of a public or private good. The subordination of purely economic considerations to health and medical values in public opinion is accentuated in the example of Medicare.

Quantification of the rate of return on human capital has little effect on government decision making. Extending social insurance of health care to the elderly, ahead of gainfully employed young adults, constitutes an irrational act in purely economic terms, but, as pointed out by John Bryant [1969, pp. 107-08], "politicians knew that such care was extremely important not only to the recipients but to the (voting age) children of the recipients." The irrelevance of cost-benefit analysis and techniques for discounting the present value of future returns of capital investment in health services is apparent, too, in the decision of numerous nations throughout the world to undertake costly public commitments to maternal and child health programs, despite anticipated low rates of return due to the lengthy lead times involved and assumptions of future employment and wage levels.

The precedence of political and social considerations over purely economic priorities is a reality confining the flexibility of government to better manage its finances by restricting public expenditures to services and individuals showing a sufficiently high ratio of benefits to costs. Reallocation of health spending away from consumption to investments aiding greater economic productivity—a not uncommon goal today among highly developed countries afflicted with declining or stagnant economies—will not occur smoothly without substantial public concurrence, especially in democracies where elected officials serve at the pleasure of the voters.

No system functions perfectly, to be sure. If anything, the frustrations emanating from the tendency of systems to resist change are magnified in the health sector. The combination of special status which health services commands in public opinion, together with the high degree of autonomy granted to physicians, and the complex interlocking of vested interests among suppliers, producers, and consumers, insulates the health field from externally imposed discipline to a greater degree than normal in other parts of the economy [Thompson, 1981; Feldstein, 1977].

Impatience for change has intensified, however, due to the unanticipated slowing of economic growth during the past decade and corresponding pressures on government to employ resources more efficiently, both because of recession-pinched tax revenues and the demands of new responsibilities for speeding and sustaining economic recovery. An air of crisis, therefore, gives sustenance to market-related solutions for badly strained public finances. The suggestion of decisive action, unencumbered by bureaucratic and regulatory expense, is, however, an illusion. Opening the health sector to unrestricted market forces is no less appropriate today than in the past.

*Social Costs of Competition*

Reforms restricting entry into medical practice and imposing uniform minimal standards in medical education and licensure were initiated in reaction to the socially harmful excesses of free market medicine prevailing earlier in this century [Flexner, 1910; Stevens, 1971, pp. 66-72]. The consequent rise in public confidence towards the ethical standards and clinical competence of medical practitioners helped to make possible the vast outpouring of political and financial support for biomedical research, diffusion of medical technologies, and patient-care amenities that have made American hospitals an object of envy in international comparisons.

Other limitations of competition underpin the origins of the Food and Drug Administration (FDA) and related regulatory federal programs in the areas of environmental protection and occupational safety and health. The public harm resulting from advertising and sale of drugs, either unsafe or nonefficacious, contributed to a gradual but steady broadening of the FDA's original 1906 mandate to investigate the safety of drugs following their entry into the market. Since 1938, drug manufacturers have been required to show proof of safety prior to marketing. Demonstration of efficacy was added in 1962. Pursuit of profit associated with product adulteration and misbranding was the stimulus for federal monitoring of medical devices beginning in 1938. In 1976, the government's power in this area was enlarged to require manufacturers to satisfy minimum safety and efficacy standards in advance of marketing. In large part because of market failures, government is today involved in health care in a big way [*Congressional Quarterly,* 1980(b), pp. 119-27].

*Negative Features of Nonprofit Competition*

The dysfunctionalities of competition are not exclusive to the quest for profits. Competition for status among nonprofit providers is widely viewed as a problem among third parties committed to curbing health costs. The negative externalities of nonprofit competition include high volumes of medically questionable or unnecessary diagnostic and treatment procedures, and noneconomic overlap and duplication of costly services [Bice, 1984, pp. 375-402; Rushmer, 1984, pp. 277-304; Jonas and Banta, 1981, pp. 331-51]. Congressional scepticism over the value of many diagnostic and treatment services performed by providers to recipients of government health care programs, e.g., Medicare, Medicaid, and maternal and child health, is behind the establishment in 1972 of the Office of Technology Assessment and such related controls as peer review of clinical decisions (Professional Standard Review organizations). Regulation of capital expansion (health planning and certificate of need) mandated in state and federal laws, and often possessing the backing of business-industrial coalitions for health cost containment, is designed to cut waste by reducing bed surplus and by promoting divisions of labor conducive to economies of scale.

Regardless of the ideological proclivities towards regulation of the political party in power, ineluctable resource scarcities and the dilemmas of financial management during periods of recession impel all payers, business and industry included, to seek greater value for their money through managerial and structural reforms. Although proponents of competition are correct in attributing much of the inflationary increases in health spending to the predilection of health professionals to pursue social equity and scientific excellence to the detriment of economy and efficiency, it does not follow that a stiff dose of market discipline is the solution [Vladeck, 1981, pp. 209-23].

Running health services more like a business, as noted by Relman, would only add to the conflicts of interest built into fee-for-service medicine [Relman, 1983, pp. 5-19]. To do so, moreover, is to ignore the lessons of recent penetrations of the commercial ethic into the health sector, including: first, the kickbacks and other incentives for ordering unnecessary tests accompanying the restructuring of medical laboratory services from professional to corporate for-profit ownership; and second, the scandals surrounding the for-profit marketing of health maintenance organizations to welfare recipients in California [Bailey, 1979; Schorr, 1978, p. 48; Committee on Government Operations, 1975].

Further insight into the inappropriateness of market solutions stems from the vacuous claims of for-profit hospital chains that they could deliver inpatient services less expensively than non-profit hospitals because of their management expertise and sophisticated financial methods. Contrary to the theory of competition, they are, in practice, more costly.

Although differences are slight in the case of bills submitted to Medicare and Medicaid, for-profit hospitals charge subscribers to private health insurance 23 percent more per day and 17 percent more on a per admission basis. For every bed-size category, for-profit hospitals have higher costs than the overall average for community nonprofit hospitals. High rates of return on equity, responsible for the popularity of their stocks among investors, are due less to efficiency than to the pursuit of such socially dubious practices as aggressive billing, creative accounting, screening out low-paying and charity patients, and loading on of services generating high profit margins [Pattison and Katz, 1983, pp. 347-53; Lewin, Derzon, and Margulies, 1981, pp. 52-8].

Rebuked by political and financial critics to manage their institutions more like a business, many nonprofit hospitals are now engaging in practices similar to those of profit-making health care corporations, with an unfortunate narrowing of the differences. It is not surprising, therefore, that at least 6 percent of the charges for services to Medicare beneficiaries are estimated by government auditors to be unnecessary [U.S. Comptroller General, 1983(b)]. The willingness of providers to abuse the system for their own economic gain is also apparent in the disclosure, reported by Joseph Califano, former Secretary of the Department of Health and Human Services, that in some of the 54 state and other political entities participating in the Medicaid program there were several instances in which as much as 25 to 40 percent of the funds paid on behalf of patients during 1976 to 1977 were for bogus procedures and drugs [Califano, 1981, pp. 136-70].

Public policy inducements for health providers to disassociate from service-ethic commitments complicate the difficulties of reconciling short-term advantages with enlightened long-term interests. Emulation of narrow business values exposes health professionals to public criticism, with adverse consequences both for themselves and broader social needs for dependable and reputable health services. Any diminution of trust in the doctor-patient relationship ties imperils the community's capability to minimize the disruptive effects of illness and disability. It is essential, therefore, that health services remain above suspicion. Findings from a recent poll of public opinion suggest that medicine and health in general are held in higher esteem than other occupations, particularly business. In the category of very-high to high integrity, respondents rank doctors ahead of businessmen by a margin of better than three-to-one and ahead of lawyers by a margin of two-to-one [Ricklefs, 1983, p. 33]. Whether public trust in medicine will persist is problemmatic if health care takes on a more commercial appearance. Government actions pushing health professionals in an acquisitive self-serving direction are counterproductive.

The latest state and federal measures to control health spending, through regulation of provider revenues, are grounded in adversarial competitive principles that provoke the distortion of health objectives for selfish ends. They spawn among providers a desperate struggle for survival in which maneuvering for financial advantage is endless. If legal, the ethical proprieties of actions such as the following are socially disturbing:

shifting of unreimbursed charges to nonregulated payers; inflating of reimbursable costs through creative accounting; overordering of money-making services; and diversifying into profitable secondary and marginally health related activities. Other defensive responses include selectivity of patients by ability to pay and by diagnosis reimbursement potential to fulfill income expectations. Ceaseless regulatory-agency counteractions against these evasive tactics invariably generate inconsistencies and contradictions which victimize the weak and damage public confidence in the wisdom and integrity of government [Battistella and Eastaugh, 1980, pp. 62-82].

**Popularity of Competitive Rhetoric**

Given the obvious disparities between theory and practice, the attention received by unadulterated competitive market rhetoric is curious. To attribute it to the influence of teachers of economics, ideologically ill-suited to deal with real-world complexities and ambiguities, is to denigrate students' awareness of contradictory evidence abounding in daily living.

To be sure, there is a hard-core of true believers in the iron law of supply and demand who possess the backing of economics' departments located in reputable universities. However, their influence for the most part has steadily declined throughout the post-war era as the gap between theory and practice has widened. Insensitivity to the opportunity costs of change and uncompromising intolerance of divergency has further relegated them to a reactionary position in mainstream politics. Incessant zeal for proselytization nevertheless has exaggerated their contributions to national health policy over the past decade, in correspondence with a deepening languor among opinion makers cognizant of the interdependence of managerial-economic efficiency and social equity. Intimidation is partly responsible for the passivity of well-informed health leadership.

Originating in the widespread concern that already unacceptably high chronic rates of increase in health spending may grow worse in future years, due to the aging of the population and escalation of voter expectations for more and better publicly-financed health care, allegations of the ineptitude of traditional service-oriented management have become vogue. Consequently, discipline born of market-place struggle for survival and bottom-line indices of managerial performance is now ensconsed in conventional wisdom as a panacea [Gray, 1983]. Conspicuously missing in such invidious contrasts is any mention of the numerous complaints against business management in thoughtful explanations of the causes of the faltering competitiveness of the U.S. economy in world trade.

The disintegration of powerful coalitions organized to take unified action within and among major interest groups further enervates the exercise of effective leadership in defense of the comprehensive purpose of health services in advanced industrial societies. More important than the specialization propagated from gains in scientific knowledge, competition for dwindling public funds has introduced a zero-sum aspect to formerly cooperative relationships throughout the health sector. Whereas health interests formerly competed with one another, competition against one another has become commonplace.

Illustrative of the devisive effects of government regulation is the elimination of long-standing cross-subsidies previously interlocking patient care with teaching and research constituencies. It is doubtful whether a single national organization can any longer hope to represent all of the nation's hospitals, due to changes in reimbursement driving a wedge among teaching hospitals, community general hospitals, and long-term care facilities. Cooperation has become rare, even among community general hospitals. Financial survival struggles divide nonprofit institutions along sectarian and nonsectarian lines. The separate agenda followed by proprietary hospitals adds to the difficulty of forging consensus among hospitals [McNerney, 1982, pp. 333-68].

The prevalence of competitive ideology in the health field also signals, in part, a yearning for escape and the return of simpler times when institutions were free to act unilaterally. Nostalgia for the romanticized past is a human response to the bewilderment and anguish stirred by unfamiliar happenings. Ideology according to George C. Lodge [1982, p. 1; 1980], "is the hymns we sing to justify and make legitimate what we are doing or perhaps what we would like to do." Although adherence to an outmoded ideology increases the difficulty of formulating new ideas appropriately attuned to new realities, it is not entirely devoid of practicality.

*Hidden Pragmatism*

Skillfully orchestrated, ideology can be a powerful force for expediting otherwise controversial change. Shared cultural ideals constitute a bond among otherwise separate interest groups. Stirrings of legendary entrepreneurial exploits and the character-building effects of unfettered competition enhance self-esteem, while befogging the senses to the substantive implications of what is actually happening. Viewed in this light, the pro-competitive strategy is akin to the pouring of new wine into old bottles.

Contrary to conjured visions of *laissez faire,* competition is a code word for rationalization or corporatization, whereby many of the freedoms and privileges long possessed by health providers and consumers are being relegated to priorities for centralized financal and managerial control. Competitive rhetoric masks the transformation of the health economy from a cottage industry, having few effective centralized controls, to a modern corporate system featuring the sophisticated financial and managerial disciplinary tools characteristic of large commercial and industrial firms. Behind the competitive banner, horizontally and vertically integrated delivery systems have made considerable progress in superseding the limited services traditionally under the control of independent small-sized providers [Starr, 1983, pp. 420-49].

Cast in the role of final arbiter, the market promotes efficiency by liberating decision makers from the constraints of public administration. Allusions to the "invisible hand" at the core of competitive doctrine help, moreover, to extricate politicians from the electoral perils of constituents seeking to personalize responsibility for hardships and inconvenience resulting from government policies. Similarly, market mythology frees government officials from having to follow the debilitating due process procedures required when the determination of winners and losers is made through planning and other public means. Health services consolidation and retrenchment is accomplished more easily if providers are allowed to fight things out among themselves according to the impersonal laws of the marketplace.

*Health-Sector Restructuring*

Not all the credit can be given to the competitive strategy, to be sure, but it does seem (in company with the side effects of regulatory controls having a common philosophical heritage in economically rational behavior) to have accelerated health services restructuring to a greater degree than likely through direct government planning. Incredibly rapid strides have been made in the consolidation of services. Nearly one-fourth of the nation's 5,853 community hospitals are now components of corporate systems, which collectively control 36 percent of all nonfederal acute beds. It is estimated that, as early as 1986, multihospital systems will possess anywhere from a 50 percent to 70 percent share of the community hospital market. In contrast, nearly all community hospitals functioned autonomously in the early 1970's [Johnson, 1983, pp. 89-109].

The trend, in many of these new systems, is to integrate community based ambulatory care services with inpatient long-term and acute care, a goal that has long eluded the grasp of planning proponents. Still more impressive, given their reputation for individualism, is the consolidation of physicians' private practices. The percentage of active physicians in some form of group practice has risen from a mere 5 percent in 1960 to approximately 25 percent today [Starr, p. 425].

Corporatization entails patterns of accountability and collective action foreign to the autonomy features of solo practice. Adjustment, therefore, entails substantial stress for both management and physicians. About one-fourth of all physicians now have some contractual relationship with hospitals; it is estimated that three out of five of these doctors are on salary. No matter how generous the conditions of employment, corporatization of medical practice signifies less individual control over such issues as hours, number of patients, and retirement age. Corporate legal accountability for quality of medical care also signifies closer scrutiny of clinical decision making. That health corporations will seek ways to modify clinical decision making to encompass managements' economic priorities is already apparent [Hull, 1984, p.33].

*Prospective Reimbursement*

Yet other radical changes are occurring behind the banner of competition. Newly introduced prospective reimbursement and related controls are impinging on the freedom of providers to set charges and subsidize high-cost, low-volume services through non-cost-related pricing, subject only to service-ethic restraints. The trend is to compel providers, beginning with hospitals and, subsequently, expanding to nursing homes and physicians, to accept either a sum fixed in advance for each service rendered, or a predetermined annual budget. Instead of being able to pass through losses in the form of higher charges to third parties, providers will be required to absorb deficits [Richardson, 1984, pp. 340-71].

Briefly stated, the aim of prospective payment is to foster greater cost consciousness. Limited at the onset to recipients of government programs (e.g., Medicare, Medicaid, and maternal and child health), private health insurance firms and self-insured employers are bound to follow suit. Failure to do so invites providers incurring losses from government reimbursement to charge other payment sources more, thereby transferring part of the burden of public financing to the private sector. Employers and the commercial health insurance industry are increasingly critical of government policies that lead hospitals to compensate for inadequate reimbursement from Medicare and Medicaid by shifting costs to private patients. These cost shifts are estimated to total $6 billion annually [Mayer and Johnson, 1983(b), pp. 20-35].

Changes in reimbursement are made more palatable by positive incentives to economize, which allow hospitals and physicians to retain a share of any savings. When combined with the power of peer review, common to group or contractural practice, prepayment consistently has been found to result in the use of fewer hospital days, as much as 40 percent, with no discernible lowering of quality of care assessed in terms of patient outcomes [Jonas and Rimer, 1977, pp. 120-63]. The intent is to encourage more effective use of resources and, in particular, to lower the amount of medically questionable or unnecessary services prevalent under fee-for-service and cost-plus payment modes.

Promotion of cost consciousness among physicians is enhanced and reinforced by the instruction of medical students in benefit-cost analysis. In a growing number of medical schools, the subject of cost-effective clinical decision making is being taught. Instead of doing everything medically possible to sustain life and health, in accordance with ancient ethical strictures, medical students are now being urged to first weigh the benefits and costs to society [Eastaugh, 1981, pp. 28-35]. This, of course, is contradictory to the patient's expectation that the physician will employ every available resource to treat his individual patient, and a source of conflict potentially inimical to medicine's larger historic role in maintaining community integration.

*Consumer Use Charges*

Chief among the changes advocated on the consumer side are cutbacks in economic security and freedom of choice of physician. On the assumption that overly generous health insurance benefits invite frivolous consumption, competitive proposals typically prescribe higher user charges in the form of deductibles and coinsurance. Abuse is seen as inevitable whenever services are provided free at the point of consumption. The impression that resources are inexhaustible is a stimulus to initiate care for many self-limiting and nonserious conditions not requiring the attention of a trained physician [McNerney, 1982, pp. 333-68].

Proponents of competition are generally undisturbed by the possibility that price and income rationing may increase future expenditures by deterring prompt diagnosis and treatment. This is based less on indifference than on awareness that only about one-tenth of all diseases can be arrested, reversed, or cured by medicine or surgery; and, moreover, that as much as 70 percent of all patient-physician contacts are for common colds, upset stomachs, and other conditions that frequently can be treated without professional care.[5] Confidence that much of the medical care consumed may not be essential is further buttressed by findings that fewer than one-third of all visits to office-based internists are for conditions classified as either serious or very serious. With respect to hospitalization, it is said that only 15 to 30 percent of emergency room visits are for urgent care, not all of which are true emergencies, in a life or death sense. Child birth is reported to account for close to 10 percent of all discharges from short-stay hospitals, whereas cancer and heart disease account for only 8 percent and 5 percent, respectively [Ricardo-Campbell, 1982, pp. 93-8].

Scepticism toward the value of routine health care also hardens many pro-competitive advocates against criticism that market rationing discriminates against the poor. With limited exceptions (notably childhood immunizations), price and income barriers are condescendingly viewed as benefiting the poor by lowering their exposure to the harmful side effects of unnecessary medical treatment. Available evidence suggests that while prices lower the utilization of the poor more than the rich, the severely ill are less likely to be deterred than the nonseriously ill [Newhouse, 1981]. On the other hand, the necessity of treatment for serious illness is acknowledged. Catastrophic insurance guaranteeing the protection of individual and family economic security for all expenditures exceeding, for example, amounts ranging from $500 to $1,000, has widespread support among advocates of market competition.

---

[5] This assertion is based on studies of primary care, such as those conducted by Fry [1966]. Findings from a number of highly industrialized countries have been compiled by Stephen [1979, pp. 11 - 4].

Proposals for broadening consumer financial responsibility for health treatment are not groundless. Properly formulated, higher consumer charges can help free government and industry to meet other important responsibilities. There is, however, a risk that consumer-use charges could aggrevate the cost problem unless certain minimum safeguards are respected: charges must be earmarked to raise health revenues; administrative costs must be minimized; payments must avoid deterring patients who, if not treated (e.g., mothers and children), will generate extra costs to the community in future years; charges must not impose the heaviest burden on the most ill people; and exemptions must be designed to avoid accentuating the poverty trap and weakening work incentives.

Price-income rationing is hard to reject if it is applied with care and selectivity. When focused on medical services of proven safety but questionable efficacy, such an approach might have the added benefit of safeguarding public health while cutting waste and raising revenues. As noted by the Office of Technology Assessment, the beneficial value of most (80 to 90 percent) medical procedures has never been subjected to rigorous standards of scientific proof, raising serious questions about the value of health spending and concerns over the safety and efficacy of the medical procedures which patients trust their lives to [Office of Technology Assessment, 1978, p. 7].

*Choice of Physician*

Contrary to the *laissez-faire* message, consumers will have less instead of more freedom of choice of physician as the substantive changes behind competitive rhetoric are implemented. There is little continuing doubt that the unlimited right of patients to seek and discontinue care from any physician is wasteful and inefficient under conditions of retrospective payment of solo, fee-for-service medical practice. As pointed out in the introduction to a collection of essays written by leading proponents of health-care competition, the freedom of choice patients with health insurance have is [Melia, 1983, pp. 788-92], "the single most important source of overspending. . . . It eliminates price competition among providers and gives patients an incentive to choose more costly care even when the gains to the patient are negligible." Thus, the goal of pro-competitive strategists is to have consumers agree in advance to receive all of their reimbursable care from a single group of providers (e.g., a health maintenance organization or a preferred provider organization) complying with cost-effectiveness standards set by reimbursement agencies.

Because of the greater economies attainable under structured forms of medical practice, employers and government are, due to economies of scale and incentives for cost-effectiveness in diagnosis and treatment, supporting innovations designed to influence consumers away from traditional types of insurance coverage, including the pocketing of a share of any savings associated with the choice of a prepayment group from an approved list. The placement of ceilings on what employers and government will pay is another inducement for "economically rational" consumers to select providers contracting to provide a range of specified services through competitive bidding and related means. Economic discipline is inevitable, it is believed, due to the financial risks for overspending which providers are required to assume under such arrangements [Enthoven, 1981, pp. 421-23; U.S. Comptroller General, 1982]. Poor persons, however, may be denied the luxury of choice, if what happened in California last year becomes a precedent for other states. Medicaid recipients in California are required to receive their health care from a group authorized to be the sole provider within large territorial and population areas established by state authorities.

*Cooptation of Private Capital*

Less controversial, perhaps, is another frequently overlooked aspect of free-market appeals—the cooptation of private capital for underwriting costly improvements in community services. Attractive tax-shelter features and favorable prospects for high rates of return on their money, at little risk, made investors eager to finance some of the obligations incurred by government in progressive social legislation to expand health-services accessibility. The inflow of private capital into the health sector, following passage of Medicare and Medicaid, helped to speed increases in the supply of inpatient services. Especially visible were the salutory effects in long-term care. Over the 10-year period beginning in the mid-1960's, the supply of nursing home beds doubled (from one-half million to one million), mainly because of government incentive to private investors [Rango, 1982, pp. 883-89]. Notorious problems of patient overcrowding and noncompliance with life-safety codes, underwent a marked improvement from the infusion of private capital. Taxpayers, too, have benefited from the easing of pressure on public budgets badly strained during the 1970's by the rare occurrence of simultaneously high rates of inflation and unemployment.

Similarly helpful has been the use of tax exempt bonds to substitute private money for government funds in meeting the capital needs of the nation's nonprofit hospitals for replacement of obsolescent physical plant and acquisition of new technologies. It was unanticipated, however, that many hospitals would incur high debt-to-capitalization ratios. Worry that high levels of indebtedness may lower their credit ratings and consequential ability to attract capital, many nonprofit hospitals are looking to the issuance of shares in emulation of the capital financing methods used by proprietory corporations. The advantage is that a hospital may go to the equity marked with one dollar and raise from 15 to 30 dollars, whereas, in the bond market, one dollar raises only two dollars.

In order to tap the equity markets, nonprofit hospitals are reorganizing themselves into complex corporate entities with profit-making subsidiaries—e.g., office buildings, contract management services, occupational-industrial medicine, transportation, illness centers, alcohol and drug abuse treatment, health maintenance organizations, emergicenter, and the like [Goldsmith, 1980, pp. 100-12]. A potential drawback to society is that the best management talent may be diverted to money-making peripheral enterprises and health care institutions may lose sight of their basic mission.

Ironically, the creative use of private capital has done more to spur than inhibit public regulation in the health sector. This was inevitable since the business of business is to make money. Lucrative tax shelters and income-enhancement opportunities have provided irresistible temptations to engage in accounting and financial practices constituting the subject of tighter government controls, especially for nursing home care. During the 1970's sensational mass-media disclosures focused public attention on numerous overtly illegal practices [Vladeck; Spitz, 1982, pp. 246-56].

Although they generate less publicity, irregularities of a morally grey nature nevertheless add considerably to the nation's health cost burden. Mergers and acquisitions provide special advantages to corporations seeking to boost reported earnings for investors. Because interest expense, depreciation, and administrative overhead are reimbursable, there is a strong temptation to claim excessive capital cost in order to maximize revenues from government health programs and private insurance companies. In analyzing the consequences of Hospital Corporation of America's 1981 takeover of the assets (54 hospitals, 18 nursing homes, and other subsidiaries) of a rival investor-owned health care corporation, the U.S. General Accounting Office (GAO) concluded that the acquisition resulted in net additional costs of roughly $55 million during the first year alone. Among two hospitals studied in depth, the overall increase in costs due to interest, depreciation, and overhead was $1 million and $300,000, of which nearly half was charged to Medicare and Medicaid and the remainder to private health insurance companies. Auditors determined that many practices did not comply with federal guidelines, e.g., extension of the useful economic lives of facilities to increase depreciated reproduction [U.S. Comptroller General, 1983(a)].

Practically minded observers nevertheless may approve the trade-offs associated with the use of private capital. There is solace in the possibility that once health services are restructured it will be fairly easy to implant a greater concern for social responsibility and patient welfare, if necessary. In any event, disputes over the role of private capital may soon become academic. The scheduled phasing out of cost-plus modes of reimbursement and discontinued assurance of high rates of return on equity, dim continuing prospects for the role of private capital in the provision of hospital and nursing home services.

## Summary and Conclusions

If the hiatus between economic doctrine and practice renders absurd the applicability of unstructured competition to the health sector, the value of ideology as an instrument for circumventing political opposition to change should be taken more seriously. Whether intended or not, exhortations to run health services more like a business have become a powerful catalyst for reshaping traditional organizational and financial arrangements outmoded by important developments in medical technology and exigencies of national economic policy.

The lifting of sanctions against the pursuit of self-interest has freed providers to compete openly with one another for scarce resources in ways which inadvertently aid the attainment of federal priorities for strong managerial direction of highly consolidated and integrated comprehensive health-services delivery networks. Recent progress in mergers and affiliations has resulted in the formation of multihospital systems, whose fiscal leverage and share of patient care services is a considerable advantage in the struggle for dominance with traditionally patterned community hospitals and independent solo medical practitioners. It is highly unlikely that comparable restructuring could have occurred in the same short time through planning and direct government intervention. The accountability and politicization characteristic of decision making in the public arena are brakes for slowing the speed of change.

Notwithstanding some notable tactical advantages, caution is advisable in the use of competition for addressing problems in a sector of the economy where experience shows that community welfare and the needs of the sick do not mix well with orthodox market principles. One of the more serious shortcomings of the competitive strategy is the philosophical bias for freeing policy from moral constraints. The sense of urgency underlying health policy deliberations heightens the predisposition to eschew any hampering of decisiveness and alacrity in pursuit of goals of cost containment and efficiency. Worry about the moral consequences of actions too often is construed by pro-competition pragmatists as a form of weakness.

Regardless of how brilliantly conceived and implemented, policies bereft of moral sensitivity hinder recognition of potentially harmful long-term consequences. This risk is inherent in the possibility that incentives for running health care organizations more like a business may succeed too well in blurring differences in the behavior of profit-making and non-profit institutions.

Expediency in response to imperatives for efficiency and economy is no virtue if mindless to community obligations for equity in the accessibility and quality of health services. It is hazardous to assume that moral purpose can be restored easily following the successful completion of restructuring. Once socialized in the culture of market competition, health professionals are unlikely to be any better disposed to withstand conflicts of interest than when subjected to the restraint of ancient ethical codes and peer pressures for socially responsible behavior.

Ultimately, a commercial approach to health care delivery is incompatible with the prevalent belief that medical practice is a privilege in which self-gain and bottom-line accounting are secondary to doing what is best for the welfare of patients and the good of the community. There are sectors of the economy in which unchecked pursuit of self-interest is an excellent guide to socially desirable action. For reasons which are described herein, the health sector is a notable exception. Pro-competitive suggestions that equity in health care delivery can be achieved without regulation are misleading and irresponsible.

## REFERENCES

Brian Abel-Smith, "Value for Money in Health Services," *Social Security Bulletin*, 37, July 1974.

Kenneth J. Arrow, "Uncertainty and the Welfare Economics of Medical Care," *American Economic Review*, 53, December 1963.

Richard M. Bailey, *Clinical Laboratories and the Practice of Medicine*, Berkeley: McCutchan, 1979.

Roger M. Battistella, "International Health Policy Trends," *Health Care Policy in a Changing Environment*, Roger M. Battistella and Thomas G. Rundall, eds., San Francisco: McCutchan Press, 1978(a).

――― and Theodore E. Chester, "The Professional Standards Review Organization Programs: A Political-Economic Assessment," *Health Care Policy in a Changing Environment*, Roger M. Battistella and Thomas G. Rundall, eds., Berkeley: McCutchan Press, 1978(b).

――― and Steven R. Eastaugh, "Hidden Perils of Hospital Cost Containment," *Bulletin the New York Academy of Medicine*, 56, January-February 1980.

Daniel Bell and Irving Kristal, eds., *Capitalism Today*, New York: Mentor Books, 1971.

Thomas W. Bice, "Health Services Planning and Evaluation," *Introduction to Health Services*, 2nd ed., New York: John Wiley and Sons, 1984.

John Bryant, *Health and the Developing World*, Ithaca, New York: Cornell University Press, 1969.

Joseph A. Califano, Jr., *Governing America*, New York: Simon and Schuster, 1981.

Committee on Government Operations, Permanent Subcommittee on Investigations, *Hearings on Prepaid Health Plans*, 94th Congress, 1st Session, March 13-14, 1975.

*Congressional Quarterly*, "Would More Competition Cut Health Costs?" *Health Policy: The Legislative Agenda*, Washington, D.C., 1980(a).

―――, "Congress Considers Major Food Law Review," *Health Policy: The Legislative Agenda*, Washington, D.C., 1980(b).

A. J. Culyer, "The NHS and the Market," *The Public-Private Mix for Health*, Gordon McLachlan and Alan Maynard, eds., London: The Nuffield Provincial Hospitals Trust, 1981.

Karen Davis and Cathy Schoen, *Health and the War on Poverty*, Washington, D.C.: The Brooking's Institution, 1978.

Marvin Dicker, National Center for Health Statistics, *Health Care Coverage and Insurance Premiums of Families, United States, 1980*, National Medical Care Utilization and Expenditure Survey, Preliminary Data Report No. 3, DHSS Pub. No. 83-20000, Public Health Service, Washington, D.C.: GPO, 1983.

Steven R. Eastaugh, "Teaching the Principles of Cost-Effective Clinical Decisionmaking to Medical Students," *Inquiry*, 18, Spring 1981.

Alain C. Enthoven, "A Brief Outline of the Competition Strategy for Health Services Delivery System Reform," *A New Approach to the Economics of Health Care*, Mancur

Olson, ed., Washington, D.C.: American Enterprise Institute for Public Policy Research, 1981.

Abraham Flexner, *Medical Education in the United States and Canada,* Carnegie Foundation for the Advancement of Teaching, Bulletin No. 4, Boston: Merrymount Press, 1910.

Paul J. Feldstein, *Health Associations and the Demand for Legislation,* Cambridge, Mass.: Ballinger, 1977.

Renee C. Fox, "The Medicalization and Demedicalization of American Society," *Daedalus,* 106, Winter 1977.

John Fry, *Profiles of Disease,* London: E. and S. Livingstone, 1966.

John Kenneth Galbraith, *The Age of Uncertainty,* Boston: Houghton Mifflin, 1977.

Robert M. Gibson, "National Health Expenditures, 1978," *Health Care Financing Review,* 1, Summer 1979.

Eli Ginzberg, "Competition and Cost Containment," *The New England Journal of Medicine,* 303, November 6, 1980.

Jeff C. Goldsmith, "The Health Care Market: Can Hospitals Survive?" *Harvard Business Review,* 28, September-October 1980.

Bradford H. Gray, ed., *The New Health Care for Profit,* Washington, D.C.: National Academy Press, 1983.

Jennifer Hull, "Hospitals and Doctors Clash Over Efforts by Administrators to Cut Medicare Costs," *The Wall Street Journal,* January 19, 1984.

Donald E. L. Johnson, "Multi-Unit Providers Are Ready to Boost Their Market Share," *Modern Health Care,* 13, May 1983.

Steven Jonas and David Banta, "Government in the Health Care Delivery System," *Health Care Delivery in the United States,* 2nd ed., Steven Jonas, ed., New York: Springer, 1981.

_____ and Barbara Rimer, *Ambulatory Care: Health Care Delivery in the United States,* Steven Jonas, ed., New York: Springer, 1977.

Herbert E. Klarman, *The Economics of Health,* New York: Columbia University Press, 1965.

Richard H. Leftwich, *The Price System and Resource Allocation,* 4th ed., Hinsdale, Illinois: Dryden Press, 1976.

Laurence S. Lewin, Robert A. Derzon, and Rhea Margulies, "Investor-Owned and Nonprofits Differ in Economic Performance," *Hospitals,* 55, July 1, 1981.

George C. Lodge, "The Uses of Ideology for Managers," *Harvard Business School Case Services,* Cambridge: Harvard Business School, February 1982.

_____, *The New American Ideology,* New York; Alfred A. Knopf, 1980.

Jack A. Mayer, ed., *Market Reforms in Health Care,* Washington, D.C.: American Enterprise Institute for Public Policy Research, 1983(a).

_____ and William R. Johnson, "Cost Shifting in Health Care: An Economic Analysis," *Health Affairs,* 2, Summer 1983(b).

Walter J. McNerney, "The Control of Health Care Costs in the United States in the Context of Health Insurance Policies," *The Public-Private Mix for Health Care,* Gordon McLachlan and Alan Maynard, eds., London: The Nuffield Provincial Hospitals Trust, 1982.

Edward P. Melia, *et al,* "Competition in the Health Care Marketplace: A Beginning in California," *The New England Journal of Medicine,* 308, March 31, 1983.

Joseph E. Newhouse, *et al,* "Some Interim Results From a Controlled Trial of Cost Sharing in Health Insurance," *Health Insurance Experiment Series,* R-2847-M.Ms., Santa Monica, California: Rand Corporation, 1981.

Office of Technology Assessment, *Assessing the Efficacy and Safety of Medical Technologies,* Washington, D.C.: GPO, 1978.

Talcott Parsons, *The Social System,* New York: Free Press, 1951.

Robert A. Pattison and Halle M. Katz, "Investor-Owned and Not-for-Profit Hospitals," *The New England Journal of Medicine,* 309, August 11, 1983.

Mark V. Pauly, "Is Medical Care Different?" *Issues in Health Economics,* Roice O. Luke and Jeffrey C. Bauer, eds., Rockville, Maryland: Aspen, 1982.

Nicolas Rango, "Nursing Home Care in the United States," *The New England Journal of Medicine,* 307, September 30, 1982.

Arnold S. Relman, "The Future of Medical Practice," *Health Affairs,* 2, Summer 1983.

Rita Ricardo-Campbell, *The Economics and Politics of Health,* Chapel Hill: University of North Carolina Press, 1982.

William C. Richardson, "Financing Health Services," *Introduction to Health Services,* 2nd ed., Stephen J. Williams and Paul R. Torrens, eds., New York: John Wiley and Sons, 1984.

Roger Ricklefs, "Public Gives Executives Low Marks for Honesty and Ethical Standards," *Wall Street Journal,* November 2, 1983.

Robert F. Rushmer, "Technological Resources for Health," *Introduction to Health Services,* 2nd ed., New York: John Wiley and Sons, 1984.

Patricia W. Samors and Sean Sullivan, "Health Cost Containment Through Private Sector Initiatives," *Market Reforms in Health Care,* Jack A. Meyer, ed., Washington, D.C.: American Enterprise Institute for Public Policy Research, 1983.

Burt Schorr, "Laboratory Kickbacks to Doctors Persist Despite Federal and State Investigation," *The Wall Street Journal,* September 26, 1978.

Bruce Spitz, "States' Options for Reimbursing Nursing Home Capital," *Inquiry,* 19, Fall 1982.

Paul Starr, *The Social Transformation of Medicine,* New York: Basic Books, 1983.

W. J. Stephen, *Primary Medical Care: An International Study,* New York: Cambridge University Press, 1979.

Rosemary Stevens, *American Medicine and the Public Interest,* New Haven: Yale University Press, 1971.

David A. Stockman, "Premises for a Medical Marketplace," *Health Affairs,* 1, Winter 1981.

Frank J. Thompson, *Health Policy and the Bureaucracy,* Cambridge: MIT Press, 1981.

U.S. Comptroller General, General Accounting Office, *A Primer on Competitive Strategies for Containing Health Care Costs,* HRD 82-92, Washington, D.C.: GPO, 1982.

————, *Hospital Merger Increased Medicare and Medicaid Payments for Capital Costs,* HRD 84-10, Washington, D.C.: GPO, 1983(a).

————, *Need to Eliminate Payments for Unnecessary Hospital Ancillary Services,* HRD 83-74, Washington, D.C.: GPO, 1983(b).

Bruce C. Vladeck, "The Market vs. Regulation: The Case for Regulation," *Milbank Memorial Fund Quarterly,* 59, November 1981.

————, *Unloving Care: The Nursing Home Tragedy,* New York: Basic Books.

John Wennberg and Alan Gittelsohn, "Small Area Variations in Health Care Delivery," *Science,* 182, December 14, 1973.

# Chapter Four

## Strategic Policy Alternatives for Health Care Provision

### GLORIA R. SMITH and PAMELA PAUL-SHAHEEN

### Introduction

In the past 25 years, a major economic concern in the United States has been the rapid and inexorable rise of health care costs. For example, in 1982, health care costs in this nation represented 10.5 percent of the gross national product—$322 billion. Health care costs are currently rising faster than inflation, at some three times the consumer price index for 1982. Since 1975, more has been spent on health care than on defense. The health care industry is the second largest in the nation behind education. By 1990, more will be spent on health care than on the entire 1980 federal budget. Health care costs are expected to reach one trillion dollars by the year 2000 [Meyer, 1984; *U.S. News,* 1983].

Given the current climate to reduce government spending and the growing concern over escalating health care costs, health care policy innovation is crucial. Actually, the problem of soaring costs is not wholly negative. Efforts to find solutions will probably compel the public and private sectors to face up to and deal with the established disincentives toward economy inherent in the health care system. Furthermore, relevant business practices, such as strategic planning and marketing, will become customary in the public sector within the next decade. One consequence will be greater public-private sector compatability due to a common problem set and a common goal of increased productivity. In addition, cost containment measures will force public agencies to target their programs more realistically because there will be fewer resources available.

Today, both regulatory and competitive approaches are being debated by health care economists [Enthoven, 1980; Feldstein, 1971a, p. 2; 1971b, pp. 854, 870; Sigelman, 1982; Vladeck, 1981; Wicks, 1977]. The advantages and limitations of regulation have been well-documented. Regulation requires some provider restraints and demands that some decision, expansion of bed capacity for example, be dealt with publicly with justifying data [Cohodes, 1982; Vladeck, 1981; Weiner, 1981]. The effectiveness of competition on cost and quality is not yet as well-established, although cost containment is one objective of regulation and competition.

A new wave of attempts to change the health care delivery system has been initiated under the mantle of cost containment. The ultimate impact of many of these, unfortunately, may be simply to hold back spending because, in general, they are not targeted at truly reforming the delivery system. Medicaid, for example, has focused on reducing benefit eligibility. Private insurers and Medicare have increased the patients' out-of-pocket expenses. True cost containment, however, is an entirely different phenomenon and may be defined as [Ginzberg, 1983] ". . . a reduced inflow of real resources into the health care system without a diminution in useful output that would adversely affect the satisfaction of patients or their health status." Thus, to accomplish true cost containment, other strategies are needed which have as their goal not only a reform of the existing delivery system but also a shift of resources from a sickness to a wellness system.

### Strategies to Reduce the Cost of Health Care

With the goal of containing health care costs in mind, five major areas for short and long-term cost containment have been identified: government expenditure policies, government regulatory policies, insurance and other prepayment mechanisms, health care delivery systems, and medical practice [Ginzberg, 1983]. All five areas are potential targets for governmental and private sector attention, and both competitive and regulatory approaches can be used in combination. The criteria proposed for assessing the values of such intervention approaches are [Luft, 1982]: "(1) The magnitude of cost savings; (2) The health effects of pursuing a particular policy; (3) Equity (including distributional effects); (4) Political feasibility; (5) Administrative cost burden; and (6) Policy flexibility (degree of rigidity)." The proposals presented here are viewed as potentially viable in terms of these criteria. Clearly, implementation of any of the strategies described in this paper should be evaluated by policymakers with regard to their integration with and impact on existing approaches, as well as their ability to reach the goals desired by policymakers.

With this as a background, let us now explore a number of policy initiatives which collectively or in part constrain current medical care expenditures, provide for development of new health care delivery strategies focusing on wellness and prevention, and encourage the creation of additional revenues to support new program development. Much of the activity undertaken in the United States is currently focused on constraining current medical care expenditures. Reimbursement for medical care costs in the United States has been handled primarily through third party payment. This insurance reimbursement mechanism puts neither the provider nor the recipient of the service at financial risk for the decisions which occur. This arrangement is now viewed as being inherently inflationary. As such, attempts are being made to add an element of risk into the insurance equation. These initiatives include the following.

1. *DRG's:* This new national initiative is currently being implemented by Medicare to cover hospital payments. It is a reimbursement strategy

based on diagnosis related groups (DRG's), a method of classifying patients by discharge diagnosis into categories that are medically similar and have approximately the same lengths of stay. These groupings include 467 diagnostic categories and can be used as a management tool to assess quality of care, and as a payment system as well. Under the system, Medicare payments will be based on the DRG classification and will be the same fixed amount, regardless of the length of stay or resources used. The payments will be phased in over the next three-year period. Since hospitals will be paid a set amount per discharge diagnosis, they will have an incentive to use medical care resources as efficiently as possible [Wilson, 1983; Minnesota Medical Association, 1983].

2. *PPO's:* In Preferred Provider Organizations (PPO's), a selected panel of physicians, hospitals, and salaried personnel enter into contracts to provide care to participating patients. The contract usually contains a fee schedule involving discounts of up to 20 percent. The emphasis is on identifying providers who are low cost, efficient in using resources, and are willing to accept strict utilization review controls with prior authorization for hospitalization. Second opinions are frequently required by the PPO before elective surgery. The PPO insures, through an economic incentive, that people signed up in the program will use these providers. If the employer has purchased the PPO, the patient gets first dollar coverage; there is no out-of-pocket cost. He may choose to go to other providers but he must first pay a deductible and coinsurance [Kimmey, 1984].

3. *Imposing Co-payments and Deductibles:* Another major strategy being considered by government and private insurers alike is the imposition of co-payments and deductibles on the consumer. These mechanisms are sometimes viewed as providing the consumer with an incentive to use health care services prudently.

Efforts are also being made to constrain medical care expenditures by expanding government regulation. Three efforts of note in this area are:

1. *Rate Regulation:* Within the United States, 25 states have adopted a variety of measures designed to directly control prices and services provided by institutions within their jurisdiction. Often targeted at hospitals, these initiatives may place defined limits on total hospital expenditures or may establish per-admission-day limits combined with strict utilization controls. Some of these initiatives are targeted at select third party payors, while others cover all forms of revenue received by the institution. All are designed to place limits on the total amount of revenue which can be received by an institution for the services provided [Berry, 1975; Cohen, 1975].

2. *Capital Expenditure Caps:* Such an initiative is designed to impose a statutorily defined annual dollar ceiling on hospital capital expenditures. Under the proposal, an annual determination would be made of the total amount which could be approved for institutional capital expenditure pro-

jects. Institutional capital expenditure projects coming in for Certificate of Need (CON) approval would be evaluated against the limit. Projects receiving approval would be credited against the limitation. Once the total number of dollars approved for expenditure had been reached, no additional projects could be approved [Wicks, 1982].

3. *CON Batching:* Currently, under existing Certificate of Need legislation, hospital projects seeking approval are evaluated for their appropriateness independent of one another. Under a batching strategy, the certifying agency would be required to review all proposals from a given area simultaneously, weighing the relative merits of one proposal against those of another.

A third area designed to constrain medical care expenditures is the development of alternative delivery mechanisms. These systems are designed to provide services similar to those generated under the fee for service system, but at lower costs. Examples of these strategies include:

1. *Hospice Care:* A hospice is not necessarily a facility but rather a program of coordinated inpatient, outpatient, and home care services which can be provided in a number of different settings. The system of support and counseling extends through the period of bereavement, when adjustments to a radically altered life-style may be required.

The focus of a hospice is to provide support services to the terminally ill (usually at lower cost), as opposed to subjecting them to a medical regimen designed to try and cure the problem. Hospice care emphasizes the *quality* of life and thus addresses itself to the alleviation of pain and other physical and emotional discomforts which dying patients experience. A hospice is most appropriately viewed as an *option* available to the terminally ill which focuses on helping patients come to terms with the prospect of death and which strives to make it possible for patients to die in relative comfort and tranquility, as free as possible from the miseries associated with their illnesses and the side effects of treatment [Office of Health and Medical Affairs, 1983].

2. *Health Maintenance Organizations (HMO's):* These are designed to provide a full range of medical and preventive services to a defined population under a capitated payment system. Recent studies suggest that HMO's are able to provide appropriate services in a cost effective manner [Luft, 1980, 1981; Gavett and Smith, 1978]. This is primarily due to built-in incentives to treat patients in ambulatory as contrasted with institutional settings. Nationally, hospital days of care used annually by HMO enrollees are half those used by the population at large with no noticeable ill effects. Additional efforts are needed in the United States, however, to assure that HMO's are able to obtain a larger market share.

Within the HMO concept, a new strategy is emerging focused on providing comprehensive care to the elderly. Known as the Social HMO, this delivery mechanism integrates the services of a HMO and a long-term care agency, utilizing a case manager to ensure continuity of care and proper resource allocations. The Social HMO features: integration of health and long-term care services, prepayment, a single comprehensive provider system, funds pooling, and a representative mix of elderly people. Its more unique aspect is that the Social HMO focuses responsibility for the coordination and supervision of a wide range of social and medical services in one organization. Revenues are generated from Medicaid, Medicare, and insurance premiums. These funds are pooled and utilized to provide appropriate care without definitional restrictions. It is anticipated that Social HMO's can address the growing needs of the elderly for integrated health and social services, effectively contain health care costs, and reduce the fragmentation of the current delivery system.

3. *Home Care:* With the relentless rise in health care costs, policymakers are turning their attention to providing incentives which allow people to remain in their homes, rather than being institutionalized. In Michigan, for example, legislation was just enacted to directly reimburse families for caring for severely mentally retarded family members. Tax incentives, tax credits, direct payment, or a deductible could be widely offered to relatives and others who care for handicapped or aged adults who would otherwise be institutionalized at great expense.

As a society, we are beginning to realize that the future of medical care and the future state of our health are not one in the same. Dramatic advances in biomedical technology, such as those which have made possible organ transplants, kidney dialysis, insulin infusion pumps, and artificial hearts are impressive achievements which can save and extend lives. They have, however, very little to do with the health status of the overall population. What is needed is a major reorientation of the health care system toward an approach which emphasizes the promotion and maintenance of health.

As most of the causes of today's ill health relate to individual and collective behavior and the physical and social environment, it is reasonable to conclude that future improvements in health status will result from changes in these areas rather than improvements in medical treatment [Hancock, 1982]. Fortunately, many are beginning to see the relevance of such an approach. As a result, many new and unique initiatives are being tried or considered in an attempt to shift collective focus to health promotion. Initiatives designed to promote health and wellness include:

1. *Worker Health Promotion:* Health promotion in the work place offers a potential which can significantly impact on health care costs by modifying behavior affecting health habits. Among the possibilities are programs for stress management, physical fitness, education on exposure to toxic substances, safety training, smoking cessation clinics, weight control, and health risk assessment and counseling. To date, corporate health programs have evidenced a good track record in behavior modification

[*Health Forecast,* 1983; Coates, *et al,* 1981; Logan, 1981]. Such programs could be greatly expanded if they were tax deductible (as is health insurance). A bill was introduced in the U.S. Senate in 1983 to provide employers with tax credits for preventive health care programs for employees [U.S. Senate, 1983].

2. *Differential Insurance Premiums:* Private insurance companies are now beginning to explore marketing alternative insurance packages which provide coverage at lower rates for people with good health habits—those who maintain normal weight, avoid smoking, use automobile seat belts, and show evidence of regular and healthful exercise. In Michigan, for example, auto insurance companies have agreed to reduce the cost of premiums for those utilizing seat belts once a mandatory seat belt law is enacted by the Michigan legislature.

3. *Mandatory Insurance Coverage:* State insurance codes could be amended to require all companies selling insurance to include certain health promotion services as part of their basic medical package. In order to avoid significant premium increases, the addition of these services could be phased in over time. That way the up front cost of adding the service would remain small but the health effects of these added services could be substantial.

4. *Personal Health Promotion:* Policymakers should look at the options available to encourage individuals to remain healthy. For example, families could receive tax rebates for purchasing memberships in physical fitness clubs or for purchasing selected sports equipment up to a specified dollar level. Individuals on government programs, such as AFDC, could receive vouchers for such memberships or purchases. Employers could be encouraged to reward employees who do not use sick days by allowing them to take additional scheduled days off as personal days or bonus vacation days. Employers could also provide financial rebates to employees not utilizing insured health care services extensively. One such program has been instituted by the Quaker Oats Company with considerable success.

5. *Public Health Promotion:* Certain health promotion programs must be initiated by state and local governments because of the scope of the population affected, the potential cost of the program, and the lack of ability of private individuals or groups to initiate the program. Proposals falling into this category which seem to be most urgent are: (a) comprehensive school health education; (b) adult health screening; (c) health education for the elderly; (d) motor vehicle accident prevention education; (e) health risk identification education; (f) enactment of mandatory seat belt laws; and (g) enactment of programs to identify toxic wastes and pollutants and remove them from the environment.

### Identifying New Revenue Sources

Although health care cost containment currently dominates the public policy debate, it is also important for policymakers to propose mechanisms for resource expansion. A number of rationales exist for this approach. First and most importantly, few involved in the effort to contain health care costs anticipate that any successful effort will result in significant savings. Rather, an effective approach will simply result in slowing cost escalation. Thus, new resource will have to be identified to initiate new programs.

Second, it is politically difficult to defund existing programs because they have entrenched constituencies. Correspondingly, it is easier to add new programs and build new constituencies. New programs, however, require new funds [Levine, 1981].

Third, during periods of recession or economic instability, there are simply more health care needs than the public coffers can meet. Private corporate and individual assistance can and should be developed to expand the resource base for health care delivery.

Finally, general public dissatisfaction with the provision of services by large-scale, traditional organizations is apparent given the latest anti-tax movement. New structures which are smaller, leaner, and easier to assess in terms of cost and impact are gaining wider acceptability. Legislators and public health executives will find the public more receptive to innovations in health care services which fit greater voter sophistication and the necessity to achieve health care goals at lesser governmental expense. One major revenue source is, of course, the tax system. Interestingly, Europeans (but not Americans) have long recognized that taxes which seem minor, or which obviously and immediately benefit the group being taxed, are rarely fought with much vigor. Also, taxes which are incrementally and very slowly increased evoke much less resistance than a single sizeable tax increase. Examples of potentially "painless" taxes which could be imposed to increase health revenues include:

1. *Tax on Hospital Admissions:* Such a tax could be minor in amount (from $1.00 to $3.00 per admission). The funds received would be available to the collecting hospital for use in health education programs which met guidelines established by enabling legislation. The virtue of this proposal, in part, is its political viability; hospitals would have an opportunity to expand into other areas of health care delivery, thus assuring their continued existence, while excess hospital capacity would be converted to other purposes, lessening the pressure on hospitals for unnecessary admissions to maintain an income flow. Further, high demand programs could be expanded, thereby increasing hospital revenues. This would be, in effect, a governmentally supported transfer of payments to subsidize entrepreneurship.

2. *Minimal Tax on Poor Health Habits:* An increase in the tax on alcohol and tobacco purchases of ¼ of 1 percent might not arouse too much antagonism, especially if the income generated supported drug and alcohol education programs in the public schools. Increases in luxury

taxes are generally supported when the proceeds are directed towards a specific purpose, rather than being deposited into the general revenue fund. Putting tax money into general accounts deprives the tax of a potentially powerful constituency (parents, employers, teachers, and so forth). Taxation, in general, is deemed as supporting government. Government is often viewed by Americans as disinterested and wasteful, but, for example, drug and alcohol education may be seen as meritorious.

3. *Unique Taxes:* Evidence is available which indicates that residents of many states and countries are willing to be taxed for provision of some health services. For example, Michigan residents seem to be willing to be taxed for a toxic waste fund. A Michigan Department of Public Health study [1982] states in part that:

> ". . . the Michigan public is concerned about the health effects of chemicals. A general profile of public expectation concerning the role of state government identifies a high level of expected protection in communities and places of work. Michigan residents do not want to compromise protection for economic growth even if protection is a tradeoff for fewer jobs.
>
> "In a climate of government deregulation, it appears that in the area of chemicals and public health, citizens are willing to make an exception to this general trend. Michigan's residents clearly expect the state to protect them from unnecessary chemical exposures."

Given this high level of public expectation, taxation programs targeted to address this or other publicly perceived problems could gain broad public acceptance.

4. *Tax Checkoff:* In 1982, a Michigan children's trust fund was established by the legislature as a permanent source of support for local programs aimed at preventing child abuse and neglect. The fund is supported by taxpayers who can donate $2.00 of their refund to the trust by checking the appropriate box on the income tax form. In 1984, another checkoff was added to the income tax form to provide a fund to preserve endangered animal species. While there are obvious limits to such an approach, it might be suitable for certain specific health promotion or disease prevention efforts.

An initiative currently under consideration in Michigan is the development of a state health foundation. The foundation would be a public-private nonprofit corporation governed by a coalition of employers, employee groups, government leaders, and consumers, with representation from the insurer and provider community.

The foundation could be charged with the organization, collection, and disbursement of donations for health in general and for selected specific purposes. It would also be legally able to receive donations from corporations and from individuals throughout the year and as a charitable donation by April 15 for the past year against state taxes, up to a selected amount. Additionally, state taxpayers would be able to direct a portion of their state taxes to support the work of the foundation. This flexibility would allow the foundation concept to be effectively marketed to that segment of the population with a high interest in health, as well as an interest in having their tax dollars directed toward specific purposes. As was stated earlier, the premise is that donations are really self-imposed taxes and taxes have never, from pre-revolutionary days to the present, been properly marketed in the United States. Tax-deductible donations, in contrast, have been remarkably successful "latent taxes" and present interesting models for voluntary resource exenditure for the public good.

## Discussion

In the current anti-government, anti-tax climate, implementation of any or a combination of the aforementioned strategies will require careful analysis. Here, the strategic planning process[1] can be useful in defining system-wide goals realistically and in allocating a critical mass of resources in a few key areas where positive results are highly probable. Existing programs can be bent toward new goals as a consequence of strategic planning and the potential of new programs can be evaluated as part of a larger, integrated whole. After critical policy decisions are made, health department managers can adapt new strategies or amend existing programs in their areas consistent with economic and environmental (including political) constraints.

Strategic planning is a process used to develop a carefully designed, unified, and comprehensive plan which guides decisions and actions so that the basic objectives of the organization can be achieved. In effect, a strategy is a fiction created so that an organization can have a better future. Strategic plans can always be adapted to new circumstances and they are useful for exploiting new opportunities. Such plans help managers to prioritize their programs, because goals and directions are clear. Effectiveness and staff satisfaction are also enhanced. Finally, resource allocation can be made based on criteria described in the plan [Glueck, 1976].

To be successful, organizations must focus outward and their managerial values must match environmental characteristics. The process of managing is really one of appropriately reacting to the complex demands of groups in the environment and within the organization. These demands result in managers incrementally adjusting objectives as well as their own aspirations in relation to pragmatic concerns. Success is a consequence of the realistic formulation of plans, structures to institutionalize plans, and effective communication and reinforcement of plans throughout the enterprise. According to Glueck [1976], "The strategic planning process will be successful to the extent that top management participates in formulating the objectives and that these objectives reflect the values of management and the realities of the organization's situation."

---

[1] For a definitive discussion of the process, see Steiner [1979].

The strategic planning process involves a number of key steps. First, a profile of the environmental threats and opportunities facing the organization is developed. Market definition and appraisal are included. If the organization is governmental, then the political sector of the environment will also be analyzed. Part of the strategic advantage profile is a description and assessment of an organization's products and markets (past, present, and future). An evaluation is made of the organization's capabilities. Frequently, an organization's product mix or marketing strategy is changed based on the strategic advantage profile.

Secondly, alternative strategies are proposed. These may be active or passive. They may be flexible-contingent or programmed, but they always define the mission of the organization briefly and simply. Grand strategies involve a choice of stability, growth, retrenchment, or a combination of these. Issues such as diversification or limitation of services are considered in light of the overall strategic approach. Strategy making (policymaking in government) occurs in the entrepreneurial (risky) mode, the adaptive mode (used in difficult environments), or the planning mode (long-term emphasis). Each has its implications for the strategic planning process [Glueck, 1976].

Third, evaluation mechanisms are identified. Evaluation is intrinsic to strategic planning because goal accomplishment levels are specified. Strategic planning, in brief, links organizational processes to outcomes through the evaluation process. Ultimately, it assists in the identification of strategies whereby the organization can reach its objectives.

**Conclusion**

As was mentioned earlier, health care cost containment measures to date have often focused on limiting access to services and/or eligibility or increasing the patient's out-of-pocket expenses. Such efforts do not, in a direct sense, address the goal of true cost containment which is to create a healthier population, reducing the need for medical care. The current environment, however, offers a unique opportunity to accomplish this goal.

First, as a public, Americans are beginning to see the true limitations of medicine. Where once it was believed medicine could find a cure for everything, individuals have now come to believe they must assume responsibility for their own health. The shift from seeking institutional assistance to greater self-reliance is evidence of this trend. Further, self-reliance suggests the population may have a potentially greater interest in maintaining health, a perspective which will support and encourage the expansion of health promotion and disease prevention programs.

Second, business and industry are now beginning to realize the need for their active participation in finding a solution to escalating health care costs. In Michigan, for example, major corporations and big labor have formed the Economic Alliance to improve Michigan's business climate. A major target of this effort is to reduce industry health care costs. This recognition may provide public policymakers with the political leverage needed to enact effective regulatory or market strategies which would be opposed by health care providers, thus making them politically unpopular.

Third, tools such as strategic planning and cost-benefit analysis[2] are tools which can be increasingly used by public policymakers to effectively evaluate options and identify alternative solutions. Greater use of those strategies will allow policymakers in the health care sector to more effectively target limited resources to meet health care needs.

Finally, the growth of corporate medicine will transform the American health care system [Starr, 1982]. Periods of massive institutional change will open doors for structural innovation, including the potential for public-private collaboration through vehicles such as the quasi-public corporation. This type of organization will be able to attract new resources through tax checkoff, foundation solicitation, and contributions from private enterprise. These revenues can be used to fund innovative projects of short duration which support health promotion and which show promise of attracting other financial support for longer periods of time. Resource expansion is essential if health care is to meet newly defined needs associated with the 1980's life-style and new structures can attract additional funds more easily than old structures can.

From a public health perspective, the current health care cost crisis offers great promise. The care of the public's health began with the prevention of disease. It has, to some extent unwittingly, evolved into the care of illness. It must return to its traditional role and place major emphasis, once again, on ways to promote and preserve health through the prevention of illness and accidents. It must also become truly public by actively involving all sectors of the population. It will take time. But it can and will be done if we are wise enough to insist that such efforts are not short-changed in favor of payments for illness care. In the long run, this is the only way we can reduce the staggering costs of such care.

---

[2] For an in-depth discussion on cost-benefit analysis, see Bloom and Berki [1983].

## REFERENCES

Ralph E. Berry, "Perspectives on Rate Regulation," *Controls on Health Care,* Washington: Institute of Medicine, National Academy of Sciences, 1975.

Bernard S. Bloom and S. E. Berki, eds., *Cost Benefit, Cost Effectiveness and Other Decision-Making Techniques in Health Care Resource Allocation,* Chicago: Proceedings of a Regional Symposium, May 19-21, 1983.

Timothy J. Coates, R. W. Jeffery, and L. A. Slinkard, "Heart, Healthy Eating and Exercise: Introducing and Maintaining Changes in Health Behaviors," *American Journal of Public Health,* 71, No. 1, January 1981.

Harold Cohen, "State Rate Regulation," *Controls on Health Care,* Washington: Institute of Medicine, National Academy of Sciences, 1975.

Donald R. Cohodes, "Where You Stand Depends on Where You Sit: Musings on the Regulation/Competition Dialogue," *Journal of Health Politics, Policy and Law,* Spring 1982, p. 61.

"Company Health Programs Pay Off," *Health Forecast,* 3, No. 2, June 17, 1983, pp. 1, 3.

Alain C. Enthoven, *Health Plan: The Only Practical Solution to the Soaring Cost of Medical Care,* Addison-Wesley Publishing Co., 1980.

Martin M. Feldstein, *The Rising Cost of Hospital Care,* Washington: Information Resources Press, 1971a, p. 2.

_____, "Hospital Cost Inflation: A Study in Nonprofit Price Dynamics," *American Economic Review,* December 1971b, pp. 854, 870.

J. William Gavett and Daniel Smith, "A Comparison of Hospital Cost Experience of Three Competing HMOs," *Inquiry,* No. 15, December 1978.

Eli Ginzberg, "Sounding Boards: Cost Containment—Imaginary and Real," *The New England Journal of Medicine,* May 19, 1983, pp. 1220-23.

William F. Glueck, *Business Policy: Strategy Formation and Management Action,* New York: McGraw-Hill Book Co., 1976, pp. 3, 6.

Trevor Hancock, "Beyond Health Care," *The Futurist,* August 1982.

James R. Kimmey, "Making Medicine Businesslike," *Monday Comments,* Comprehensive Health Planning Council of Southeastern Michigan, January 2, 1984.

Charles H. Levine, *Managing Fiscal Stress, The Crisis in the Public Sector,* Chatham House Publishers, 1981.

A. G. Logan, B. J. Milne, C. Achber, W. P. Campbell, and R. B. Haynes, "Cost-Effectiveness of Worksite, Hypertension Treatment Program," *Hypertension,* 3, No. 2, March-April 1981, pp. 211-18.

Harold S. Luft, "Assessing the Evidence of HMO Performance," *Milbank Memorial Fund Quarterly,* 58, Winter 1980.

_____, *Health Maintenance Organization's Dimensions of Performance,* New York: Wiley and Sons, 1981.

_____, "On the Potential Failure of Good Ideas: An Interview with the Originator of Murphy's Law," *Journal of Health Politics, Policy and Law,* 7, No. 1, Spring 1982, p. 75.

Jack A. Meyer, "Economics: The New Factor in the Delivery of Health Care," *Update,* 16, No. 1, January 1984.

Michigan Department of Public Health, *Michigan Opinion on Chemicals and Health,* 1982, pp. 3-4.

Minnesota Medical Association, "A New Reimbursement System, DRGs are Coming," August 1983.

Office of Health and Medical Affairs, "Hospice: A Comprehensive Care Alternative for the Terminally Ill," *Issues in Health Policy,* Michigan Department of Management and Budget, No. 3, May 1983.

Daniel W. Sigelman, "Palm-Reading the Invisible Hand: A Critical Examination of Pro-Competitive Reform Proposals," *Journal of Health Politics, Policy and Law,* 6, No. 4, Winter 1982.

"Soaring Hospital Costs, The Brewing Revolt," *U.S. News and World Report,* August 22, 1983.

Paul Starr, *The Social Transformation of American Medicine,* New York: Basic Books, 1982.

George A. Steiner, *Strategic Planning,* New York: The Free Press, 1979.

U.S. Senate, 88th Congress, 1st Session, S. 1618, July 14, 1983.

Bruce C. Vladeck, "The Market vs. Regulation: The Case for Regulation," *Health and Society,* 59, No. 2, 1981, pp. 209-23.

Stephen M. Weiner, "On Public Values and Private Regulation: Some Reflections on Cost Containment Strategies," *Health and Society,* 59, No. 2, 1981, pp. 269-95.

Elliot K. Wicks, "Why Normal Supply/Demand Economics Don't Fit Health Care Costs," *Michigan Medicine,* May 1977, pp. 230-34.

_____, "A State Limitation on Capital Expenditures by Hospitals Can Help to Contain Rising Hospital Costs," *Issues in Health Policy,* Office of Health and Medical Affairs, Michigan Department of Management and Budget, No. 1, June 1982.

Peter A. Wilson, "Hospitals and DRGs," A briefing paper prepared for the Michigan Hospital Association, July 1, 1983.

# Part Three

The Caribbean Experience

# Chapter Five

## Economic Challenges in Puerto Rico and the Caribbean Community

### CARLOS ROMERO-BARCELÓ

The Caribbean is on the threshold of a potentially very promising new era, both in economics and in social justice. In Puerto Rico, hard work by the people, combined with the opportunities offered by our American citizenship, have—in only a few decades—converted an island of despair, disease, and depression, into the region's undisputed leader in terms of economic development, participatory democracy, and individual creativity.

Like many of its Caribbean neighbors, Puerto Rico has had to confront such obstacles as a very high population density; a total lack of income from mineral resources; a plantation-style agricultural economy; geographic isolation; and a long history of colonialism.

Despite those enormous handicaps, Puerto Ricans since World War II have succeeded in building a technologically sophisticated, industrialized society.

The children of sugar-cane cutters are today assembling heart pacemakers and computer components. And sons and daughters of underpaid piece-work seamstresses have become doctors and teachers and entrepreneurs.

Given the challenges Puerto Ricans have had to overcome, including the *still* unresolved political status dilemma, it goes without saying that the island has *not* been able, in so brief a span of time, to yet achieve full equality with the world's most advanced societies. Nevertheless, a trail has been blazed that is recognized as exceptional throughout the Caribbean and Latin America. And today Puerto Rico stands ready to lend its talents, and experience, in helping its neighbors to achieve greater progress in the years ahead.

On its own, as well as in collaboration with the U.S. Agency for International Development, Puerto Rico has already furnished professional and technical assistance to such countries as the Dominican Republic and Jamaica. In these and other lands, Puerto Ricans can and will play a uniquely valuable role; because they speak both Spanish and English; because they come from a similar culture, with similar geographic conditions; and because they have already met and surmounted many of the same problems that their neighbors are confronting today—problems as

63

fundamental as roadbuilding and flood-control, and problems as complex as designing tax incentive packages and industrial promotion programs.

The Caribbean Basin Initiative (CBI) is only now beginning to be implemented. But the author has consistently given the concept his strong personal support. Indeed, he supported it even before the President formally announced it in February 1982.

There were some people in Puerto Rico—and indeed, there still are some—who objected to the CBI, on the grounds that it would weaken Puerto Rico's competitive position in the region. The author regards such views as extremely short-sighted.

A prosperous, democratic Caribbean is important to Puerto Rico, and to the entire free world, for many reasons. International security considerations are, of course, among those reasons. And so too are fundamental humanitarian considerations.

Where Puerto Rico is concerned, however, another factor enters the picture as well: Puerto Rico stands to benefit enormously from every improvement in regional stability and regional economic growth.

Its neighbors do not constitute a threat to Puerto Rico economically: Puerto Rico is *decades* ahead of most of them, and by the time they catch up to where it is now, Puerto Rico shall have advanced still further.

Far from constituting a threat, the increased well-being of its neighbors offers Puerto Rico an *opportunity*. Caribbean Basin exports have increased *seven-fold* in just the last 10 years, reaching an annual volume that now exceeds $700 million. Assuming that its neighbors grow more prosperous under the CBI, their purchasing power will increase commensurately, and Puerto Rico will, therefore, gain the opportunity to greatly *expand* its level of commercial interchange with countries throughout the area.

Moreover, as a part of this process, Puerto Rico can and should become the principal base of operations for a wide variety of regional *service industries:* transportation and communications; warehousing and distribution; repair and maintenance; banking and finance; translation and data processing; research and development; conferences and conventions; and advanced education and technical training.

Today is a moment of excitement and expectation throughout the Caribbean Basin. One is urged to pay close attention to developments in the coming years, and to lend support, wherever possible, to an effort which offers new hope to millions of people, in a vitally important region of the world.

In the late 1930's, Puerto Rico was widely regarded as "The Poorhouse of the Caribbean." Living conditions were as bad as, or even worse than, the living conditions that prevailed on the most poverty-stricken of the neighboring islands. The life expectancy was only 46 years.

Today, by contrast, the average life expectancy is in the range of 74 or 75 years, which is actually higher than in some parts of the U.S.

In the span of just a couple of generations, and *without* receiving the same level of federal funding that the states receive, Puerto Ricans have completely reversed *centuries* of inadequacy in the health care field.

Needless to say, accomplishments in this regard have attracted international attention. This is one of the many areas in which Puerto Rico stands ready to assist the U.S. government in the Caribbean outreach program.

This author's administration, with outstanding supervision from Dr. Jaime Rivera-Dueno, Secretary of Health throughout the author's seven years as Governor, has devoted special attention to two items of particular interest.

One area is preventive medicine. The other is what one might call the "democratization" of health delivery services.

Prevention programs have included injury as well as illness. Puerto Rico was the first United States jurisdiction, for instance, to implement a mandatory no-fault auto accident insurance system.

On the medical front, meanwhile, physician-training and public health curricula have been restructured in order to place increased emphasis on *preventing* illness—including drug and alcohol addiction. At the same time, laws have been enacted to ensure that every school student in Puerto Rico is inoculated against *seven* different diseases.

Primary care instruction, for future doctors and para-professional personnel, includes training in nutrition, emotional adjustment, and life-style evaluation. In other words, preparation is by no means limited to clinical analysis or the diagnosis of illness: in addition to those skills, personnel are taught to reach out further, and to treat the patient as a *whole person* and member of society.

As the cost of medical care continues to escalate dramatically, the savings generated by *keeping people healthy* will more than compensate for the investments made in the prevention of illness—especially when one factors into the equation the human suffering and the lost productivity that illness causes.

What has attracted the most interest outside of Puerto Rico, however, has been the program to "democratize" medical services. Here, the goal is twofold: first, to guarantee high-quality *care* to all citizens, whether they be rich, or middle-class, or poor. And second, to minimize *costs* by effecting economies of scale.

What the administration is endeavoring to do is to eliminate the wasteful and often inequitable situation wherein communities are served by *two* sets of hospitals, with a duplication of equipment and personnel, much of which is not fully utilized.

What is referred to is, of course, *private* hospitals for those who can afford to pay, and *public* hospitals for those who cannot. Too frequently, the limited resources of the government make it extremely difficult to provide first-class treatment, 24 hours a day, every day, in conventional public hospitals.

In Puerto Rico, over the past half-dozen years, the government has been constructing and equipping modern *public* hospitals, and then contracting with *private* health-care organizations, to have *them* administer and staff the facilities.

The terms of such contracts oblige the private corporations to provide full and complete service to medically indigent patients, with the government picking up a reasonable share of the bill for those services. Simultaneously, patients who can pay use these same facilities, under a fee structure set by the management firm.

Under this system, everybody in a community receives the same quality of care, and the cost to the government is significantly reduced. The concept of "democratized" medical care offers great promise, not only in Puerto Rico but as an idea that can be applied in other places as well.

# Chapter Six

## Democratization of Health Services in Puerto Rico

### JAIME RIVERA DUENO

## Introduction

The foundations of Puerto Rico's present public system of health were laid some 40 years ago when tuberculosis, malaria, and gastroenteritis were decimating a population of which general mortality was 18 of every 1,000 citizens and infant mortality was 113 of every 1,000 live births. The first 10 causes of death were all infectious or parasitic diseases and the average Puerto Rican had a life expectancy of 46 years.

The action plan developed then was innovative and daring. Without interfering with the private practice of medicine, the government undertook responsibility and control of health services by establishing a public system, initially centralized and later regionalized, through which prevention efforts and treatment reached the community by means of a service unit in each town and several hospitals strategically located throughout the island. A network of public health units, health centers, and district hospitals began dispensing services for immunization, nutrition, hygiene, maternal infant care, and detection of infectious diseases, among others.

As a result of improved health services and living conditions, Puerto Rico's demographic statistics showed dramatic improvement during the brief historic moment that saw the island change from an agricultural to an industrialized society. By 1980, general mortality was down from 18 to 6 per 1,000 population, infant mortality had gone from 113 to 18 per 1,000 live births, and life expectancy had risen from 46 to 74 years, one of the highest in the world.

Originally, the regionalized system of health was harshly criticized by groups in private practice, but the results attest to the efficiency of the effort. The results also point to some of the changes that shaped the reality of the present decade. During that stage of progress, Puerto Rico underwent demographic, socioeconomic, and political changes that in turn mandated changes in the regionalized system of health.

There was a population increase from 1.9 million to 3.1 million, with a consequent surge of large metropolitan areas and suburbs. There was an increase in commercial and industrial activity. An extensive network of new highways linked isolated communities with urban centers, making it possible to move patients from local to regional units of service. Large hospitals were built in readily accessible cities (Caguas, Bayamon, Maya-guez) and a plan for construction of intermediate hospitals in other stra-tegic points (such as Yauco, Guayama, and Humacao) was carried out.

These last 10 years also saw the swift adoption of sophisticated tech-nology for handling patients, a condition which threw the cost of medical services into an upward spiral which is yet unchecked.

Longevity and different life–styles brought about new health problems. At present, only one of the first 10 causes of death, pneumonia, is of infectious origin. The rest are chronic conditions such as cardiovascular diseases, diabetes, homicide, suicide, and others directly linked to rather new life–styles.

In terms of health services, these factors, combined with changes in the world economy, rendered the public system of health less and less compet-itive, despite growing budgetary allocations.

The tight fiscal situation was limiting the Puerto Rican Health Depart-ment budget to basically a maintenance effort, reducing the scope of exist-ing programs, and curtailing implementation of new ones. Public hospi-tals were overcrowded and some, which are also teaching institutions, had lost accreditation due to deficiencies. Meanwhile the occupation rate was extremely low in the health centers in each town, but they still had to operate with a budget to cover the hospitalization services they were called to provide. Medical and paramedical resources were unevenly dis-tributed: while San Juan had a doctor for every 250 population, there were towns like Maricao, for instance, that had no one to tend a 14,000 population.

While fiscal reality hampered the system, the demand for services grew by leaps and bounds due to increased unemployment and the consequent reduction in coverage by group and prepaid medical insurance plans. (At present, it is estimated that 64 percent of Puerto Rico's 3.1 million popu-lation is medically indigent, or dependent upon the government for its health services.)

Despite efforts to provide good health services to all the population, Puerto Rico had wound up with a dual system: quality care for the paying patient and deficient services for the medically indigent dependent on pub-lic service.

To bridge the gap, or better yet, to make health services democratic, the quality of public services had to be made equal or better to that of private practice. The traditional options did not provide efficient answers to cur-rent problems. Once more innovation was called for. The established patt-erns had to be modified or replaced, a course of action that is invariably termed "controversial" by most and "essential" by very few.

### The Blueprint

Adequate legislation and the results of several pilot projects allowed the Secretary of Health to design and begin implementing a plan for change that has five salient points:

1. Shift emphasis from curative to preventive medicine, considered the most efficient strategy in dealing with chronic conditions which, like in Puerto Rico, can be traced to life–styles.

2. Implement an Area System in which health services are divided into three levels: preventive at the local level, curative at the secondary level in area hospitals, and highly specialized at the tertiary level or medical centers. In addition to being a service pattern, the Area System is also an administrative tool to control cost and quality: general services are distributed, while specialized and therefore costlier services are concentrated.

3. Improve deployment of medical and paramedical personnel through a compulsory year in public service established by law. A positive side effect of this requirement has been retention of some 43 percent of this personnel in the public system.

4. Reestablish the accreditation of public hospitals.

5. Make public hospitals more competitive, if necessary by converting them into community hospitals.

The objective of this five–point plan is to have one type of medicine practiced in Puerto Rico, of *equal quality for indigent and non–indigent patients.*

### Levels of Service (The Area Concept)

The concept of "areas," considered a development within the concept of regionalization, consists of establishing an intermediate or secondary level between the primary or local level and the tertiary or regional level.

To do this, the island was divided into six health *regions,* each served by a tertiary hospital.

Each region was divided into *areas* comprising three or five towns (see Figure I). Existing health facilities and the potential each community had for attracting health professionals were considered to determine the seat of each area.

The towns in each area have primary institutions that provide mainly preventive services. Hospitalization is not included, except in those towns where its geographic location (like the off–shore island of Vieques) mandate it. Primary institutions with no beds are called Diagnostic and Treatment Centers. Those with hospital beds are called Health Centers.

At the *primary level,* services are provided by health teams that are the patient's access to the system. The patient is then referred to secondary or tertiary levels, depending on his or her condition (see Figure II).

The *secondary level* consists of an intermediate or area hospital with up to 150 beds. Patients with no complications are referred to this area, which provides services in all basic specialities: pediatrics, medicine, obstetrics, and surgery. There are also specialized out–patient departments. The health professionals at the hospital can be deployed to the

FIGURE I

DEPARTMENT OF HEALTH
*GOVERNMENTAL REGIONS AND AREA HEALTH SERVICES*

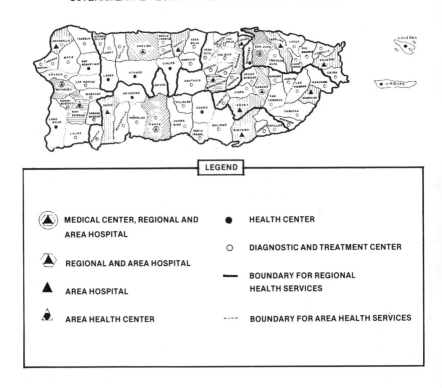

FIGURE II

# AREA CONCEPT

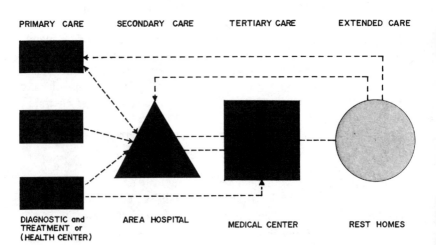

local level when necessary. In addition, the secondary level is to develop training programs for medical and paramedical personnel geared towards preventive and secondary medicine.

The *tertiary level* is made up of the regional hospitals and the medical centers. It has sophisticated equipment and specialized personnel. A patient who is treated at the tertiary level is eventually referred back to the secondary or primary level for follow–up.

A *supratertiary* level has been developed during the last three years and has been located at the Puerto Rico Medical Center. This site will be the only one to house the most expensive services, which have been organized into specialized units, such as a Cardiovascular Center, a Burn Center, Neonatology Center, Neurologic Center, and others.

## Hospital Conversion

Turning over public and private hospitals to independent firms specializing in hospital management is a growing trend in the United States, Europe, and the Middle East. The firms are getting high efficiency at a lower cost.

Puerto Rico decided to go the same way as a means of making some public hospitals more competitive, to better control expenditures for service, and to free the Health Department from some of the service duties that hamper its supervisory role.

It is, in fact, the same system that the Government of Puerto Rico has been using for decades with other properties, such as hotels and factories.

What is being done is turning government–built hospitals over to private management firms or non–profit boards for operation. The government pays for the medically indigent, the privately insured or wealthy pay for their own services. All use the same facilities, equipment, and personnel. All receive the same type of service because they are not segregated within the facility. The government retains quality control powers.

For the time being, the concept is being employed in areas where there are no private hospitals. The purpose is not to compete with private medical practice but to combine private and public resources for quality service to all.

The development and operation of the concept is not as concise as its description.

## The Concept

The Health Department enters into an agreement with a corporation that agrees to provide all health services to the medically indigent population and to comply with Health Department requirements for service. These services are provided for a fixed sum negotiated on the basis of the medically indigent population to be served, a system called "capitation."

Since the amount is negotiated independently of the amount of services to be provided, the corporation is taking a financial risk. It will have to cover its budget through fee for service charges to a paying clientele (see Figure III).

FIGURE III

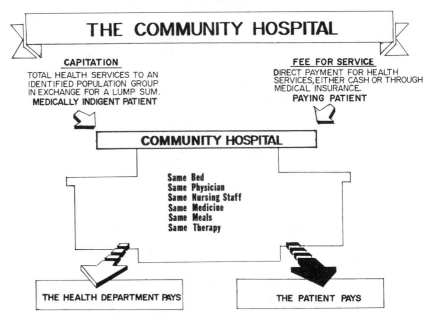

The corporation has fiscal and administrative autonomy. The day–to–day business at the hospital is the same as at a private institution. Medical and supplementary services can be subcontracted to group practices which also agree to serve the medically indigent for a fixed sum. In exchange, they can see their private patients at the hospital. This arrangement provides the hospital with a varied clientele and patients are rendered services according to their medical, not economic, condition.

### Safeguards and Conditions

In order to implement this concept, it was necessary to:

—Set conditions to guarantee compliance with the governmental commitment of quality, quantity, and access of service for the medically indigent.

—Determine the requirements to be met by interested parties.

—Establish safeguards to protect the operation's fiscal integrity, government property, and the rights of public employees if the conversion were made in an operating public hospital.

—Design an adjudgement procedure that could not be tampered with.

—Try out the concept.

### Tryout and Implementation

The first hospital conversion essayed under the present reorganization of the system was at the Yauco Area Hospital, dedicated in 1979 under management of a community board of directors. The board became a non-profit public corporation to run the hospital.

Improvement in both quality and access to service was evident right away, during the first year of operation. In addition, the hospital recovered $3 million.

The positive results in Yauco paved the way for the subsequent conversions.

*Requirements and Conditions*

A corporation interested in running a public hospital has to meet a total of 35 requirements and conditions which cover 10 basic points. The corporation must:

1. Commit itself to always give first priority to the medically indigent.
2. Give evidence of administrative capacity and experience.
3. Prove that it is financially sound.
4. Submit a performance bond of $1 million or more.
5. Submit a payment bond of at least $500,000.
6. Agree to several quality control audits a year.
7. Agree to several internal fiscal audits a year.
8. Agree to an independent fiscal audit at the end of the fiscal year.
9. Agree that a percentage, open to negotiation, of any resulting profits will be set aside for hospital improvements and that another percentage will be allocated for an employee productivity bonus.
10. Agree to retain regular employees. Under this system, no permanent employee loses his or her job. Most are kept on, but under the supervision of the corporation that takes over, although the Health Department continues to pay their salaries. The total thus paid is deducted from the contract payment to the corporation. A small number of regular employees are relocated within the system. Temporary employees become corporation employees, with an immediate salary increase because the company has to pay minimum federal wages.

*Advantages*

Improvement in working conditions and salary, and the productivity bonus for employees, are but a fraction of the advantages that have resulted from this system. Several benefits, some of them intangible, can be quoted for each of the parties involved.

*Employees*

It has been noticed, for instance, that employees develop a more positive attitude towards their work and a sense of belonging towards an institution that is no longer lost in the vastness of bureaucratic anonymity that is the public system of health.

*Hospitals*

—Faster capital improvements.

—More and better equipment.
—Less administrative bureaucracy.
—Computerized systems.
—Better levels of occupancy.
—Better maintenance.
—Renewed accreditation.

*Health Department*

—Savings.
—Improvement of its supervisory role.
—Better quality control.
—Ability to concentrate more efforts on preventive medicine.
—Capacity to concentrate more efforts on mental and environmental health.
—Improvements in the health system (referrals, primary medicine).
—Cost containment.

*Patient*

—One type of medicine.
—Access to new services.
—Better quality of service.
—Specialized services around the clock.
—Access to more qualified professionals.
—Less waiting time.
—More and better support services (labs, X-rays, anesthesia).
—Fewer referrals to tertiary levels.
—Semi-private rooms.
—Closer-to-home hospitalization.

*Achievements*

One type of medicine for all, where those who can pay do so, but those who cannot still get good quality health services. In short, *Democratic Medical Services.*

**Summary**

The Health Department has been involved during the last eight years in an all-out effort to restructure its services towards a more efficient use and equitable distribution of limited resources and facilities, a more realistic approach to prevailing health problems, as well as an overall improvement in quality.

The comprehensive plan has shifted emphasis from curative medicine, organized services into levels determined by their frequency of use, complexity and cost, insured availability of personnel by demanding one year of public service from medical and paramedical disciplines, and made public hospitals more competitive, in some cases by turning them over to private management.

This system also results in cost containment with generalized services provided island-wide and increasingly specialized, and therefore costlier, services concentrated at convenient geographic locations.

Adequate distribution and uniformity of quality is sought through a compulsory year in public service, which insures availability of necessary personnel, and through more competitive public hospitals. This competitiveness is being achieved in some cases through a new modality of management.

What is being done is turning government-built hospitals over to private management firms or non-profit boards for operation. The government pays a lump sum for the medically indigent of the area, the privately insured or wealthy pay for their own services. All use the same facilities, equipment, and personnel. All receive the same type of service because they are not segregated within the facility. The government retains quality service to all.

Results so far consist of marked improvement in quality and access of service, better working conditions for employees, and cost containment. The social objective of this effort is one type of medicine for all.

# Chapter Seven

## Puerto Rico — A Microcosm of Health Care Models And Theories

### REINALDO A. FERRER

### Introduction

Throughout history, health care models and theories have been linked with the socio-economic conditions of specific groups of people and the quantity and quality of their health care services have reflected these conditions. As expected, they have changed from one historical period to another as the problems of providing services changed and demanded new solutions.

Puerto Rico's health care models and theories reflect pluralistic approaches that have been taken by the public and private sectors to safeguard the health and welfare of the people, and the search for health care models with egalitarian features with respect to the availability, accessibility, variety, quality, and quantity of their health care services. They have some of the elements of the health care models through which health services are organized, financed, managed, and provided to people through the world today: public assistance, free enterprise, social insurance, and universal service. Public assistance predominates and others play subordinate roles.

### Public Assistance Model

Over 60 percent of the population depend, for the most part, on health services provided free by the commonwealth and municipal governments and financed with general revenues. These services are provided by salaried personnel within a regionalized system of public hospitals, health centers, and dispensaries controlled and managed by the Puerto Rican Department of Health. The regionalization health care model was developed in 1956 to bring about the integration of all governmental health and welfare resources into a system that would provide integrated health and welfare services in a progressive institutional order, within a defined geographical region. Experience has shown the integration concept to be philosophically desirable but not achievable in practice. Some municipal health and welfare resources remain out of the system, as well as the welfare resources and services of the commonwealth government.

The regionalization model is viewed by some in the private sector as the vehicle through which the commonwealth government will in time make all health services a public benefit within a system of socialized medicine.

The model has been unable to marshal the economic resources needed to provide a minimum set of health services of uniform quality at the primary, secondary, and tertiary institutional levels. Patients often bypass the primary and or secondary levels of services, aided by a means test theoretically applied to determine eligibility, but taken for granted in every day life. It continues to operate side by side, not in coordination but in competition, to the disadvantage of the private, free enterprise health care model. Recently, some features of this model have been incorporated in the area and regional hospitals. It is difficult to visualize, at this time, the future cost effectiveness of this move or its impact on the quantity and quality of services at these institutions.

**Private Health Care Models**

About 40 percent of the people receive health care in the private sector through health insurance plans, labor and industrial health care plans, cooperatives, and with direct out-of-pocket expenditures from physicians in private practice, private profit and not-for-profit hospitals, health centers, and dispensaries. Some people use private health care models for conditions that are treatable on an ambulatory basis, are covered by their insurance plans, or require a small direct out-of-pocket expenditure. For a condition requiring inpatient hospital care, public hospital facilities are often used when the condition is not covered by the insurance plan or coverage is limited.

The bulk of ambulatory health care is provided by physicians in private practice. Estimation of the number of physicians' offices is not possible, as many physicians have several offices. Some offices are well equipped, others have a minimum of equipment. Individual private practice is predominant, although there is a growing tendency for physicians to establish their offices in a particular building, but without group practice arrangements.

**Other Health Care Models**

Some individuals receive part or all of their health care in models with social insurance features, where benefits are related to special conditions and available in specific facilities. Workers are covered by and receive work related medical care through a system of compulsory insurance required of all public and private employers managed by the Puerto Rican State Insurance Fund. Services are available island wide at dispensaries operated by the fund, in private hospitals and other facilities under contract, and at the fund's own hospital on the grounds of the Puerto Rico Medical Center.

Other individuals receive ambulatory and inpatient health care through membership in private, not-for-profit health care associations with features found in Health Maintenance Organizations. Two of these associations own and operate their own general hospitals. Veterans and members of the armed forces receive the bulk of their care in facilities of the United

States government and in private facilities under contract.

Proposals have been made, studied, considered, and discarded to move away from the present combination of public assistance and free enterprise health care models to a universal insurance model found in Great Britain, New Zealand, and Russia.

Except for veterans and members of the armed forces, Puerto Ricans receive their inpatient hospital care in 82 general hospitals with a total bed capacity of 10,212, of which 41 are governmental with 5,394 beds and 41 are private with 4,818 beds. There are also nine special hospitals with a total bed capacity of 2,366, of which six are private with a bed capacity of 893 and three are governmental with 1,493 beds. There are 3.1 general hospital beds per 1,000 population, of which 47 percent are private and 53 percent governmental. There are 0.7 special beds per 1,000 population, of which 64 percent are government owned and 36 percent privately owned. Of the 41 private general hospitals, 13 are not-for-profit and 20 are accredited by the Joint Commission on Accreditation of Hospitals; of the 41 governmental general hospitals, only eight are accredited by the commission. Only one private special hospital is accredited by the commission.

In Puerto Rico, like the United States, the determination of general hospital bed needs remains a controversial subject. The manipulation game between authorized physical bed capacity and daily operational bed capacity produces general hospital beds figures which, like the weather, change on a daily basis. Another complication is the often low utilization of governmental general hospital beds, with an average daily occupancy rate of 53 percent, and the high utilization of private general hospital beds, with a daily occupancy rate of 84 percent. In both governmental and private general hospitals, the higher the bed capacity, the higher the daily occupancy-utilization rate. Of the general hospital beds controlled by the Department of Health, about 566 are in local health centers with hospital units of less than 50 beds and an average daily occupancy rate of 40 percent.

The low utilization of governmental general hospital beds is ascribed to inadequate financing, staff shortages, and low productivity. High utilization of private hospital beds is ascribed to availability and higher staff productivity because of better wages and working conditions, although a high rate of unnecessary admissions for diagnostic studies or surgical procedures is given also as a reason for the observed high utilization rate.

There is agreement that Puerto Rico has an excess of general hospital beds, but there is disagreement as to whose beds are in excess, private or public. The total, island wide, general hospital beds needed could be somewhere inbetween the 9,000-11,000 range. Puerto Rico has some very good private and public hospitals but, like elsewhere, assurance cannot be given that all the people can receive inpatient hospital care in safe, well-maintained, well-equipped, and adequately staffed facilities.

## Health Care Expenditures

Puerto Rico does not have a Health Care Statistics Center for the routine collection, tabulation, analysis, interpretation, and publication of health care statistics. Data on health care expenditures are available on a piecemeal basis and their collection, analysis, and usage in this paper are like Swiss cheese; full of very large holes. Health care expenditures, by source, given for fiscal year 1982 represent this author's estimates.

With respect to health care costs, Puerto Rico has not been immune to the national and international disease of constantly increasing costs. From 1970 to 1980, health care costs are estimated to have risen 100 percent and 34 percent for the years 1978-1982, equivalent to an 8.6 percent annual increase in costs. Total health care expenditures, by all sources in fiscal year 1982, amounted to over $1.2 billion or slightly over 10 percent of Puerto Rico's gross national product of over $12.6 billion for that year, and a $394 annual per capita expenditure. Similar figures in the United States, for the same year, are health care expenditures of over $332 billion, representing over 10.5 percent of the gross national product and a $1,365 per capita expenditure in health care.

The breakdown of the $1.2 billion health care expenditures, by source, is estimated in Table 1.

### Table 1
### Puerto Rican Health Care Expenditures
### Fiscal Year 1982

| Source of Expenditures | Total | Percent |
|---|---|---|
| Commonwealth and Municipal Governments | $334,081,959 | 27.0 |
| Federal Government, excluding Armed Forces | $309,447,185 | 26.0 |
| Private Health Insurance and Out-of-Pocket | $558,490,000 | 47.0 |

Constantly increasing health care costs and expenditures are of real concern to the general public, local, commonwealth, and federal governments and to existing health care insurance plans, labor, industry, and private health care organizations. This concern is manifested by the many studies proposed and undertaken to identify the reasons for higher expenditures and costs, by the clamor for effective control measures, and recognition of the need for better means for financing needed health care.

Some of the factors which affect health care expenditures and costs are well-known. Other things being equal, the operation of a small hospital is more costly per patient day than a large hospital. Hospitals have certain fixed expenditures which cannot be reduced as the occupancy rate goes down. Operational costs increase with each additional service a hospital is expected to provide. Other factors which contribute to increased costs and expenditures are higher staff salaries and shorter working hours per week, greater quality of care, increase in average length of hospital stay, inflation, governmental and professional requirements and controls, increase in the population seeking hospital care, and the image of the health care facility in the community.

**Health Care Personnel**

No model for providing health care can be better than the professionally trained personnel who render the services. Quality health care is impossible unless the model has adequate financing to recruit and retain in service needed qualified personnel to work in properly located, equipped, and maintained facilities as part of an organization providing needed health care under an efficient and effective administration committed to high standards of professional performance.

The private and commonwealth-municipal health care models have been slow in upgrading the salaries and working conditions of health care personnel. Inadequate financing is most often given as the reason why health care personnel are being paid low wages. In recent years, there has been steady migration of health care professionals to the United States, attracted by higher salaries, better working conditions, and fringe benefits. Shortages of qualified health care personnel remains a problem within the health care facilities of the municipal-commonwealth health care model. Other health care personnel problems are geographic maldistribution, minimal career opportunities, and professional frustrations.

**Conclusions**

The preceding sections have summarized the organization, administration, facilities, financing, costs, and personnel of Puerto Rico's health care models. Statements have been made regarding old and new emerging problems and deficiencies. It is the author's conviction that good health for 3.2 million people is an achievable goal and that the steps will be taken to bring this to fruition in the years ahead.

Puerto Rico, land of many people, over 900 per square mile, is today a modern, bustling society with a growing middle class dependent on a high technology economy. This change has taken place during the last four decades. It must give the people the confidence, technical know-how, and experience to move ahead in search of health care models. Effective and efficient utilization of health care resources can result in the provision of a defined minimum of good health care, below which no one should fall. This must be accomplished at the local community level, where health services will reach and affect the daily lives of the people.

Chapter
Eight

Puerto Rico's Changing
Health Care
Environment

JESUS M. RODRIGUEZ

Policymakers are managers, whether it be the management of information, knowledge, or institutions in the private and public sectors, including
government and its multitude of services. Their actions and decisions are,
therefore, deeply influential and perhaps the implications are not appre-
ciated to the fullest extent because of the highly complex and stratified
working environments that may well isolate managers from the ultimate
recipients of their decisions. Therefore, one must always search for a
broader perspective because policymakers deal in people and the quality
of life for society.

The most obvious reality now, both in the continental U.S. and in
Puerto Rico, is that a very difficult transition period is being experienced.
The past decade has been one of crisis and, in economic and political
systems, these long cycles of crises provide a transition to new ways of
political and economic organization. It is not by chance that the recurrent
theme is reindustrialization, a conflictive process that affects every conceivable economic and social activity with extensive political repercussions. The transition is far from over and one can foresee that, in spite of
short-term recoveries and adjustments, the cycles of crises are not complete, although the fundamental stepping stones for new and long-lasting
economic systems have been laid. Computerization, linked to new forms
of automation that redesign whole industries and create an even tighter
network of economic interactions on a social scale, seems to be the most
important symptom of a new economy at the present. But, inevitably this
trend poses immense problems. One has only to consider the rate of
unemployment to realize this.

Structural or long-term unemployment is a very important reality.
Many jobless people cannot go back to their past jobs simply because
those jobs no longer exist. The structure and elements of the labor market
are changing and with them, the function of the worker and his qualifica-
tions. For those who retain jobs, the urgent tradeoff is whether to retrain
or to wait and be phased out into stagnant redundancy.

There is no doubt that people are Puerto Rico's prime resource. But in
order for people to function in a productive manner, it will be important
to establish the necessary links among the different professionals that

83

comprise the modern health care team. That, specifically, is the greatest challenge for health administrators, and leadership is the key to success.

These are, in general, probably the most important tendencies which will have unforeseeable consequences in the transformation of policy and in management. Unless one is able to cope with the already existing crisis in management, in the formulation of policy, and in the management of that policy, even greater political and economic problems will be created. This could very well be seen as a crisis in itself; a possible crisis in the management of a crisis. In a sense, what has been called the fiscal crisis of the state is part of this conflictive shift in the recognition and importance given to divergent social, economic, and political priorities.

It is obvious, when one looks at the relationship between Puerto Rico and the mainland, that these tendencies do not unfold at the same rate, consist of the same elements, or have the same effect. These differences are very important. The problem is not one of size or availability of resources, but of a real dependence that the Puerto Rican economy has developed historically upon the economic development of the mainland United States. The two are closely bound by the same processes, yet, at the same time, share different economic autonomies. This is, of course, not unilateral. In some aspects, creative solutions have been found for similar problems that could well be adapted to mainland realities. Some health care solutions that fit into this overview have been recognized by the federal authorities.

Capital formation in Puerto Rico is subdued and is part of the process of American capital investment on the island. This investment is cyclical and has been the basis for drastic economic changes in this century. In less than a century, changes have been made that other countries have taken centuries to perform. One rarely knows what to expect from this economic interchange because it tends to be a function of the capital needs of the mainland economy.

The demographics of this reality are devastating, not only in terms of migrant Puerto Rican labor and the formation of a stable ethnic minority of Puerto Ricans on the mainland, but also in terms of a large number of unemployed people on the island. Each major economic shift provoked in Puerto Rico by the investment strategies of mainland capital unleashes major social reorganization. The current problem is determining where the health care industry fits in the present transition and in the new economies that are painfully and slowly emerging.

A product of that change is Puerto Rico's present-day health care system, with almost 200 hospitals; multiple diagnostic and treatment centers; specialized ambulatory care models; a strong pharmaceutical, patient-care product and equipment industry; and a third party coverage system similar to the United States. The complexity of growth and change presents a challenge to Puerto Rico.

Today, Puerto Rico's epidemiology is a totally different picture than it was in the 1940's. As in other countries, health is affected by chronic illness, such as cerebrovascular disease, cardiovascular disease, trauma, stress, cancer, and other conditions that require different methods of care. The result has been a transformation of the traditional health care system.

The health care industry, in itself a growth sector, will be profoundly reorganized over the next few years. In this, too, Puerto Rico and the United States are unavoidably linked. The question is how this change will affect the economy both in the short run and in the long run, and how Puerto Rico may obtain the optimum benefit as part of an economic transition that, in general terms, is shared by both economies. There is no question that the ultimate goal is to maximize the efficiency and the quality of health care, while, at the same time, making health care services available at a reasonable cost to the consumer. The Puerto Rican health care system requires special attention because it is distinctly apart, without being separate from the United States.

To meet this changing environment requires strong leadership by those who must design and implement sophisticated financial, inventory, and staffing models. Leadership takes on a special emphasis when one addresses such issues as productivity, motivation, coordination, and evaluation of people in a health care setting. Puerto Rico is also faced with mounting pressure from physicians for staff privileges in hospitals, personnel demands for higher wages and fringe benefits, and consumer demands for greater accountability.

Health care administrators and political leaders need to provide and coordinate sensible solutions to these problems. This will take a team effort in order to permit comprehensive solutions to complex problems. Strong leadership must be a primary concern if Puerto Rico is to continue to grow and develop.

# Part Four

The Medicare Challenge

# Chapter Nine

## Reforming the Medicare System

### JOHN M. VIRGO

### Introduction

Health care delivery in the United States has undergone dramatic changes over the last 10 years. The Medicare system was created in 1965 to provide universal health coverage for those 65 years and older. This bold concept has been marred over recent years by escalating costs that have far outstripped the expectations of Medicare's developers and supporters.

By 1985, Medicare had become one of the fastest growing parts of the federal budget. Medicare payments were $3.6 billion in 1965; $10 billion in 1970; and will be an estimated $70 billion in fiscal year 1985. With a projected deficit of over $63 billion by 1998, it was evident that universal health coverage for the elderly had a price tag that could debilitate the economy in the not-so-distant future.

Questions about the fundamental objectives of Medicare, its financial drain on society, whether it should survive, and what form its future should take abounded in the political arena. The Reagan Administration's response was the implementation of a new and controversial payment system for hospitals, with future extension to physicians. This incursion into the reward system of hospitals and physicians has established battle zones in an area of reasonable tranquility since 1965.

First, this chapter will consider the historical circumstances leading to the development of the new prospective payment system. Next, it will describe the new system and reasons behind its implementation. The impact on manpower in the health care sector is analyzed, including a possible stimulus to further unionization. Cost-shifting is then considered, followed by an analysis of numerous responses by hospitals to limit the negative impact of the prospective payment system. Finally, the future of Medicare and a number of alternative strategies are considered.

This chapter is designed to provide a basis and general overview for the following chapters on the new prospective payment system. These chapters give various perspectives about the system from professionals who have designed and are responsible for its implementation, from those who have evaluated it, and from those that would suggest other alternatives. The following chapters accentuate the complexity of the social, economic, and political dynamics impacting today's health care sector.

## Historical Development

A study of the evolution of the Medicare system is necessary to understand the changes or, more specifically, the reasons for the changes being
made in the program.

The Social Security Amendments of 1965 created a program designed
to meet the growing problems of providing health services for the elderly.
Although the Medicare program was considered to represent a radical
change in traditional methods of providing health care, the idea evolved
over a number of years [Virgo, 1984, pp. 49-59]. Government-sponsored
insurance programs had been in existence for some time and had surfaced
as major political issues during previous presidential campaigns.

Programs developed during the Kennedy and Johnson Administrations
led to the addition of Title XVIII to the Social Security Act. Title XVIII
provided insurance benefits under two separate but closely related programs. Medicare Part A is the Hospital Insurance Trust Fund which provides payments primarily for hospital benefits, skilled nursing care, and
home health care following hospitalization. The cost of Part A in 1984
was approximately $45 billion. Social Security beneficiaries who reach age
65 are automatically entitled to Part A insurance. It is a pay-as-you-go
system which is financed by universal mandatory contributions of 1.3 percent of the first $37,800 of annual earnings [Subcommittee on Health,
1984, p. 1].

The cost of Medicare hospital benefits per capita increased by 178 percent from 1967 to 1982 [Peterson, 1982, pp. 34-8]. Between 1985 and
1998, expenditures for Part A are projected to grow at 12.4 percent each
year, but revenues from currently scheduled payroll taxes will only
increase by 7.9 percent [Subcommittee on Aging, 1984].

Medicare Part B (Supplemental Medical Insurance Trust Fund) pays
for doctors' fees, diagnostic services, and some outpatient services. This
coverage is provided under a voluntary program to which beneficiaries
may subscribe. Twenty-five percent of the trust fund is financed through
monthly premiums of $14.60 from enrollees. Federal general revenues
make up the remaining 75 percent. The estimated cost of Part B in 1984 is
$21 billion. Part B is the fastest growing major domestic program, with
expenditures between 1984 and 1985 estimated at 16 percent [Subcommit-
tee on Aging, 1984]. Figure I shows the sources and applications of Medicare funds.

The intent of this initial legislation was to pay all costs of program
beneficiaries. The program would pay actual cost when incurred, regardless of how widely that cost might vary from institution to institution.
Existing patterns of third party reimbursement were to be followed. (A
third party payor is an agency that contracts with hospitals and patients
to pay for the care of covered patients.) Use of intermediaries (organiza-

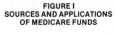

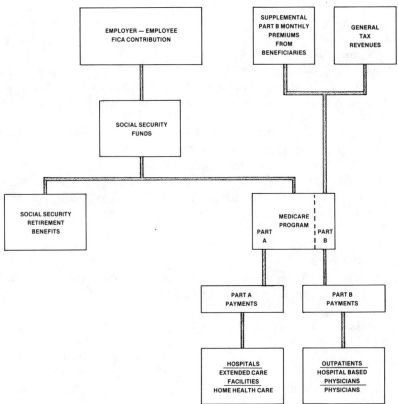

*Source:* Peat, Marwick, Mitchell & Co., *The Financial Management of Medicare.*

tions that receive billings from hospitals and make payments on behalf of the payor for covered services) was specified as an alternative to central-ized government control. The program was to provide a review structure (including due process and appeals procedures) and issue all regulations necessary to implement congressional standards through the Secretary of Health, Education, and Welfare (now Health and Human Services [HHS]).

Administration of the Medicare Program is the responsibility of the Secretary of Health and Human Services. Specific responsibility for administration is delegated to the Social Security Administration and sub-delegated to the Bureau of Health Insurance. The Medicare Bureau of the Health Care Financing Administration (HCFA) has the following respon-sibilities: (1) to establish coverage and eligibility policies; (2) to develop health quality and safety standards; (3) to define services that contractors and states are to perform; and (4) to develop and manage agreements with contractors and states.

Public Law 92-603 was signed into law on October 30, 1972. This legislation redefined reasonable costs as well as expanded Medicare entitlement. Prior to this enactment, the Medicare program paid for services rendered to beneficiaries on the basis of reasonable cost. Reasonable cost for such services was determined by HHS regulations. These regulations established methods to be used and actual costs to be included in determining reasonable costs. Public Law 92-603 included several provisions modifying the statutory definition of reasonable cost and the basis on which payment would be made for services rendered to Medicare beneficiaries.

The Secretary of HHS was authorized to set prospective limits on reasonable costs by first grouping providers (hospitals) in various service areas, and then estimating the cost of delivering efficient patient care. Payment to providers for higher charges to Medicare beneficiaries than regular charges to other patients for similar services was prohibited. Beginning December 31, 1973, reimbursement was limited to the lesser of customary charges or reasonable costs.

This legislation extended hospital insurance (Part A) benefits to disabled persons under age 65. Part A benefits were also made available to persons under 65 who have been medically determined to have chronic renal disease, subject to certain other specified conditions [Peat, et al, (a), p. 6].

The retrospective cost reimbursement system had many shortcomings. Proposals for replacing it with an alternative payment system started to receive increased attention by the federal government. Attempts to control Medicaid outlays had not been successful and the hospital industry's shortfall in reimbursement was quickly growing. Private payor subsidies of Medicare and Medicaid doubled from $1.5 to $3 billion during 1976 to 1979 [Caufield, 1981, p. 18].

In an attempt to influence Medicare use of hospital services and cost shifting to the private sector, the Omnibus Reconciliation Act of 1981 (P.L. 97-35) was passed. Medicare providers were required to file cost reports within 90 days of the end of the reporting period. These cost reports compute the actual cost of services provided to determine the final reimbursement settlement. This act changed the cost reporting forms used by providers and the treatment of certain items for Medicare. It increased hospital coinsurance and deductible amounts under Part A and Part B.

Historically, hospitals were reimbursed at 80 percent of reasonable costs for Part B services plus 20 percent of charges from patient billings [Kerber, et al, p. 5]. The total of these two amounts generally exceeded actual costs. Reimbursement for hospital Part B services was limited to reasonable cost by this act. Outpatient reimbursement was limited to amounts no greater than the cost of similar procedures in a physician's office. Access to books and records of subcontractors who had contracts with providers for longer than 12 months or more than $10,000 was mandated.

In 1982, extensive changes to Medicare were enacted through the Tax Equity and Fiscal Responsibility Act of 1982 (TEFRA). It substantially modified the way hospitals are reimbursed by expanding reimbursable cost limits to cover all reimbursable hospital inpatient costs, establishing limits (target rates) on the rate of increase in reimbursable hospital inpatient costs, and transitioning the Medicare reimbursement program to a prospective payment system (PPS). TEFRA changed reimbursement from an implicit per diem to an explicit per case basis. Case-mix was also incorporated into the payment system [Virgo, 1984, pp. 141 - 45].

TEFRA was a two part Medicare strategy to reduce its financial liability to hospitals. First, a peer group ceiling attempted to reduce costs below current levels for hospitals with costs high relative to peer hospitals. Peer groups were determined based on hospital bed size and whether a hospital is located in an urban or rural area. During the first year of implementation, the ceiling was set at 120 percent of peer group mean cost per discharge. The ceilings for the second and third years were set at 115 percent and 110 percent, respectively.

The second phase of the strategy utilized a target rate to reduce the rate of increase of all hospital charges. These target rates would be published quarterly and set at the market basket index, plus one percent. During the first two years, only 25 percent of costs in excess of the target rates would be reimbursed. After that, no costs in excess would be reimbursed. However, a hospital below the target rate would be payed the lesser of 50 percent of the difference between operating costs and target cost or 5 percent of the target costs.

Historically, the government has used its discretionary powers to limit the cost of the program by restricting or eliminating reimbursement of costs actually incurred in the care of patients or by transferring administrative costs attributable solely to program participation by providers. The Social Security Amendments of 1972 provided the only major expansion in Medicare that was adopted during its history to date. TEFRA merely bought some time for the system [Stromberg, et al, p. 41].

## The Prospective Payment System

TEFRA required the Secretary of HHS to develop a prospective payment system (PPS). The Secretary reported to Congress in December 1982; by April, 1983, prospective payment was embedded in law [Lave, 1984, p. 63].

It was apparent that without the legislation of the Social Security Amendments of 1983 (P.L. 98-21), the hospital insurance trust fund was headed for severe economic problems. A $7 billion deficit was projected for 1988, growing to a $63 billion deficit in 1995. For the period of 1988-1995 alone, the cumulative deficit was expected to be over $310 billion

[Grimaldi, 1983, p. 47]. With health care costs rising at more than 18 percent per year since 1970 and the federal government paying approximately 30 percent of the national health care bill, Congress adopted a new system for hospital reimbursement.

During 1983, the Prospective Payment System (PPS) was introduced, bringing an end to cost-based reimbursement. The overall goals of PPS are as follows: (1) assure equitable payment to all hospitals; (2) encourage efficiency of operations; (3) simplify the payment and reporting process; and (4) maintain both accessibility and quality of care for Medicare beneficiaries [Peat, et al, (b), p. 44].

PPS classifies all patients into one of 468 diagnosis-related groups (DRG's). The 468 DRG's were developed from HCFA's 1981 Med Par file (a sample of 20 percent of Medicare patient bills) and are based on the Uniform Hospital Discharge Data Set, considering principle diagnosis, significant secondary diagnosis, surgery, age of patient, complications, comorbidities, and discharge status [Virgo, 1984, pp. 150-63].

For fiscal years 1984 and 1985, the PPS must be "budget neutral" [*Federal Register,* 1983, p. 39755]. This means payments may not be greater or less than the amount that would have been paid under the previous law. In an attempt to handle atypical cases, outlier payments (for unusual lengths of stay or costs) are restricted to 5 to 6 percent of total projected DRG-related payments. This reduces basic DRG rates in order to achieve budget neutrality.

PPS offers two methods of payment. Payment may be made on either actual bills submitted by the hospital or may be made in the form of prospective interim payments (PIP). PIP estimates total reimbursable cost for the year and periodic level payments are made to the hospital based on that estimate.

All hospitals participating in Medicare will be paid a specific amount per discharge based on the case's DRG for inpatient services provided. A three year phase-in period will shift payment rates from being based on an individual hospital's own reasonable cost to being set on a national basis. Beginning November 15, 1984, hospitals are required to have an agreement with a Utilization and Quality Control Peer Review Organization (PRO) to review admission patterns, length of stays, validity of diagnostic information, and quality of services on an ongoing basis.

The evolution of PPS will be guided by studies and reports provided for in the law itself. The Prospective Payment Assessment Commission (PAC) was established when the new Medicare prospective payment system was enacted by Congress. It was charged with conducting studies and advising the Secretary of changes in both DRG categories and payment rates for each category. The independent body is responsible for identifying medically appropriate patterns of health resources use; assessing safety, efficiency, and cost-effectiveness of new and existing medical and surgical procedures; and establishing a payment inflation index for years beginning on or after October 1, 1986.

The Social Security Amendments of 1983 have not yet been fully judged. It is predicted that PPS will not have a significant impact until it is fully operational and hospitals have implemented cost-effective management [*Federal Register,* 1983, p. 39807]. The government believes that the benefits of PPS, when recognized, will be substantial. It will restructure economic incentives facing the health care system to establish market-like forces. Hospital cost increases will be restrained, thus preserving Medicare trust funds. PPS will help hospitals identify what services they do (and do not) provide efficiently.

PPS is viewed as a "risk-benefit" system. A hospital that treats a patient for less than the diagnosis-based payment rate will benefit; one that cannot deliver the service for less than the rate will lose from PPS. It gives hospitals incentives to produce care efficiently; it does not motivate beneficiaries (patients) to consume care more efficiently, because additional cost sharing is not required. Thus, it attacks the rising cost problem only on the supply side, i.e., hospitals and providers.

From the date of its institution, the effects of Medicare have been monitored throughout the health care system. In 1966, predictions about Medicare and its relationship to hospitals ranged from complete government control of hospitals to a financial gravy train for the hospitals themselves. Some even predicted that hospitals would take over Medicare and mold it to fit their needs [Somers and Somers, 1967, p. 1]. It was furthermore believed that a flood of elderly patients would inundate hospitals, causing a severe shortage of beds and manpower. Many of the changes expected by hospitals in response to Medicare legislation have come about, while others have been unrealized. Major areas of concern for hospitals were the effects on bed occupancy, manpower, services, and costs. The recent changes in Medicare's programs have brought all of these issues back into the forefront.

In 1966, within six months after the institution of Medicare, the proportion of hospital beds occupied by the elderly increased from 25 percent to 30 percent of the total census. Demographic changes have, and will continue to have, a significant impact on Medicare costs. When the program was started in 1966, 9.4 percent of the population was 65 years or older. By 1982, it had grown to 11.6 percent and in the year 2000 it will be up to 13.1 percent.

In addition to the increase in the number of elderly admitted to hospitals, the length of stay was also extended. Both these changes were attributed to Medicare. Length of stay, as well as type, quality, and intensity of medical care a patient receives is often influenced by the insurance he carries. The individual who has minimal insurance may seek outpatient services, or request a minimum stay, even when hospitalization is required. Thus, when it is noted that hospitals did show an influx of elderly in beds occupied, it can be attributed to the quality of insurance provided by the government's Medicare program.

The recent changes in the Medicare program and the newly instigated PPS are having an effect on the number of admissions and discharges, and length of stay of the Medicare patient. The average length of stay has dropped and Medicare admissions have leveled off. By October 1984 the average length of stay for all hospitals was 9.0 days, down from 9.6 days in 1983. But for those hospitals under prospective payment the average length of stay was only 7.5 days. According to the American Hospital Association, admissions also decreased by 3.4 percent in the first quarter of 1984, compared to the same time period in 1983. This can be compared to a 1.6 percent increase in admissions for the first quarter of 1982 [Richards, 1984, p. 76]. With shorter length of stay and lower admissions, average hospital occupancy rates fell substantially from 77.4 percent in the first quarter of 1983 to 71.9 percent for the same period in 1984.

"Reasonable costs" was the original definition of amounts to be paid to hospitals. The wording allowed for *ala carte* payment to be made as long as the method of treatment and items included for payment were justifiable. Not only were direct costs included, but indirect costs as well [Somers and Somers, 1967, p. 158]. Even at the time this wording was developed there was the realization that problems could occur in the years ahead. Therefore, the wording of the original open-ended Medicare regulation left no incentive for cost control by the Medicare provider.

From 1966 to 1982, cost of the Medicare program grew to the point where reimbursements increased 20 percent annually [Lave, 1984, p. 63]. The costs became unpredictable under the system. In 1965, improving the health care system for the elderly was the overriding concern but, by the 1970's, cost containment had become most important. In 1965, the estimate for Medicare payments had been $3 billion and the actual payment was $3.6 billion. By February 1970, projections were that the fund for Medicare payments would be exhausted by 1973, without corrective action. To offset this shortfall, larger amounts taken from the employers' payroll deductions have gone into Medicare [Campbell, 1971, pp. 30-2]. According to Robert Teitleman [June 1984]:

> "Since the 1960's hospitals have grown fat off of a system of private and public reimbursements that rewarded the wasteful and punished the efficient. Even the hospitals knew that the 15 percent annual increase in costs that has been the norm couldn't be blamed entirely on expensive technology and inflation. So when Congress moved to end the gravy train in April 1983, by limiting hospital reimbursements, hardly a whimper was heard from the health care industry."

Medicare hospital expenditures are currently more than $3 billion a month, compared to $3 billion for an entire year at the time of Medicare's inception [Grimaldi, 1983, pp. 46-52]. The recent PPS was designed to temper this runaway Medicare spending.

To offset the drop in revenues due to Medicare, hospitals may attempt to generate additional income with an increase in admissions and discharges. Many hospitals may be motivated to discharge patients prematurely and thus generate several hospital admissions for multiple problems in the same patient, to profit from the DRG system.

However, interviews with leading hospital officials in the Midwest suggest that premature discharges will not occur in most hospitals. It was generally felt that the patient is not aware that there has been any change in Medicare payment related to the care he or she receives. Hospitals have no intention of discharging patients who are still in need of hospital services. Most administrators felt that only the marginal or borderline hospital patient would be discharged a little sooner than before. Medicare patients are usually reviewed when the time limit allowed by Medicare approaches, but no patient will be discharged prematurely. However, multiple sequential admissions for different ailments are taking place at many hospitals. Medicare administrators, therefore, will be reviewing admissions and discharges, comparing historical data with current data, and assuring themselves that no gross abuse is occurring.

Hospitals have also responded by laying off staff members, closing sections of hospitals, reducing inventory supplies, comparing physicians with their peers, and introducing benefit-cost analysis.

**Manpower Needs**

The change in bed occupancy rates created by Medicare may have also created changes in the demand for manpower in the field of medicine. In 1965, there was a national shortage of qualified health care employees. At that time, predictions were that it would take an additional 10,000 health professionals per year for the next ten years to erase the skill shortage [Somers and Somers, 1967, p. 96].

The introduction of the original Medicare legislation intensified the problem. It not only increased bed occupancy, but also upgraded the quality and intensity of services most patients were entitled to receive. For example, many patients covered by Medicare who were previously ward patients became entitled to semi-private rooms. Medicare standards also required a professional nursing staff 24 hours per day. Hospitals not complying with this standard were ineligible for Medicare reimbursement. Thus, hospitals made considerable effort to upgrade their staffs. However, when bed occupancy decreased, hospitals often found themselves temporarily overstaffed, thereby creating a manpower waste. Because of the professional shortage, however, hospitals were fearful that staff members would find other places of employment unless promised a specified number of hours. In addition, this costly inefficiency was exacerbated by the long overdue trend to improve pay and working conditions for health care employees.

By the end of 1984, the bed shortage and manpower shortage had remarkably changed. Length of stay decreased, causing bed occupancy to decline. Many hospitals found themselves overstaffed on a regular basis.

Their administrators attribute some of these changes to the new Medicare payment procedures. But a review of the facts suggests that Medicare may not be the main culprit for today's hospital unemployment and high ratio of part-time employees.

By 1982, the utilization of federal funds to educate nurses and thus overcome the nursing shortage caused a flooded job market [Teitleman, July 2, 1984, p. 68]. Thus, recent Medicare changes represent only a small contributing factor. Most hospital administrators interviewed agree that the nursing surplus today cannot be blamed on Medicare. The problem really lies in the fact that employers are increasingly requiring employee deductibles for health care benefits. In addition, the two back-to-back recessions of 1980 and 1981-82, along with the high unemployment levels for the past several years, have combined to cause the drastic reduction in hospital admissions experienced in 1984 and 1985.

The recent Medicare changes were necessary because of the rapid cost increases in hospital services—an increase of 38 percent per year [Johnson, 1983, p. 33]. In spite of the other variables, most believe this rise can be attributed to the cost-based system of Medicare. Since the system paid the hospital after the fact, based on costs, it provided no incentive to control costs, no rewards for efficiency, and required a costly regulatory process to monitor the entire system. As early as 1970, a report by the Senate Finance Committee claimed that "increased costs to Medicare is indicative . . . of a serious lack of effective utilization and cost controls in administering the Medicare program" [Campbell, 1971, p. 62].

In 1982, according to the American Hospital Association, the rate of admissions and total inpatient days declined for the first time. In spite of this, some hospitals are still adding beds and are eagerly developing expensive medical technologies without knowing if financial support will materialize. The consensus by critics of the health care system is that hospitals think the government will not let a hospital go bankrupt. Such an assumption, however, is hard to justify, based upon available HHS data.

Since the implementation of DRG's, a large number of hospitals reduced their work force. For example, in the first quarter of 1984, there was a 0.5 percent decrease in the level of full-time equivalent workers in community hospitals nationwide. Some hospitals have laid off up to one-third of the staff. Others are eliminating and combining positions in an attempt to drastically reduce costs to offset the drop in occupancy rates. Between 10-15 percent of all hospital laid off workers in 1983; estimates are that between 30 - 40 percent of hospitals will have layoffs in 1984-85. Figure II shows the full-time equivalent employees from the first quarter of 1979 through the first quarter of 1984.

In addition to layoffs, hospitals are reducing hours of full-time workers, suspending wage increases, changing pay scales, reducing or freezing time off, increasing health insurance deductibles, and increasing health and life insurance premiums. These tactics decrease worker satisfaction and job

FIGURE II

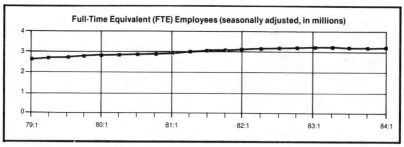

Source: Richards (1984)

security [Baird and Baird, 1984, pp. 52 - 4].

Tables 1 and 2 compare worker attitudes towards benefits and job security, both before and after implementation of DRG's. Employees consistently responded less favorably in all areas after the hospital came under the new payment system. There was also a perception that competition with other departments in the hospital had increased, cooperation had decreased, and understaffing in one's own department was higher.

Changing attitudes due to layoffs, reduced wages, hours, and benefits will have an impact on hospital employees' desire to unionize. The United

## TABLE 1

### Attitudes Toward Benefits

| Survey Item | Pre-DRG mean | Post-DRG mean |
|---|---|---|
| Do you think that the organization has a good total benefits plan? | 3.53 | 3.15 |
| Do you like the life insurance plan? | 3.89 | 3.47 |
| Do you like the medical care plan? | 3.83 | 3.24 |
| Do you like the vacation plan? | 3.89 | 3.71 |

*Note:* Mean sources based upon a possible 5.00. A score of 1.00 = extreme dissatisfaction; 3.00 = neutrality; and 5.00 = extreme satisfaction.

*Source:*Baird and Baird (1984).

## TABLE 2

### Feelings About Job Security

| Survey item | Pre-DRG mean | Post-DRG mean |
|---|---|---|
| Do all departments or work groups in the hospital try to cooperate with your work group? | 3.48 | 3.21 |
| Is there adequate staffing in your work group? | 3.26 | 2.95 |
| Do you feel that you will keep your job as long as you do good work? | 4.17 | 4.04 |
| Do you clearly understand the pay scale for your job? | 3.37 | 3.18 |
| Do you think that pay increases are given fairly here? | 2.88 | 2.74 |

*Note:* Mean scores based upon a possible 5.00. A score of 1.00 = extreme dissatisfaction; 3.00 = neutrality; and a 5.00 = extreme satisfaction.
*Source:* Baird and Baird (1984).

Food and Commercial Workers Union, the Service Employees International Union, and a half-dozen other major unions are actively trying to take advantage of the workers' concern for job security and reduced wages. Since only 15 percent of health care workers are unionized, compared to 20 percent of the rest of the labor force, there is substantial room for organizational efforts. The Labor Department estimates that the current health care labor force of six million will increase to nine million by 1995.

With the recent growth of large hospital chains, unionization drives at the national level are starting to take place. Major unions are targeting the health care field and are planning to spend millions of dollars to organize unions over the next several years. No longer can hospital administrators take comfort in past attitudes by workers that union affiliation was unprofessional. Lack of job security is quickly eroding those feelings.

### Cost-Shifting

Changes in Medicare will be far-reaching, and will not stop with modifications in hospital procedures and expenditures. The DRG plan, like any cost control program, could limit the ability of the health care industry to adapt to changing circumstances. An example is the practice of cost-shifting. All hospitals have a number of uninsured patients. Many of these become bad debts or charity cases. Charges applied to those who are self-pay, as well as covered by third party insurers (such as Blue Cross) contribute to overcoming the cost burden of these cases. The cost-based reimbursement plan of Medicare indirectly assisted these cases as well, because the hospital was able to cost-shift many of the losses.

PPS includes no factor for a cost-shift of this nature for the average hospital. Currently, the only provision for this type of payment is in an adjustment made to teaching hospitals which have an unusually high percentage of indigent patients [Lave, 1984, p. 69]. Non-teaching hospitals, however, also provide these services on a smaller scale; at present, no provision is afforded them by PPS. "If this situation is not altered, non-teaching hospitals may find they can no longer provide such services" [Johnson, 1983, p. 33].

Furthermore, the Medicare payment may be less than actual costs. This will cause more overbilling to self-pay and commercial patients. Hospitals with high Medicare case loads may not be able to cost-shift the load. Johnson [1983, p. 33] states, "...the probability for these hospitals is that those patients not on Medicare will look for other suitable medical services." Based on these observations, it is likely that the effects of the changes in Medicare payment will filter to many individuals throughout society. If so, pressure may be applied for the inclusion of a provision with a payment factor for indigent cases. On the other hand, other third party insurers may institute a plan similar to the PPS of Medicare.

It is not unusual for hospitals to cost-shift $200 or more per day, per patient, to self-pay and other insurance carriers. The result is that other insurance carriers might well initiate a system similar to PPS. However, payment systems of this sort do not mean that the hospital cannot bill the patient for the difference in payment and charges. The payment structure would be new for all parties concerned. This does not mean, however, that the hospital will not be able to recover costs. Currently, Blue Cross makes payments based on a different rate structure than self-pay or Medicare. The possibility exists that this type of discrimination will be extended to other carriers.

The use of a national average cost may also create problems for some hospitals. Lave [1984, p. 71] asserts that when looking at averages and the actual rates for other services in cities in the northeast, it should be noted that these cities consistently pay more on the average than cities in many other regions of the United States. This situation necessarily brings up the question of the quality of hospital services.

The new ceiling on Medicare payments may save billions of dollars; but the counter-argument is that it may not enable hospitals to stay abreast of new technologies. As it stands, the new program allows for a 1 percent increase due to new services, new personnel and upgrading of equipment;

the old program allowed for a 3 to 4 percent increase per year [Grimaldi, 1983, p. 48]. Most supporters of the new Medicare system state that the quality of hospital service need not diminish. The problem is learning to trim away the excess and to become more efficient. Another positive outcome is that elaborate and expensive diagnoses of iatrogenic problems and illnesses may be reduced since patients may no longer receive unnecessary services.

## Hospital Responses

Adaptive responses by hospitals to the changes in Medicare reimbursement abound. Today, hospitals are concerned about efficiency and service contraction. The recent effects of PPS have caused some hospitals to close wings. Others may close completely as length of stay continues to decrease and hospital occupancy falls. Table 3 lists some of the most significant responses.

One of the greatest concerns of the responses in Table 3 is that some hospitals may transfer or refuse certain types of Medicare patients. Other hospitals may find it less expensive to refuse Medicare patients altogether. The result would be a two-class medical system where public and private patients are separated by facility or treatment. Medicare's recent freeze of physicians' Medicare fees also functions to direct medical care into a two-tier system. More doctors will become unwilling to treat Medicare patients. Furthermore, hospitals may become more specialized and use a product line approach to management and planning.

Governmental administrators intend for PPS to work and are extending it to other segments of the health care sector. On July 1, 1984, a 15-month freeze was imposed on Medicare's prevailing fees paid to physicians [HFM, August 1984, pp. 1-3]. Failure to comply carries a possible penalty and exclusion from Medicare for up to five years. The system of incentive and penalty provisions in the program is intended to encourage the physician to accept the Medicare assignment.

Of course, it is always possible for PPS to fail. If so, the alternative may be a simple payment rate, per case, based on costs to the hospital, or arrangements may be made with certain hospitals to provide services to Medicare recipients. However, a provision of this type will accelerate any trend toward a two-tier medical system. Specified locality for receiving medical attention would also obviate any freedom of choice in selection.

## Future of Medicare

When reviewing the Medicare system, it is difficult to forecast or make predictions about its future. In view of the historic cost of Medicare, it was necessary to institute a plan to contain costs if a national health plan for the elderly was to remain intact. With a larger percentage of the population moving into the Medicare age group, it is unlikely that the demand for this service will disappear. The most feasible change would be to

## TABLE 3

**Hospital Responses to Prospective Payments**

- Decreasing services provided to patients.
- Increasing preadmission testing and shifting collection to secondary carriers.
- Shifting laboratory testing out of hospitals.
- Phasing out cross-subsidized services such as nutritional counseling and health promotion.
- Selecting only the relatively inexpensive patients and transferring more acute patients to another institution.
- Using discharge-readmission or discharge-transfer tactics to reduce average length of stay per DRG.
- Decreasing length of stay for particular diagnoses.
- Increasing case-mix management by improved medical record coding, without necessarily treating more severely ill patients.
- "DRG creep" — placing patients in DRG's that will pay more than the illness deserves.
- Choosing surgical over medical patients.
- Shifting costs to non-Medicare patients.
- Cost-consciousness lectures to physicians.
- Comparing physicians with their peers.
- Revoking staff privileges of physicians who overuse resources.
- Increasing the decision making role of physicians.
- Increasing outpatient treatment.
- Establishing "self-care" units.
- Starting low-overhead satellite businesses (emergency centers; home-health care services).
- Sharing of specialized services and costs with other hospitals within a local or regional area.
- Reducing new technological equipment purchases.
- Increasing use of generic products.
- Decreasing supply inventories.
- Increasing bargaining on supply contracts.
- Increasing marketing and promotion.
- Reducing room rates.
- Increasing economies of scope.
- Increasing economies of scale.

(Table 3 continued)

- Decreasing staff.
- Decreasing wages.
- Reducing or freezing time off.
- Increasing insurance deductibles and premiums.

---

advance the eligible age past the current age of 65. Another alternative to the current system would be to turn the Medicare system into a closed system by enrolling the Medicare beneficiaries into a managed health delivery system. Lave [1984, p. 30] describes this type of arrangement as one whereby Medicare would pay a specified amount for all health services supplied by that organization.

The Medicare patient seems to care most about the integrity of the program over the long run and the out-of-pocket cost to the recipient. Various groups, such as the American Association of Retired Persons (AARP), have launched major public relations and lobbying efforts to cut the rise in health care costs. These groups attribute to these rising costs the fact that Medicare deductibles and co-insurance have risen in every year since the inception of the Title XVIII program. Congressman Claude Pepper, Chairman of the House Subcommittee on Health and Long Term Care, has held public hearings throughout the country for providers, consumer groups, and recipients.

The end results of these activities lead to the conclusion: The federal government will not abandon the Medicare program and the program will continue, even though the recipient may receive care in a different manner than before, and may be required to participate more in the cost of care. Abandonment of the Medicare program would be, according to Representative Pepper, "a major breach of contract with millions of workers who have paid for 10 or 30 or 40 years into the Social Security System, and will be retiring in the future" [Cunningham, 1982, p. 88]. In a presentation given before an Illinois Hospital Association Seminar on Peer Review Organization (PRO) contracting, October 24, 1984, the HCFA Midwest Deputy Director stated, "While we talk about cost containment, we realize that technology and quality of care is paramount. We will not abandon the best care possible for the Medicare recipient" [Ill. Hosp. Assn., 1984].

Alternative methods of care for the Medicare recipient are also being addressed [Virgo, 1984, pp. 57-9]. For example, approximately 60 percent of the inpatient hospital expense of the Medicare patient is in the last two months of a patient's life. Thus, the federal government has recently embarked on a significant program to decrease the cost of care for terminal patients through a hospice approach, whereby terminal patients are allowed to die without heroic efforts on the part of providers. Section 12 of TEFRA requires that any patient entering a hospice-type situation relinquish other Medicare benefits.

TEFRA also requires that hospitals contract with a PRO for review of the treatment of Medicare recipients. This will further lead to different forms of care. For example, in Illinois, 299 common surgical procedures must now be performed on an outpatient basis, unless specifically approved in advance by the PRO.

It is interesting to note, however, that even with legislative changes in the method of providing care, during the first 10 months of the PPS there were 9.7 million Medicare admissions to acute care hospitals. This represents virtually no change from the previous year [HCFA, 1984].

Significant changes in the way services are provided under the Medicare program will occur in the future. These changes will include different forms and philosophies of treatment, additional cost-sharing, and perhaps some types of care which may somewhat dilute the recipients' freedom of choice of provider and site of care.

As a basically federally funded and administered program, Medicare falls prey to the politics of the decision-making power structure. In 1965, improving access to the health care system was a major concern of public policymakers. By the mid-1970's cost containment became the over-riding concern.

The problem hospitals are now facing is a growing partisanship with respect to health policy issues. Previous bipartisan congressional leadership has led to, for example, the Medicare PPS and HMO option passage. The 1984 election year has strengthened partisan loyalty. Criticisms from congressional Democrats and associations representing the elderly stifled a HHS proposal to increase co-payments for Medicare beneficiaries. This politically volatile proposal could have saved $765 million in 1985.

The Kennedy-Gephardt Bill (S.2424), introduced in March 1984, provided the Democratic response to the Medicare crisis. The bill called for an all-payer plan with comprehensive, systemwide restructuring of health care financing. According to its sponsors, taxes would not be raised and benefits would not be cut. Hospitals and physicians would have federally mandated admission caps, states would be encouraged to create cost-containment programs, and fixed payment rates would cover all inpatient services. Physicians practicing in hospitals would be paid based on the prospective payment system.

The bill is considered a redirection of policy. Democrats are more willing to place the burden of health care costs on industry and to regulate the health care sector. Republicans are more inclined to ease the burden of industry, increase competition, and shift more of the health care costs to beneficiaries.

However, election year partisanship will wear off. Controversial decisions are typically avoided by politicians during an election year. Politicians' slowness to act to correct the Medicare trust fund imbalance since the early 1970's reflects their political commitment to the elderly and, therefore, their need to postpone, as long as possible, any bad news for this constituency [Subcommittee on Health, 1984, p. 18]. Since it could affect how much the elderly will pay for health care, changing the Medicare system entails playing with political dynamite; not changing it is analagous to nesting on a political time bomb.

The 1985 fiscal budget of the federal government proposed a total Medicare and Medicaid budget of $92 billion, considering $939 million in cuts. Most of these cuts will affect physicians. HHS also wants to gradually increase the amount beneficiaries pay for Part B premiums and index the Part B deductible to a Medicare Economic Index. According to a staff member of the House Ways and Means Committee [Donosky and O'Shea, 1984, p. 1]:

> "Politically, the decision has been made. We nicked the patients in 1981, we got the hospitals in 1983, and now it's the doctors' turn."

Since it is certain that Medicare will survive in some form, the four basic options available to ensure its future are: (1) cut back benefits to enrollees; (2) cut back payments to providers; (3) implement beneficiary cost-sharing; and (4) increase co-payments and deductions. Most alternatives to Medicare or solutions for Medicare's problems stem from these four basic options, either individually or combined.

The Congressional Budget Office's annual economic forecast, released in February 1984, made the following recommendations for Congress to consider to offset the projected Medicare deficit (Table 4).

## TABLE 4

### 1984 Recommendations by the Congressional Budget Office

- Freeze physicians' fees paid by Medicare.
- Limit Medicare's reimbursement to physicians for inpatient medical care.
- Adopt fee schedules for physicians.
- Limit increases in Medicare's prospective payment rates.
- Increase the hospital insurance payroll tax.
- Expand coinsurance for hospital care.
- Tax some employer-paid health insurance.
- Increase cost sharing through the hospital deductible.
- Require all payers to limit hospital payments.
- Reduce Medicare's payments for direct medical education expenses.
- Disallow reevaluation of hospital assets under Medicare.
- Limit Medicare's payments for excess hospital admissions.

- Include nursing home and home health payments in Medicare's hospital payment rates.
- Increase the premium of Medicare's Supplementary Medical Insurance (SMI) program.
- Increase the SMI deductible.
- Establish tax premiums for "Medigap" policies.

---

*Source: FAH Review,* March/April 1984 (p.48).

The National Citizens' Board of Inquiry into health in America recommended a national health care plan in a two-volume report entitled, *Health Care U.S.A.: 1984.* The plan would be modeled after Canada's system, which is publicly financed and operated by the provinces. (For a detailed explanation of Canada's system, see Chapter 2 by Malcolm Taylor in this book.) The Board also encouraged states to establish their own cost control plans under federal guidelines and to set statewide limits on cost increases. Extending a PPS to all doctors and hospitals was also recommended.

The Advisory Council on Social Security concluded an intensive 15 month study on Medicare, which was released in March 1984. (Otis R. Bowen, chairman of the Council and Thomas R. Burke, the Council's executive director, explain the major findings in following chapters.) Only a few of the Council's major recommendations are summarized here.

The Council recommended: (1) Raising the age of eligibility from 65 to 67 in incremental steps between 1985 and 1990; (2) Increasing federal excise taxes on alcohol and tobacco; (3) Taxing employer-paid health insurance benefits; (4) Rearranging Part A and Part B benefit structure; (5) Decreasing of Medicare's support of medical education; (6) Encouraging the enrollment beneficiaries into Health Maintenance Organizations and similar plans; (7) Developing fee schedules to replace the reasonable charge system; (8) Establishing fee schedules for physicians; and (9) Establishing "means testing" by tying benefits to a beneficiary's financial status.

Some of the Council's recommendations started to be implemented within a few months after its March 1984 report. The 1984 freeze on physicians' fees is considered a transitional measure until legislation is passed bringing physicians under a DRG system. Incentives have been added to encourage physicians to accept Medicare assignment. Those accepting assignment agree to accept Medicare payments in full, without additional billing to the beneficiaries.

On January 1, 1985, the Medicare deductible that a patient must pay before being admitted to a hospital increased from $356 to $400. After the first 60 days of hospitalization, the patient must pay $100 per day, up from $89 per day. The monthly premium to ensure treatment in the physician's office has also risen and will continue to rise until about half of the cost of supplementary insurance (up from about 25 percent) is paid by the patient.

From February 1, 1985, Medicare was authorized to pay, in advance, the yearly enrollment fees of patients who enroll in an HMO. For an average monthly fee of $54 for individuals and $172 for families, the patient is covered for all visits to a group of physicians and for hospital costs. Since physicians in an HMO have higher incomes when costs are kept down, HMO physicians are 40 percent less likely to send a patient to the hospital than other physicians. Even more traditional third party payors are now starting to establish their own HMO's.

Margaret Heckler, Secretary of Health and Human Services, has recommended that the federal tax on cigarettes, which is scheduled to drop from 16 cents to 8 cents in Fall 1985, be kept at its present level. The additional $1.7 billion per year in revenue would be given to Medicare to help offset the depletion of the fund.

Linking doctor and hospital participation is the only feasible way to control costs and ensure that doctors will continue to treat Medicare patients, according to Jack Christy, lobbyist for the American Association of Retired Persons (AARP). The AARP advocates forcing hospitals that want Medicare dollars to require doctors who use their facilities to accept Medicare-set fees. Opposition was voiced by the AARP (as well as by other groups) against the Advisory Council's recommendations. It felt the study was too restrictive and did not address the forces behind increasing costs. The recommendations simply shifted the costs back to the taxpayers, consumers, elderly, and health providers, according to the AARP.

The American Medical Association (AMA) is conducting a $3 million study, scheduled for completion in 1985, that will contain AMA proposals for altering the Medicare system. Because of the inevitability of significant future changes, the AMA wishes to be an active participant in suggesting what direction those changes should take.

Another alternative would be to privatize Medicare through the use of Medicare IRA's. Proponents of this alternative assert that the level and scope of old age health insurance would then be a result of rational choices by individuals, rather than political choices that are often irrational.

Under a Medicare IRA, tax incentives would be given to establish health-bank IRA accounts. Built-up funds in these accounts could be used to pay for private health insurance and other medical expenses when a person retires. The underlying concept is that Medicare could then be substantially privatized. (For a more detailed explanation of this approach, see Chapter 12 by Richard W. Rahn in this book.)

**Conclusion**

Political implications ensure the existence, in some form, of the Medicare programs. However, the survival of the program will surely be accompanied by dramatic changes, some of which have already been implemented, in the way these programs are carried out. These changes will affect all portions of the health care delivery system: providers, government, payors, and recipients.

Providers will be looked upon to furnish services in a more efficient, cost-effective manner and to provide alternative forms of delivery, such as enhanced outpatient procedures and hospice-type programs.

Beneficiaries will be required to participate more in the cost of care by means of higher deductibles and co-payments and will be forced to forego certain rights, such as complete freedom of choice of type and provider of treatment.

Lastly, government will be forced to examine its role as a provider of all things to all people. The government faces hard choices in the areas of possible means tests for Medicare beneficiaries and the providing of adequate funds to perpetuate an efficient system of quality care for all Americans, without resorting to the use of multi-tiered delivery systems or health care rationing.

Fundamental ethical issues must also be addressed. Questions of who gets medical care, what is quality of life worth, who should live and who should die, and how much cost should be shared and by whom, set the framework for a national debate transcending benefit-cost analysis and marginal cost theory. Behind the numbers are living human beings whose dignity and self-esteem must be protected.

The consideration of the Medicare program and its associated effects on runaway health care costs provides an excellent example of society's concerns and demands which cause governmental intervention in the market mechanism and a resulting dramatic adjustment in the health care industry. The economic, social, and political interactions are varied and complex. The end result will provide a graphic example of pluralism in a democratic and free market oriented society.

## REFERENCES

John E. Baird and Linda A. Baird, "Prospective Pay Abruptly Changes Workers' Feelings About Jobs, But Shift Isn't All Bad," *Modern Healthcare*, September 1984.

Michael D. Bromberg, "Partisanship and Health Policy," *Federation of American Hospitals Review*, September/October 1984.

"Business Outlook," *Modern Healthcare*, January 1984, pp. 103-06.

R.R. Campbell, *Economics of Health and Public Policy*, Washington, D.C.: American Enterprise Institute for Public Research, 1971, pp. 30-2.

Stephen C. Caufield, "Cross Subsidies in Hospital Reimbursement How Will New Health Proposals Affect Cost Shifting?," *HFM Journal*, October 1981.

Robert M. Cunningham, Jr., "Social Security Must Change," *Hospitals*, 56, No. 24, December 16, 1982.

Lea Donosky and James O'Shea, "Doctors' Bills Bitter Pills for Medicare," *Chicago Tribune*, January 22, 1984.

*Federal Register*, 48, No. 171, September 1, 1983.

Paul M. Grimaldi, "Prospective Payment Scheme Overhauls Financial Incentive," *Hospital Progress*, August 1983, pp. 46-52.

R. L. Johnson, "Shooting Oneself in the Foot: Congress May Re-Create Two-Tier Care," *Hospital Progress*, December 1983, pp. 32-9.

Health Care Financing Administration Background Paper, *Prospective Payment System Monitoring Activities,* October 1984.

Illinois Hospital Association, Seminar on Peer Review Organizations, Sangamon State University, Springfield, Illinois, October 24, 1984.

Kerber, Eck, and Braeckel, *Medicare Seminar,* Vol. I, pp. 1-10.

Judith R. Lave, "Hospital Reimbursement Under Medicare," *Healthcare Financial Management,* July 1984, pp. 62-74.

Peat, Marwick, Mitchell, and Co., (a), *The Financial Management of Medicare,* Vol. I, pp. 1-22.

_____ , (b), *Prospective Payment System (PPS).*

P. G. Peterson, *Social Security: The Coming Crash,* New York Review of Books, December 2, 1982.

*Proceedings of the Conference on the Future of Medicare,* Subcommittee on Health of the Committee on Ways and Means, U.S. House of Representatives, February 1, 1984.

Glenn Richards, "Layoff Wave Rolls Through Industry," *Hospitals,* August 16, 1984.

H. M. Somers and A. R. Somers, *Medicare and the Hospitals Issues and Prospects,* Washington, D.C.: The Brookings Institution, 1967.

Special Committee on Aging, U.S. Senate, 1984.

R. Teitleman, "Taking the Cure," *Forbes,* June 4, 1984, pp. 82-91.

_____ , "Labor Pains," *Forbes,* June 4, 1984, pp. 82.

"Update," *Healthcare Financial Management,* August 1984, pp. 1-3.

John M. Virgo, *Health Care: An International Perspective,* International Health Economics and Management Institute, 1984.

# Chapter Ten

## U.S. National Health Policy: A Federal Perspective

### CAROLYNE K. DAVIS

### Introduction

The United States, from a federal perspective, is embarking upon a landmark period in health care reform. It is an era where soaring health care costs are beginning to price health care out of the range where it can be afforded by all Americans. Nonetheless, the government is charged with coming up with policy alternatives which will correct the situation and maintain a viable, cost-effective health care system whereby all Americans can receive quality health care at a reasonable cost.

The objectives of this paper are several fold. It is first intended to review the initiatives that have been undertaken for reforming the federal sector of the U.S. health care system, and second to analyze their impacts. Of necessity, some of the impacts will be conjectural in nature in that the outcomes that are anticipated are a function of the incentives inherent in the current and proposed health care initiatives. Also, the numerous reforms which have been instituted will be discussed, the results to date described and the conceptual framework into which the various initiatives fit explained. In some areas the evidence is more conclusive than in others, however, the preliminary movements within the health care industry over the past few years have been described by several industry observers as no less than revolutionary.

### Background

When the Medicare program began in 1965, the Congress elected to provide payment for services to hospitals based on a retrospective cost reimbursement system. Although everyone recognized the lack of proper incentives in such a system, there was no other viable system which could have been implemented. The drafters of the original Medicare program had to choose between payment by individual hospital charges or payment of costs as defined by Medicare. The latter was selected because it seemed to be the more fiscally responsible decision, but the choice resulted in enormous increases in hospital costs over the last 17 years. Over that 17 year period, hospital costs have increased at a rate 2½ times the consumer price index. The effects of that increase on the health care industry and the economy in general cannot be overemphasized. A review of the data is

111

enlightening, if not startling.

- In fiscal year 1967, only 17 years ago, the Medicare program's total inpatient hospital expenditures were $2.4 billion. In fiscal year 1984 the United States will be spending almost 1½ times as much in each month and almost $42 billion for the year.
- While the overall CPI has increased 200 percent since fiscal year 1967, the index for inpatient hospital room care has increased by 588 percent.
- Health care expenditures represented 10.8 percent of the gross national product in fiscal year 1983 up from 6.4 percent in 1967.
- In 1983, the nation spent $355 billion or approximately $1,500 per person on health care.
- By 1990, total spending is projected to increase to $690 billion and consume 12.3 percent of the gross national product.

The impact of these increases in health care costs have been devastating to the Medicare Hospital Insurance trust fund. It is estimated that by the mid-1990's we will be spending more than the revenues flowing in to that trust fund creating a potential for insolvency if we do not act to reduce these enormous outlays. With this as the backdrop, Congress passed the Tax Equity and Fiscal Responsibility Act (TEFRA). The Act provided for a cost limits payment system for hospitals to attempt to slow expenditures in the hospital arena.

The Tax Equity and Fiscal Responsibility Act of 1981 also provided an opportunity to address the inequities of cost-based retrospective reimbursement when it required the Department of Health and Human Services to develop and submit to Congress a proposal for a Medicare prospective payment system for hospitals.

This request could not have been made to a more receptive Administration. The Reagan Administration was already examining alternatives to the highly inflationary, heavy-handed regulatory payment methodology being used by Medicare. This confluence of purpose between the Executive and Legislative branches of the government presented an opportunity not to be ignored.

The Administration reacted quickly and defined six overall policy objectives that the proposed Medicare system would have to meet. It would have to:

- be easy to understand and simple to administer;
- be capable of being implemented in the near future;
- be predictable in terms of government outlays and predictable for hospitals in terms of their Medicare revenue;
- establish the federal government as a prudent buyer of services;
- provide incentives for hospital management flexibility, innovation, planning, control, and efficient use of hospital resources; and

- reduce the cost reporting burden on hospitals.

Drawing on 10 years of experience in the Health Care Financing Administration's Office of Research and Demonstrations, the choices were reasonably clear. Many types of prospective payment (setting rates of payment ahead of time) had been tested. Lessons learned from these early demonstrations allowed an accurate selection of the best prospective payment system to initiate nationwide. Individual hospitals budget review systems were not advisable since they were too labor intensive, did not provide sufficient management flexibility, clearly would not be simple to administer, and would need additional federal staff to manage such a system. The system of total capitation that had been tested in an area of up-state New York was feasible but failed to meet one of the major policy objectives. It would have been extremely difficult to implement quickly on a national basis. Consequently the choices were narrowed to either a per admission system similar to the one operated in New York State or a Diagnosis Related Group (DRG) payment system similar to the one which was being tested in New Jersey. The conversion from TEFRA to either of these systems would not be difficult. The decision for a Diagnostic Related Group payment system was made by Secretary Schweiker primarily because it was recognized that resource allocation varied by the type of case being cared for in a hospital and was a simple system for them to administer. Competitive bidding, while of philosophical interest, was simply not feasible at that time, but had clear potential for future development utilizing DRG's as a bidding mechanism.

**Federal Health Care Initiatives**

*Prospective Reimbursement*

In October 1981, the U.S. government enacted a new system for reimbursing hospitals. Termed prospective payment with DRG's, this system was in lieu of the existing retrospective cost reimbursement system and proposed to reimburse hospitals according to a nationwide schedule of rates for Medicare patients. This new system is being phased in and will be fully operational at national payment rates in three years. It includes the following features:

1. Hospitals are to be paid on the basis of output. When fully operational, Medicare will have implemented separate urban and rural national price schedules for each type of patient based on a DRG patient classification system.

2. The prospective payment system recognizes existing differences in area wage costs, but all hospitals in an area will receive the same payment for the same service.

3. The issue of implementing this system using a single national payment rate created significant concern among, and pressure from, industry representatives. The hospitals felt that Medicare should provide a phase-in period to allow them more time to adjust to the

new system. Responding to these arguments, Congress mandated that during the 3-year transition period each hospital will be paid a blended rate developed from the prospectively-determined rates which are projected forward based on a percentage blend of each hospital's own costs, its regional average costs, and national average costs for each DRG.

In the fourth year, rates will be based solely on the urban or rural national rate. Congress did, however, also require a report by the end of 1985 on the feasibility and impact of eliminating or phasing-out the separate urban and rural rates.

4. Payment rates will cover all operating costs. Congress agreed with the department's recommendation that initially, capital and medical education costs would not be included in the prospective rate, but would be paid separately. However, the Health Care Financing Administration is required by Congress to study and report on how capital-related costs can be incorporated into the prospective payment system and it specifically legislated that any capital costs obligated after the passage of the new law may be or may not be recognized and/or paid according to a different method.

5. Teaching institutions receive a special adjustment to recognize individual hospital differences in indirect costs due to approved teaching activities. The adjustment is based on the ratio of interns and residents per bed.

6. Special provisions are made for outlier cases with extraordinary lengths of stay or cost. Congress mandated that the outliers would be defined so that total payments for these cases could not exceed 5 to 6 percent of total payments.

To date, the prospective payment reimbursement system has been working with surprising results. As noted earlier, it has been called truly revolutionary by many experts in the field. The total impacts of this system are probably difficult to assess accurately at this stage since the system has not become fully operational. However, it has provided several positive externalities from an economic point of view. One of these positive externalities has been the realignment of the medical record function in hospitals. Prior to the introduction of this new system, medical records were often relegated to the basement of a hospital. With the introduction of prospective payment hospitals were quick to realize that the DRG system is a product line accounting system with each DRG composed of direct and indirect patient care in their expenditures as products. The federal government is no longer paying for a heterogeneous day of care but rather for a specific type of care and payment levels were adapted to the types of care provided. This has set the stage within the hospital industry, one of the largest industries in the United States, for the movement to other even more imaginative forms of reimbursement.

Some refinement of the system still needs to be done. Reviewed separately, some components such as outpatient payments, payments for rehabilitative and psychiatric services, and payments for physicians' fees need to be analyzed for their eventual inclusion into hospital-specific components, or what is referred to as DRG's. Also, for lack of a federal alternative, medical education expenses and capital expenses continue to be paid on a cost pass through basis. The Department of Health and Human Services is currently studying methods for incorporating these two components within the output related payment system. Needless to say, this will require a rigorous technical analysis since medical education and capital costs account for a significant portion of hospitals overall reimbursements, and to be equitable, it is essential that they be fairly and judiciously integrated into the system. To give but one example, it has been found that in many of the very large teaching hospitals, the federal government is currently paying more in the Medicare program for medical education expenses than it is for the individual health care provided to its beneficiaries per DRG payment.

Because the original law did not ensure hospitals that they may not retrospectively disallow capital expenditures incurred between the time the prospective payment legislation was enacted and the time that a report to Congress on how to incorporate capital was completed by the Department of Health and Human Services, the health care industry overall is being very cautious in analyzing its capital acquisitions policies. Expensive new pieces of equipment are being screened to see that they are truly needed and for the first time there is concerted movement toward a joint sharing of large items such as nuclear magnetic resonance machines (NMR's). In the past these larger expense items were automatically purchased because they were a cost pass through to third party cost reimbursement payers. Previously, hospitals, in order to acquire prestige and attract more and better physicians purchased every new equipment item without regard for the operational costs. Now because of the awareness of the operational cost to maintain these expensive acquisitions, communities are beginning to seek joint purchasing of these items leading to more planning to meet its community's needs. All this has a positive impact on federal and other third-party payer reimbursements. It has, however, a negative effect on the hospital supply manufacturing industry which must now concentrate on marketing their equipment and supplies through emphasis on productivity and cost benefit analysis to the institutions.

It might be asked what is the impact of prospective payment to date? One of the most notable trends is the length of stay which has dropped from 9.9 to 7.5 days per hospital admission.

Hospital administrators and board members who are business-oriented in their outlook are putting a basic fundamental knowledge of economic theory to work in the hospital arena for the first time in several decades. An awareness of fixed costs and price per unit are causing trustees and hospital administrators to question whether or not infrequently performed procedures should be continued or whether joint planning efforts should be initiated among multiple hospitals within the same locality so that high cost low volume procedures of several individual hospitals can become the high volume low cost procedures of one hospital.

The fact of the matter is, despite much rhetoric to the contrary, the quality and cost effectiveness are not opposing choices but rather complementary goals. To the extent that hospitals specialize in certain procedures they tend to become more cost-effective in performing those procedures and do them at a lower cost than hospitals which perform them with less frequency. To use an extreme example, were this not the case we would be having cardiac catheterizations and organ transplants being done at many more institutions than is currently the case. In a word then, low cost is in no way synonymous with low quality and, in fact, the exact opposite is frequently the case. One need only look at the data to see this is true. The number of readmissions is lower in hospitals which have higher volume of specified procedures than in those hospitals that do fewer of those procedures. This is true not only of community hospitals but also large teaching hospitals. As with the Industrial Revolution in the United States we are embarking in the health care industry upon a period of increased specialization. As economists who have read Adam Smith's *The Wealth of Nations*, the health industry in the United States might now be likened to the analogy of the pin factory in preindustrial England.

Based on the evidence to date, it would seem that a clear pattern is emerging for hospitals to begin concentrating on those types of care with high volume, high quality, so as to promote greater overall specialization within the industry.

*Professional Review Organizations (PRO's)*

Any economist is quick to realize that the total revenues accruing to a new institution or any business entity is the product of the price times the quantity. With a prospective payment system such as is currently being implemented for Medicare, the federal government has a potential liability if any given health care provider increases their utilization *unnecessarily* so as to increase their total revenue. The federal government was not unaware of this potential downside risk and for this reason professional review organizations were enacted to work closely in each area to maintain close surveillance on providers to ensure that inappropriate admissions did not occur and also to ensure that the quality of care did not suffer under the reimbursement system.

These professional review organizations will be in addition to the existing mechanisms in place in hospitals which have review committees to oversee DRG utilization by unit, by physician, and by departments. Since prospective payment came on-line hospitals have been closely examining and comparing costs associated with various DRG's. Those physicians with patterns of care that consistently create outliers are counseled by their peer committees and corrective courses of action are suggested. In addition to the professional review organizations that are in all fifty states and U.S. territories, the Health Care Financing Administration is carefully monitoring both volume and quality of care being provided by different hospitals. This evaluation is being undertaken to determine if there has been any adverse reaction to the reimbursement system, and if so, what has been the extent and direction of that action. As noted previously, volume changes are certainly a risk area to Medicare under the DRG system. Although there is no current evidence of the existence of a problem, indeed the overall admissions to hospitals dropped significantly during the first year of implementation of the prospective payment system, alternative methods for providing disincentives for increased volume are still being examined within the construct of the overall system.

While incentives are certainly inherent in the prospective payment system for physicians and hospitals to control the length of stay and ancillary usage, a phenomenon current statistics are tending to bear out, PRO's are, nonetheless, being charged with ensuring that the quality of care is maintained and unnecessary utilization patterns flagged for corrective action.

The fundamental responsibility of the PRO's will be to examine patterns of treatment by physicians within a DRG and this should, in time, lead to less divergence in standard practice patterns within hospitals. Ideally, hospitals will use these analyses to increase their productivity and consequently, their financial viability. Hospitals are going to be forced to make conscious decisions between continuing to subsidize nonprofitable DRG's and working with nearby facilities to create more specialized and productive facilities.

One of the primary areas that the PRO's will inevitably address is the discrepancies that currently exist between providers in different geographical areas. Lengths of stay and the considerable differences in the number and types of procedures being given to similar groups of patients will come under closest scrutiny. In a recent study published in the *New England Journal of Medicine* it was found that in two localities within the same state different providers were performing as much as 77 percent more procedures of the same type as other localities in the state not distantly located. Throughout the history of the Medicare program great discrepancies have existed between the utilization patterns in the eastern United States and the western states of the nation. PRO's will be charged with exploring the underlying reason for these discrepancies and initiating recommendations for corrective action in those areas where there is believed to be significant variance from accepted protocols of care.

Thus, it can be seen that when the professional review organizations become fully operational true competition among hospitals for admissions is clearly on the horizon and should promote the provision of high quality services at the lowest possible prices. Consolidation of hospitals and the formation of multihospital systems should also become more prevalent. Many hospitals may move to provide more out-patient care through vertical integration with other providers such as home health agencies, skilled nursing facilities, clinics, and ambulatory care centers conveniently located in large metropolitan areas.

We are confident that maintenance or improvement in the quality of care will clearly result from the new reimbursement system when coupled with operational professional review organizations in every geographic area.

In order to improve the quality of care being given by different health care providers PRO's are being charged with reviewing mortality rates and readmission patterns among all providers in order to assist in ensuring continued delivery of high quality care to all beneficiaries.

The role of the Professional Review Organization and its charter from the Health Care Financing Administration is not merely to ensure continued delivery of high quality care but also to upgrade the existing quality of care. The health industry, not unlike the steel, auto and other large industries in the United States has ample room for productivity improvements. Productivity improvements in the health industry can be measured by an improved product which in this instance is increased quality of care. There are many measures of quality of care that PRO's will be using to evaluate the performance of hospitals within the United States. A listing of all of these is outside the scope of this paper, however two examples are cited: (1) the number of needless invasive procedures that are performed on patients, and (2) reducing avoidable post-operative complications and infections associated with surgeries.

In general the prospective payment coupled with the safeguards embodied in the professional review organizations that will oversee the administration of the program have now put in place a totally new reimbursement mechanism that will provide proper incentives and safeguards for ensuring a more efficient, cost effective overall health care delivery system.

*Health Maintenance Organizations (HMO's) and Competitive Medical Programs (CMP's)*

A number of initiatives have recently been enacted which are designed to strengthen and increase competition within the health care industry. These initiatives center around the refinements which have been enacted in the HMO programs and the provision for establishment of competitive medical plans. As one keen industry observer noted, "We are right smack in the middle of a structural revolution involving providers. And that revolution is about to heat up in a way that will make the transition from cost reimbursement to DRG's pale by comparison." In the 1984 Deficit Reduction Act provisions were enacted to authorize Medicare reimbursement to prepaid health care providers on either a reasonable cost basis or under a risk reimbursement basis. Prior to 1972 Medicare payment to

HMO's was made on the basis of the cost to the organization for providing a specific service to beneficiaries. In 1972 the law was amended to authorize payment to HMO's on a capitation basis which is consistent with their mode of operations. It provides that an HMO may enter either a reasonable cost contract or a risk sharing contract. Under a reasonable cost contract payment is made to an HMO, on an interim basis, using a monthly capitation fee. At the end of the contract year payments are adjusted to equal the reasonable cost of the covered services furnished by the HMO's to Medicare enrollees. Under a risk reimbursement, however, an HMO receives monthly payments at an interim per capita reimbursement rate. Final reimbursement is based on a comparison of the HMO's cost for furnishing services to its Medicare enrollees with its adjusted average per capita cost (AAPCC). The AAPCC is the average cost of furnishing services to Medicare beneficiaries who have the same characteristics as those enrolled in the same geographic area as the HMO. If the risk-based HMO's costs are less than its AAPCC it shares the savings with the Medicare program. The HMO may receive savings up to 10 percent of AAPCC.

Now what does this portend for the evolution of a national health care system? The developments to date suggest the entire industry is realigning itself into what have been called "total care systems." Providers are evolving into what has been described by some as hybrid health care organizations. That is, large investor-owned and not-for-profit hospital chains are acquiring HMO's and related health care providers and are beginning to offer continuity of care that will utilize the full range of providers associated with that institution including home care services, episodic hospital care and even long term nursing home services. These are taking the form of preferred provider organizations and in the future will probably evolve into insurance companies buying hospitals and related health care providers and offering competitive medical plans from which the public may select. This is competition in its truest form. The incentive is there for efficient management for if the HMO or CMP is able to deliver services at prices that are less than its agreed upon price it can share the savings. On the other hand if this cost exceeds the agreed upon price the provider will be at risk for those added costs. A full spectrum of care will be offered not only to Medicare but to other purchasers of health insurance such as large corporations, labor unions and the like. We are now beginning to see a rapid expansion and proliferation within the United States, of risk based HMO's and competitive medical plans. Within the next 3 years it is conservatively anticipated that 600,000 Medicare beneficiaries will enroll in these capitated, prepaid health care systems.

Certain classes of purchasers, particularly large purchasers, are going to be attracted to entities that provide the most comprehensive quality of care at the lowest possible price. Health delivery functions and insurance functions may well be blended in the future. We can see these developments are currently evolving within the United States and one can only conjecture as to the direction in which national health care policy will finally evolve when all of these forces work themselves out.

## Summary

From the preceeding it should be evident that there is occurring in the United States the gradual evolvement of a market oriented health care system. In the short time since the enactment of prospective payment we have seen remarkable changes in our health care delivery system. We have also witnessed accomplishments in the last few years unlike what we have been able to achieve in the previous 17 years. Health care, the fastest growing industry in the United States, is being transformed through the powers of competition into a more cost efficient, higher quality system. This is not being done by regulation ala government fiat but rather by market oriented forces being let loose by the government to do their thing. In the author's tenure as Administrator of the Health Care Financing Administration she has observed remarkable changes and never ceases to be encouraged at what the future holds forth when the industry is encouraged and proper incentives are provided.

# Chapter Eleven

## Medicare Benefits and Financing

### OTIS R. BOWEN

## Introduction

Medicare is the nation's largest federally financed health insurance program serving approximately 30 million elderly and disabled Americans. One of the most successful social programs, it has provided basic protection against the costs of health care for a significant portion of the population. However, the continued escalation of health care costs and an increasing elderly population have placed extraordinary demands on the program and its resources that were not anticipated when the program began in 1966. If Medicare is to continue to meet the needs of elderly and disabled citizens, prompt action is required to restore its financial position.

When the Advisory Council on Social Security was appointed in September 1982 by the then Secretary of Health and Human Services, Richard Schweiker, it was directed by its charter to place particular emphasis on a review of the Medicare program. This was the first Council to address itself primarily to Medicare. Prior councils had devoted most of their considerations to the social security monthly benefit programs, the Old Age, Survivors, and Disability Insurance programs.

The Council took its charter very seriously, devoting more than a year to intensive deliberations, involving 14 meetings and eight public hearings. The public hearings were held in cities throughout the United States, including San Francisco, California, Evanston, Illinois, St. Petersburg, Florida, and New Brunswick, New Jersey. The Council has developed a series of recommendations which are designed both to alleviate the financial problems currently confronting the program and to improve its responsiveness to the needs of program beneficiaries.

The Council is making 26 different recommendations. Due to time constraints, it was not possible to address every health care issue that probably should have been addressed. It has, nonetheless, developed a plan for rescuing the financially burdened Medicare program. The Council does not claim that this is a perfect plan or the only plan, but an agenda that will hopefully facilitate discussions on this important national issue. The extensive staff work should be of assistance to those who will continue to address this problem, a problem that is very quickly going to confront the

entire country, particularly the elderly and disabled Americans who are
served by the Medicare program.

To put the problem in perspective, the Council adopted a working
assumption that the hospital insurance trust fund would experience a
cumulative deficit of $200 to $300 billion by the end of 1995. This estimate
was based on information provided by the 1983 Annual Report of the
Medicare Board of Trustees, estimates issued by the Congressional Budget
Office, and additional information provided by the Health Care Financing
Administration's (HCFA) Office of Financial and Actuarial Analysis.
Although some recent estimates indicate that the point of insolvency may
be delayed a few years, the time frame in which action is necessary is
already close at hand.

The Council's recommendations are categorized into six general areas:
financing, eligibility, benefit structure, reimbursement, issues general in
nature, and issues deserving further study. This paper highlights some of
the more significant recommendations of the Council.

## Benefit Structure

In addressing the benefit structure of the Medicare program, the Council's principal objectives were: to provide improved catastrophic protection
for all beneficiaries; to simplify, as much as possible, the benefit package;
to incorporate reasonable cost-sharing by beneficiaries; and to identify
ways to alleviate the financial crisis facing the hospital insurance trust
fund.

The Council is recommending a restructure of the Medicare package.
The revised benefit package is designed to accomplish the stated objectives
and to do so by using traditional health insurance concepts that spread
the risk and liability for increased costs across all beneficiaries who will be
eligible for the improved benefits recommended.

A variety of cost-sharing approaches were reviewed that provided for
increased coinsurance during shorter, more typical hospital inpatient stays
to finance improved catastrophic protection and produce savings for the
trust fund. The major problem with these approaches was that the
improved catastrophic benefit protection that would be made available to
all would be financed only by a minority of the beneficiary population
who actually use inpatient services.

Instead, the Council recommends that a new basic Part A hospital insurance protection be provided to all beneficiaries, based on the payroll or
self-employed tax contributions they make during their working years.
For those who elect only Part A hospital insurance, this new benefit
would provide unlimited days of inpatient hospital care, 100 days per year
of care in a skilled nursing facility, and all of the currently offered home
health and hospice benefits. A per admission hospital inpatient deductible,
as currently computed, would apply but for no more than two admissions
in a year. Further, a daily coinsurance equal to 3 percent of the deductible

would apply to all days used, with the exception of the day of admission when a deductible was collected. The current 12.5 percent coinsurance on the 21st through 100th day of care in a skilled nursing facility would continue to apply.

With this as a basic restructure, the Council further recommends that all beneficiaries who elect Medicare Part B, supplementary medical insurance, (about 95 percent now do) automatically receive, for an additional annual premium, an improved Part A benefit. The improved Part A benefit would eliminate liability for the daily 3 percent coinsurance on hospital inpatient days and the 12.5 percent coinsurance on applicable skilled nursing facility days of care. In effect, the beneficiary's cost sharing liability would be limited to the admission deductible and a maximum of two such deductibles per calendar year.

An additional premium amount, estimated to be approximately $98 in 1985, would finance the costs of catastrophic protection and the cost-sharing limits and would also provide additional program revenues that will help to alleviate the growing deficits in the hospital insurance trust fund. Under this plan, the improved Part A benefit would be supported by the substantial majority of all beneficiaries, not just those who require and use inpatient hospital services in a given year.

The Council also recommends a plan for providing improved catastrophic protection for Part B supplementary medical care expenses. The unpredictable and potentially substantial cost sharing that can occur under Part B of the program was a frequently cited concern of beneficiaries at several public hearings that the Council conducted. Under the Council's plan, the beneficiary electing Part B would have the option—it would not be required as part of the Part B election—to purchase a supplemental plan that would establish an annual dollar limit ($227 per year in 1985) on their cost-sharing liability for approved Medicare Part B charges. The premium for this protection, assuming that a substantial percentage of Medicare beneficiaries opted for it, would be approximately $150 per year in 1985.

In summary, under the Council's recommended restructure plan, all beneficiaries eligible for Part A hospital insurance would receive catastrophic protection. For an additional $98 per year premium in 1985, those beneficiaries enrolling in Part B would also be relieved of liability for cost sharing beyond the inpatient deductible.

Beneficiaries who also elected the optional Part B supplement would limit their cost-sharing liability under Part B. Although such beneficiaries would experience an increase in the Medicare premiums they now pay of approximately $250 per year, the Council estimates that beneficiaries who supplement their Medicare coverage with private "Medigap" insurance (over 70 percent do so now) will actually realize a net savings in the cost of their health insurance protection. Most Medigap policies are priced for $300 to $600 per year, with those at the higher end of this range being typical.

The net effect on the Part A trust fund of the above recommendations over the next 10 years is estimated to be approximately $38 billion. This includes some $25 billion in additional revenues and $13 billion in reduced expenditures.

With respect to other benefit structure issues, the Council also endorses the concept of voluntary vouchers, since it perceives that this would enhance competition in the health care field. However, precautions should be taken to ensure that coverage would be at least as comprehensive as current coverage and that use of the voucher be entirely voluntary. Voluntary vouchers are estimated to cost approximately $50 million to implement.

Also, the Council is recommending that the Part B deductible be indexed to the Consumer Price Index. That is, when the social security benefits are increased, the Part B deductible, which is currently $75 would also be increased by the same percentage. Indexing of the Part B deductible would have no impact on the hospital insurance trust fund shortfall. However, if begun in 1985, the supplementary medical insurance trust fund would realize accumulated savings of approximately $680 million by the end of fiscal year 1989.

### Reimbursement

A second major group of recommendations of the Council addresses Medicare reimbursement policies. The Council endorses the concept of prospective payment and did so prior to the enactment of the Social Security Amendments of 1983. The Council recommends, however, that the rate of increase in DRG payment be limited to the hospital input price index, and not the hospital input price index plus 1 percent, as is currently in the law. It is estimated that restricting the increase in DRG's to the hospital input price index would save some $34.5 billion by 1995.

A major recommendation, which may prove to be controversial, would eliminate Medicare's reimbursement for medical and other professional health education expenses incurred by hospitals. It is the belief of the Council that it is inappropriate for a health care program, designed to provide care for elderly and disabled Americans, to be subsidizing such education expenses. The Council fully recognized the importance of medical education and the need for continued federal support; however, it believes that these costs should be funded through other federal, state, or local programs and not by the Medicare program.

Another significant recommendation of the Council, which is not expected to generate any savings but is a consequence of the extensive testimony the Council heard throughout the United States, concerns Medicare's physician assignment policy. The Council is recommending that physicians annually be given the option to either elect to participate, or not to participate, in the Medicare program. Those physicians who elect to participate would agree to accept Medicare payment as payment in full and not bill the beneficiaries for the difference between their charges and what Medicare considers reasonable and allowable (customary, prevailing, and reasonable charges). If a physician does not participate, the Medicare payment will be made to the patient who will then be responsible for paying the physician's entire bill. A physician would be given the option to elect to participate; however, he or she could terminate the participation agreement by providing Medicare with 180 days notice.

In return for agreement to participate, the Council further recommends that HCFA publish local directories of participating physicians in every major locality. The directory would identify, by medical speciality, those physicians who have agreed to participate in the program. As added incentives, Medicare would allow for batch billing or subsidized electronic billing by participating physicians and would provide for electronic funds transfer of payments to provide a more predictable cash flow for participating physicians.

## Financing

Under the category of financing, the Council opposes increasing payroll taxes beyond currently legislated levels to pay for the projected deficit in the Medicare trust fund. However, it does endorse the taxation of a portion of employer provided health insurance, similar to the proposal submitted by the Reagan Administration last year. The Council does not view revenue raising as the primary benefit of this proposal. Rather, Council members believe that, over the long run, consumers will choose more cost-effective types of care, thus decreasing the overall rate of growth in health care costs.

A majority of the Council also recommends increasing the federal excise tax on alcohol and tobacco products. The rationale for this latter recommendation is the increasing evidence that these two products cause significant increases in health care expenditures and, if additional revenues are needed, current excise taxes should be increased and earmarked to the hospital insurance trust fund to help solve the Medicare shortfall. Those who oppose such increased excise taxes emphasize the negative affects on the industries involved and point out that such taxes have traditionally been the prerogative of the states as a source of revenue. In the final analysis, however, the Council believes that some additional source of revenue should be identified and that an increased excise tax is the least objectionable of the available alternatives.

## Eligibility

The eligibility recommendations include, perhaps, the most controversial recommendation of the Council, advancing the age of eligibility for Medicare from age 65 to age 67 over the next five years. If implemented, this recommendation would produce about $75 billion in Medicare savings over the next 10 years.

Since the Medicare program began, the average life span has increased more than three years. This increase in life expectancy has major implications for the Medicare program. The steady decline in the ratio of workers contributing to the trust funds to beneficiaries collecting benefits will continue. The expanding population, combined with the increasing longevity of that population, places a particularly severe financial burden on Medicare as health care costs increase with age.

The Council recognizes that recent changes in the age of eligibility for cash retirement benefits will be implemented over a 40-year period. However, the Council believes that to continue to have a viable Medicare program, more immediate changes in the age of eligibility for Medicare are necessary.

### General

Finally, the Council endorses the concept of "advance directives" or "living wills" which are currently recognized by law in 14 states. The Council called for a study to look at the impact on health expenditures in those states having such laws and encouraged other states to adopt similar legislation. Living wills would prevent unnecessarily heroic measures being taken in the terminal days of life. Eleven percent of Medicare expenditures are spent in the last 40 days of life and some 25 percent of Medicare expenditures are incurred by patients in the last year of life. The Council fully recognizes that this may be a controversial recommendation; however, the Council unanimously endorsed it. Personal experiences in losing a loved one and thus knowing the enormous costs that were incurred in terminal days prior to death contributed to the Council's decision.

### Further Study

In addition to its formal recommendations, the Council did identify several issues which it viewed as deserving of future study by the Department of Health and Human Services. These subjects include some suggested alternatives for a longer term restructuring of the Medicare program and development of incentives for younger workers to save toward health care expenses during retirement years.

The Council recommendations just reviewed would, if enacted, eliminate the financial burden of the hospital insurance trust fund. If those recommendations, whose savings or revenues have been quantified, were to be implemented promptly, the trust fund would be fully solvent in 1995 with a moderate reserve to guard against contingencies. Those recommendations which have not been quantified represent, in the Council's view, viable alternative sources of revenue in the event of delays or failure to adopt portions of the quantified package. Additional recommendations not discussed here would not have significant financial impact on the programs, but are designed to improve the administration of Medicare and its responsiveness to the needs of its beneficiaries.

In conclusion, the author should like to add that the Medicare Program is on the verge of having to confront significant financial difficulties, if it is to remain solvent through the next decade. The financial woes of the program are confounded by the fact that it is an enormously complex program and solutions are going to be difficult to construct. Certainly, this is a program that is totally ill-suited to quick-fix solutions. Action must begin soon to develop viable solutions in order to salvage this financially burdened program so that America's elderly and disabled can be assured of continued high quality health care.

# Chapter Twelve

## Long-Term Proposal for Restructuring Medicare

### RICHARD W. RAHN

### Prologue

The costs of the Medicare program are recognized to be out of control. The Congressional Budget Office estimates that, under present conditions, the Health Insurance Trust Fund alone will have a deficit in the range of $200 to $400 billion by 1995. The fundamental problem with the program is that it has caused a new national ethic to develop. That ethic, in essence, is "all Americans are entitled to all the medical care they perceive they need, regardless of their ability to pay." Even though such a belief may be a humanitarian notion, it is economically and fiscally unrealistic.

In times past, people had an incentive to have children, in part to be cared for in their old age and provide needed medical care. Essentially, they had a social contract with their children to provide for their care and schooling until adulthood and, in turn, to be provided for during their retirement. With the development of the Old Age and Survivors Assistance and Medicare programs, part of the incentive to have children was reduced since the government, that is, everybody's children, would be paying for their upkeep and medical bills during their retirement years. As the economic benefit of having children declined, the cost of having and educating children continued to rise rapidly. Hence, there became a strong disincentive to have children, which contributed to our very low and declining birth rate. Both Old Age and Survivors Assistance and Medicare programs were, and still are, based on the assumption that the population would continue to grow rapidly and life expectancies would not increase dramatically. These assumptions are questionable at best, and in fact, the nature of the programs encourages the undermining of these fundamental assumptions.

The only alternative to an extraordinary tax burden being placed on relatively few workers as a result of the low birth rate, combined with an ever increasing number of retired persons, is to establish a mechanism and incentives for people during their working years to set aside sufficient funds to provide for their living expenses and medical needs during their retirement years. The development of the universal individual retirement accounts in the 1981 tax act was a giant step in this direction. However, it did little to alleviate the growing Medicare problem.

129

The basic notion inherent in the passage of Medicare was that there were adequate medical care facilities in existence at the time the legislation was passed, and that the law providing Medicare was to allow people to purchase already existing goods and services. The fact of the matter is that since the entry of the government into Medicare in 1966, which was further extended to Medicare, Part B in 1973, the cost of medical care services has increased by 291 percent. This compares to an increase in the price of all items, less medical care, which rose by 198 percent in the same period.

In order to provide for these ever growing medical needs during the retirement years, the savings rate needed to be greatly increased and control gained over the growing cost of medical programs. A partial solution to the cost control problem is to increase cost sensitivity on the part of the recipients. Economists have known for hundreds of years that free goods would be overly utilized. In essence, much of medical care to the elderly is now a free good and, as a result, it is both excessively utilized and inefficiently allocated. This is not to argue that increased price sensitivity on the part of participants would ever be sufficient to bring cost totally under control. However, by increasing the price sensitivity of medical care, particularly for long-term and chronic illnesses, people will have incentive to switch to lower cost alternatives, such as home health care, nursing homes, and so forth, rather than being forced to choose the high cost alternatives; e.g., staying in the hospital. Also, individuals have different levels of preference regarding the desirability of health care. The present system allows the elderly relatively little trade-off among forms of medical care and other goods and services. Both quality and quantity of care are now prescribed to a much greater degree than most individuals would choose.

Finally, as a result of private pensions, government transfers, and income security programs, the after-tax incomes of the elderly have more than reached a parity with working Americans. In addition, the assets held by the elderly are considerably larger than those held by the average working American. The fact is that most retired people do not have medical expenses in any given year sufficiently high to give them a greater degree of hardship than if those same medical expenses were incurred by a working person, nor are these expenses sufficiently high to cause a significant decline in their actual standard of living.

These facts indicate that appropriate public policy should be to expect the elderly to provide for a larger portion of the growth in their medical expenses, rather than increasing taxes on the less affluent working age population. However, if the elderly are going to be expected to pay more of their own medical care cost, they also should be provided the means by which to increase their savings during their working years.

**The Proposal**

This proposal is designed to allow an orderly process of restructuring the Medicare system that will both require and enable individuals to make provisions to pay for the bulk of their own medical care bills, other than those attributable to catastrophic expenditures. The system is designed to be phased in over a 30-year period. It is also designed to reduce the anxiety senior citizens have about the possibility of being confronted with medical expenditures beyond their means to pay for them. The system would involve the following components:

1. The current Medicare tax, for both employers and employees, would be frozen at present levels.

2. A universal "health credit account" would be established for all working Americans, including their non-working spouses, for the purpose of providing an amount of money for the purchase of basic expected medical care during a normal retirement period. In addition, working Americans would be encouraged to set up a tax deductible health bank Individual Retirement Account (IRA) which would allow them to set aside funds in addition to the government established health credit account, up to a specified dollar level each year. The Internal Revenue Service would send a statement annually to all taxpayers which would specify the value of their health credit account. The value will be equal, accumulated yearly credits which would be specified by Congress, plus the average government T-bill rate compounded, in effect, an implicit interest payment. No actual funds will be set aside. It will be an accounting entry only. Upon age 59½ or any year thereafter, the participant would be able to draw upon the balance of the health credit account for the purchase of medical insurance or actual medical care.

Those who choose to establish their own IRA health bank account, in addition to the health credit account, would be able to withdraw funds at age 59½ for medical insurance or medical care, or continue to allow the funds to grow and begin withdrawals any year thereafter. Individuals would be encouraged to establish IRA accounts in order to purchase more medical care during retirement years, with less financial hardship and to offset possible hardships occurring because of unanticipated extended illness periods.

The current Medicare tax will be used to provide benefits for current beneficiaries and for those who retire in the next few years, and over time it will be used increasingly to fund the health credit accounts.

Beginning in 1986, deductibles for Medicare payments will be gradually increased over a 30-year period, until Medicare pays for only catastrophic care, which would be defined on an individual basis, such as costs that exceed "X percent" of after-tax yearly income. The actual level will depend upon the growth in value of the health credit account, and the rise in the cost of medical care. However, even the catastrophic care would be coupled with some minimal co-payment, such as 10 percent, to ensure continued cost sensitivity on the part of the patient and patient's family. This should reduce over-utilization of heroic medicine and encourage use of living wills. The cost of the current medical care program will fall, and the resulting revenue, after the catastrophic program costs, will be applied to the health credit funds.

### Financial Effect

The health credit account will have no immediate financial effect on federal budget outlays and the deficit. However, over time, it will increase government liabilities and will affect, depending on the health credit account level, actual outlays which would be funded by the existing HI payroll tax and, perhaps additionally, by expenditure reduction or some increase in other taxes.

The health bank IRA tax deduction will cause a reduction in federal tax revenues, depending upon the amount of the allowable deduction and the utilization rate. Hence, the deficit will be enlarged, but at the same time, private saving will be increased. This increase in national saving is likely to more than offset the revenue loss, thus reducing rather than increasing "crowding out."

Provisions could be made to enable holders of health bank IRA's to make deductions for medical insurance or medical care during a period of unemployment. Like the existing IRA accounts, holders of these accounts would be able to withdraw them for other purposes, provided they paid the tax penalty.

### Benefits of the Proposal

1. It would, for the most part, solve both the short and long-term financing problems of Medicare.

2. Over the long run, workers would be able to get coverage under the new system for substantially less than under the current system. Under current law, the HI tax rate will probably have to climb over 10 percent. But the new system could avoid this tax increase. These savings arise primarily because workers under the new system receive the benefit of the increased production and full market returns generated by their health bank IRA investments.

3. Further substantial cost reductions should be realized because the new system allows far wider scope for the operation of private market incentives:

(A) It would increase competition in the medical sector by allowing private insurers and providers to compete for coverage of retirees. This competitive pressure would likely lead to the development and adoption of institutions with better cost controls, such as HMO's.

The competition would increase pressure for development of lower cost medical procedures.

(B) Workers who choose to pay medical expenses directly out of funds accrued in their health banks would have a powerful incentive to conserve medical resources, because they personally will retain the savings. Such conservation would also lead to reductions in medical prices and costs because of reduced unnecessary demand. Workers will also have an increased financial incentive to maintain good health habits.

4. The new system will also sharply increase workers control and choice over medical coverage. The system would be diverse and flexible, allowing workers to choose from a myriad of options in the private marketplace the coverage best suited to each of them individually. Workers would choose the mix of institutional coverage and personal financial responsibility they desire. They would also have increased freedom to choose their retirement age, with earlier retirement allowed, and no penalties for later retirement.

5. The new system would provide essential government aid that people need—catastrophic coverage for the elderly, to protect against highly expensive long-term incidents, and supplements for those without sufficient resources to pay for needed medical services. But the new system would, at the same time, maximize the role for the private sector within a framework enabling people to develop the resources to pay for private sector services.

6. The new system would also reduce the anticipated growth in government medical spending over the long run, with most elderly medical coverage provided through the private sector, in a much less expensive fashion.

7. As a side benefit, the reform is likely to increase national savings substantially, due to the funds stored away in the health bank IRA's. This will result in increased capital investments, jobs, and economic growth.

In return for these benefits, the costs of the reform seem well worth it.

# Chapter Thirteen

## An Alternative for Restructuring Medicare

**THOMAS R. BURKE**

An alternative long term proposal for restructuring Medicare would retain some of the basic concepts included in the Rahn proposal, but the Individual Medical Account (IMA) purchased by individuals would provide for catastrophic coverage, with Medicare continuing to cover basic health care needs. The current Medicare benefits would be maintained, but Part A and Part B would be combined with all such expenses financed, as Part A is at present, by a payroll tax paid during one's working life. However, the basic cost-sharing under Medicare would be modified to provide for a flat percent coinsurance on *all* medical expenses an individual incurred during a given year up to a catastrophic cap.

To insure against catastrophic expenses every individual, at age 52 or 55, who would be potentially eligible for Medicare, would be required to begin paying into an IMA, which would be maintained by the government. All contributions to the IMA would be deductible from gross income for income tax purposes. For married couples, the IMA could be a joint account with a composite rate for married couples where both are employed and an individual rate for a single family wage earner. The amount to be contributed could be a specified flat amount or varied according to income.

When an individual became eligible for Medicare, the IMA would be available to cover catastrophic expenses arising from payment of the coinsurance. Catastrophic expenses would be defined along the lines outlined in the initial proposal, namely, a cap at 15 to 20 percent of one's after-tax income in any given year. The IMA would then be available to pay medical expenses that exceeded that cap.

By making the catastrophic coverage a function of one's income, the proposal would automatically reflect income differentials among the population at large. Once an individual had incurred catastrophic expenses, i.e., had incurred medical expenses equal to the determined percentage of income, he or she would draw on the fund in his or her IMA to pay for these catastrophic expenses. If an individual did not incur substantial catastrophic expenses during his or her retirement years, then upon death the contribution remaining in the account that he or she had made to the IMA, less interest, would accrue to his or her estate. Any interest that had accrued from his or her remaining contribution would be transferred to a government "catastrophic health care bank." This health care bank would fund the catastrophic expenses of those individuals whose medical care costs exceeded the amount they had accumulated in their IMA's. For example, low income individuals, with a small retirement income, may incur catastrophic expenses that exceeded the value of their IMA. To protect such individuals once they had drawn down their IMA, the government health care bank would fund those expenses in excess of their IMA.

Under this proposal, persons who do not fully exhaust the IMA would obtain a tax break during their high earning years in return for the foregone interest in their retirement years. In most instances, the tax credit would exceed the interest income foregone during retirement years.

This would be an equitable approach. Individuals with very high income in retirement would have catastrophic expenses paid from the IMA only when a higher dollar limit had been reached. Low income individuals, on the other hand, would be eligible for catastrophic coverage when a smaller proportion of medical expenses had been incurred, since catastrophic would be defined as expenses in excess of a designated percentage of one's after-tax income. As with the initial proposal, this proposal would have to be phased in and it would be several years before it would become fully operational.

Although this approach does introduce the concept of means-testing in the Medicare program, it is an approach which is not in anyway unique and does not depart from the current income tax structure. It would insure that elderly Americans who have adequate financial means to pay for a greater portion of their health care expenses would do so without unreasonable hardship. Those with lesser means would pay a lesser share of their costs; both would be protected, through their IMA and government health bank, against catastrophic illness costs.

To be successful, this would have to be a mandatory program where all elderly Americans who have attained a designated age would be required to contribute to an IMA. In effect, they would be required to invest some portion of their income during their working years to provide protection against catastrophic health care expenses they may incur in their retirement years. In a sense, they are purchasing a health insurance policy, but for which their investment, less interest earned, is refundable if not used.

Although this proposal does not alter the responsibility of Medicare to pay for basic health care needs of the elderly, it does remove from Medicare a significant portion of the costs currently incurred, namely catastrophic expenses.

This proposal is offered as a suggested area for further exploration for a long term alternative to the current Medicare program.

**Benefits of the Alternative Proposal**

1. Although under this proposal only catastrophic expenses would be funded by the IMA and Medicare would continue to cover basic health care costs, it would still remove a substantial portion of the current Medicare costs. The flat percentage coinsurance on all Medicare services would produce these savings. The more excessive health care expenditures would be shifted from the Medicare trust fund to the individual IMA and if that was exhausted to the health care bank.
2. This alternative would continue to instill cost-consciousness on the part of the health care consumer since the individual would be liable for a specific percentage of covered medical expenses he or she incurred until out-of-pocket expenses exceeded the designated percentage of the total retirement income.
3. The Medicare benefit package could be adjusted in the future depending on actuarial experience. Should the Medicare trust fund, which would be supported by FICA taxes paid over one's working years begin to accumulate a large surplus, the benefit package could be expanded or the taxes reduced until some actuarially sound level were reached. In effect, the removal of liability for catastrophic care costs from Medicare could allow for broader or additional coverage of needed health care services.
4. The use of "living wills" would be encouraged since beneficiaries would realize that if extraordinary measures were taken on their behalf, the cost of such measures would be paid from their IMA account resulting in the depletion of the estate eventually payable to their survivors.
5. Many of the benefits identified in Richard Rahn's paper would also apply under this alternative.

# Part Five

Strategic Planning

# Chapter Fourteen

# Strategic Planning for Health Care Systems: Quantitative and Qualitative Methods

## LYNDSEY STONE

In an information society, technology performs tasks that people could not do or which would otherwise be performed so slowly that there would be little rationale for going about the work at all. Technology indicates feasibility and technology alters social and economic systems with its introduction and widespread use. Problems arise with industrial-age technology in health systems analysis which one must wrestle with in order to solve data management problems. Quantitative information tends to be task-specific, yet policymakers are expected to leap from the quantitative to the qualitative without formal analytical techniques to bridge the gap between statistics and meeting more abstract human needs.

Further problems cloud the application of quantitative policy analyses to real-world policymaking. According to Bloom and Berki [1983, p. 38]:

> "Analysts may argue that the moral and ethical issues are more tractable at the macro, or policy, level because they are made in terms of statistical lives— unseen, unidentified patients—as opposed to the micro level, where decisions are made in terms of individual patients. But when groups of beneficiaries become real and present in the decision-making process by representation, or when their plight is translated by the media into identifiable individuals or groups, the moral and ethical issues become as sharp and salient as they are at the micro, or direct patient, level. In fact, translating statistical entities into real entities, thereby giving voice to the statistical person or firm, is one of the vital functions of interest groups. Therefore, at whatever level decisions are made, their impacts are in terms of who benefits or who pays; it is useful to carefully and explicitly enumerate who gets what as well as why, how, at what cost, and with what effects."

Impacts are often problematic to estimate in an information society. Communications are often rapid, graphic, and brief, with formats determined by equipment. Messages are compressed, decoded, and synthesi⌐ Interpretations require technicians. Rapid analysis and evaluati⌐ validity of messages occurs in a complex economic, polit⌐ milieu [La Conte, 1982, pp. 2–4]. Complex message⌐ decision-makers are asked to make even mor⌐ pace with the computer [Toffler, 1980]. ⌐ usage of computerized policy analyses, re⌐ of analyses available. Their objections sh⌐ understood fully, because not all consequenc⌐ analyses will be regarded as positive, especi⌐

141

spective.

1. *Decision makers attempt to minimize uncertainty.* Analyses highlight areas of uncertainty, sometimes making decision making more difficult. Elected officials are usually concerned with programmatic or political effects of alternatives; these can rarely be stated completely or accurately with a high degree of certainty.

2. *Systematic analyses illuminate economic questions and those of efficiency, but they do not address the issue of equity.* Equity in the distribution of rewards and costs to politically viable groups are of immediate importance for political survival. The uncertainty is great when quantitative analyses attempt to address the impact on powerful constituencies.

3. *Much information produced by policy analyses is not deemed useful or desirable.* Decision makers have a high preference for closure on any single issue so that they can move on to other issues on the political agenda. According to Stephen C. Crane [Bloom and Berki, 1983, p. 56]:

> ". . . policymakers make their political 'profit' on the decisions they reach, not necessarily on the time spent in reaching those decisions. Sometimes, information can get in the way of making a decision quickly or of making a decision at all. This can occur because of the additional time required to conduct an analysis or because the analysis produced may introduce new issues or actors who complicate the process of negotiation and consensus-building. This fact may account for the cool reception that policy analysts sometimes receive when they venture forth into the political world of health policymaking."

4. *Conflicting findings or recommendations frequently result from multiple analyses, causing difficulty for policymakers.* Greater time is necessary for data–based policy, involving a wider range of options and, further, support and opposition for each alternative may require both time and internal conflict.

5. *The growth of analysis, as a basis for policy decisions, may force interested groups with lesser resources out of the decision–making arena entirely.* Many analyses are presented by special interest groups vested in the policy outcomes. Enormous resources may increasingly be necessary to produce persuasive analyses, weighting decision making toward those with better staffs, information, and organization. The end result (and a perverse one at that) may be a dramatic increase in the cost of political participation (restricted entry into an already limited political marketplace) [Bloom and Berki, 1983, pp. 55–6].

Health care leaders in all countries are, nevertheless, heavily impacted by many characteristics of the information society. For example, technology has encouraged the growth of huge data banks with enormous amounts of relevant and irrelevant information on the cost and effectiveness of health care system policies. There frequently seems to be no way to refine and coordinate vast amounts of micro–level data collected by a variety of health care businesses and interest groups. The U.S. government sometimes sends a message to an industry, such as health care (for example, DRG's), which forces more intelligent use of computers.

Automated merging of clinical and financial information would not have occurred in most American hospitals prior to the Tax Equity and Fiscal Responsibility Act of 1982 [Nathanson, 1983, pp. 58–60]. Thus, policy analyses are forced by federal law requiring quantitative data of a more sophisticated type as a condition of survival.

In the final analysis, DRG's have probably added impetus for hospitals to engage in strategic planning activities. In a more competitive environment, where analyses of external conditions and markets must occur with more depth and frequency, long–range strategic financial planning is probably necessary to compete effectively. Previously, hospital planning usually meant "bricks and mortar" and took the form of construction strategy. In other businesses, strategy typically involved examination of threats and opportunities in relation to the firm's strengths and weaknesses. Strategic alternatives were devised to creatively enhance the success of the business enterprise in its marketplace [Jones, 1981, pp. 23–9].

Traditional strategic planning has finally taken hold in hospitals, where it has been utilized to design ambulatory care delivery systems [Meiselman, 1982, pp. 7–21] and to evaluate the potential for diversification [Wolford, 1981, pp. 31–43]. Cost and rate control issues require hospitals to analytically examine their product mix, rather than merely noting bed size, location, and teaching or other programs [Silver, 1981, pp. 57–67]. As hospitals begin to offer a broader range of in– and outpatient services, accurate measurement of case mix may be crucial to financial success and to the refinement of measures of efficiency and effectiveness.

The big business of medicine is being revamped by a new medical–industrial complex, increasingly dominated by nationwide multihospital, for–profit corporations. These corporations operate at the forefront of the information technology which allows them to understand their own internal and the external environment. Their market niches have been defined by the corporate ability to make financial predictions and to align costs to remain in the black [Newsweek, October 31, 1983]; smaller competitors, operating at a financial loss and in the absence of accurate and meaningful data, have become the mausoleums of the traditional health care system.

The computerized management information systems which have, so successfully, supported consolidation of multi–hospital systems, provide models for computerized application to system–wide strategic planning. But problems abound in the conceptual and operational ends of development and use of nationwide health management systems. Strategic management of health systems encounters the following problems:

1. Juxtaposed qualitative and quantitative methodologies to deal with political–financial variables;

2. Policy alternatives with economic, social, and political constraints;

3. A patchwork of local, state, and national data collection requirements to extract meaningful information for decision making;

4. Different frames of reference between policymakers and management information system analysts;

5. Integration of policy, planning, and resource availability into flexible, adaptable, and responsible national health plans;

6. The tendency of the human mind to simplify and of decision makers to support the rational mode while using the intuitive mode;

7. The sheer variety of quantitative techniques makes choice among them difficult, especially when decision makers distrust quantitative methods; and

8. Different local, statewide, and national strategic health care goals reflecting economic, geographic, and life–style differences.

Each of these problems should be considered separately, and carefully understood, because they must be resolved in order to workably plan for health care systems which are strategically designed and not merely politically dictated.

1. *Quantitative and qualitative methodologies in relation to political–financial variables:* A veritable army of quantitative techniques are available, including linear and non–linear programming, networks programming, integer programming, queuing analysis, forecasting, Delphi and nominal group processes, gaming, bargaining analysis, decision analysis, and simulation and Markov decision analysis. All of these are time–consuming, complementary, expensive, and complex means of dealing with predictably uncertain aspects of the future. Simpler methods, such as cost–benefit analysis (CBA) and cost–effectiveness analysis (CEA), are more widely known and more easily used [Bloom and Luft, 1983, p. 38]. Available qualitative strategic planning processes include contingency planning and alternative future scenario generation.

Typically, the strategic planning process is largely conceptual in its nature, with numerical anchoring points, which, when reached, indicate that decisions should be reviewed for goal accomplishment or shortfall. The same or an alternative scenario is accepted and contingencies which do occur change the nature or scope of the plan. For example, if a substantial rise in smoking occurs nationwide for five years, indicating that the cost of this increase will be $5 billion in the next 25 years (future scenario), then more extreme legislation to combat the problem and a public education program costing $1 billion over five years (contingency planning) is indicated.

Quantitative and qualitative methodologies can be integrated carefully and simply if a country determines its five to ten health care priorities and plans only for them; targeting allows in–depth analysis and monitoring, with presumably easier generation of funds to address changes in variables associated with the magnitude of a single health problem. The difficulty is that problems occur in the policymaking process. The public's interest in health problems is changeable over the years. Some problems are solved, whereas others linger or increase in visibility and prevalence. Flexibility of financial resources to meet strategic planning goals is almost unheard of in the public sectors of democratic nations, posing a problem requiring political solutions. In brief, for strategic health care planning to be effective, the methodologies employed must take into account and, in turn, influence funding policies and practices.

2. *Policy alternatives with economic, social, and political constraints:* Policy alternatives have differential costs which are financial, life–style, and human, as evaluated from different political positions. Each group in a democratic society uses data under somewhat different ground rules, valuing policies in a different heirarchy of preferences. Policy alternative assessment is itself difficult to judge in terms of its merit, making the public and policymakers frequently suspicious about the outcomes. People are more or less willing to modify their behavior to reach health goals, making policy alternatives more or less feasible over time, e.g., smoking cessation, weight control, and so forth.

3. *A patchwork of data collection systems:* Enormous quantities of data are collected by local, state, and federal governments to justify expenditures on health care. Each level of government and program administration is financially and historically "invested" in these data. Frequently, the data remain unprocessed or cannot easily be converted for management decision purposes. Yet it still seems to be difficult for administrators to give up the inflow of reassuring paperwork or to exchange its safety and predictability for program budgeting with performance standards. To fuel a national strategic planning process, key figures and ratios utilizing the same service categories and measures of effect (both process and outcome) will have to be devised and marketed through legislative initiatives.

4. *Negotiating between policymakers and management information systems (MIS) specialists:* Policymakers are mostly concerned about feasibility, while MIS people look for the optimal. Policymakers use MIS for consciousness–raising, whereas MIS specialists would like to see decision making based on their analyses. Luft states, for example, that [Bloom and Luft, p. 23]:

> "Cost–benefit and cost–effectiveness analyses are pernicious, they assault our notion of democracy, and they are confusing and misleading. Further along the continuum are those who believe these analyses have little or no impact (which is probably what most people believe). On the positive side, these techniques can raise consciousness concerning issues these individuals had not considered and can assist in making decisions."

5. *Integration of policy, planning, and resource availability:* Policy and planning are difficult enough, but resource allocation has staggering problems attached to it—political and managerial. According to Henry A. Foley [Bloom and Luft, p. 47]:

> "Resource allocation in an environment of scarcity requires creative decision makers, a competent management team to implement decisions, and a network of leaders and media representatives to make the public aware of the benefits of these decisions."

Foley cautions about the public–private resource interplay, stating that [Bloom and Luft, p. 53]:

> "As long as the purchasing power remains separate in the states or in the country as a whole we will see the private sector expenditures increase one year and the public sector the following years, then vice versa, as in other Medicaid programs. Governments, employers, or employees who pay for medical services must be able to negotiate in a price–competitive environment."

Competition is essential for optimal resource allocation to implement policies and plans. The national patchwork in many countries defies logic and resists order. A rational strategic planning process requires both!

6. *Simplifying decision making for rationality and the use of intuition*: Decision–aiding techniques for large, complex decision problems can provide descriptions of the power and limitations of policy alternatives. These techniques are essential for quantitative and conceptual descriptions of the operation of a health care system. The dilemma is described in this way by Piershalla [Bloom and Luft, p. 29]:

> "First, many decisions involve large, complex processes. Second, our ability to handle complexity is limited. Third, the time we have to make decisions is often limited, and we are usually involved in many major activities. Fourth, considerable time and money are frequently required to gather most of the information needed to make a decision. Finally, many decisions involve future, uncertain events.
>
> "As a consequence, decision makers tended to make simplistic decisions that were based on a simple model of cause and effect and on possible consequences, with few data. These decisions were rarely made to optimize goals, but rather to satisfy lesser criteria of feasibility. Furthermore, the decisions were often made incrementally rather than comprehensively. The results were usually decisions of lower than optimal quality."

The intuitive mode may suggest variables and their relation to each other, and quantitative techniques can refine impressions with data and also spin out the financial cost of alternative solutions to national health problems.

7. *Choosing among quantitative decision support techniques:* Each technique is more or less appropriate, depending upon the specific problem set. Quantitative decision support systems can be briefly defined in conceptual terms so that policymakers understand what they can and cannot do. When policymakers are at least minimally literate in the use of computers, they can ask basic questions about what a technique is suited for. By refining the policy problem for MIS specialists, suitable analyses can be negotiated by the parties.

8. *Accommodating different local, statewide, and national strategic health care goals:* Any strategic planning for the country's health system must be flexible and adaptable, accommodating local, state, and regional health problems. This is no more difficult than strategic planning for decentralized nationwide and multinational corporations. A formula is devised which allows for state and, through the state, local participation

in resource allocation. For example, if cancer is more prevalent in northeastern states and toxic waste disposal problems are more common in the upper Midwest, then each state or region could shift funds within established service categories.

Hospitals have already integrated estimation and simulation tools for the development of systematic plans and marketing strategies to face an uncertain, rapidly changing environment. Expected changes include the nature and delivery of services, organization and financing, regulatory involvement and emphasis, and changes in population and patient-age distribution [Freeberg, 1981, pp. 32-48]. DRG-based cost accounting and managerial control offers the opportunity to examine case-mix as part of planning and budgeting, which makes possible integrated nationwide health care strategic planning [Thompson, et al, 1979, pp. 111-25].

A conceptual process has been proposed which ties strategic planning to management control [Anthony and Reece, 1975]. The process described in Figure I has been applied to strategic planning, programming, budgeting, and control in health care organizations [Vraciu, 1979, pp. 126-49]. Corporate objectives and strategies, based on external information, affect and are affected by programming, which in turn drives budgeting. Additional external information feeds into the budgeting process and the controlling function fits the budgeting method and procedures. External information is brought to bear upon the controlling function which feeds into programming. The feedback loop involves reporting and analysis of internal and external information. Issues of service mix, production efficiency and effectiveness, and capacity can be dealt with in this relatively simple model.

Some cautions are necessary as the level of analysis is moved from hospitals to health care systems. Strategic planning and management controls should flow from program categories (such as Medicare and Medicaid) which will be relatively stable politically, and which have considerable financial impact upon budget and management control procedures throughout the country's health care system. Requiring a few crucial figures nationwide allows a country's government to exercise enormous influence upon health care delivery, provided that the correct pulse of health system functioning is selected. In the United States, it is hospital costs which have risen most in the past decade and it is the physicians who are most responsible for generating those charges, but who are least aware of the actual expenses generated by their actions. DRG's force hospitals to hold physicians responsible for their styles of practice.

In brief, strategic planning is not about keeping track of everything possible one might want to know; it is about careful selection of a crucial variable (for example, diagnosis related groups) which has a substantial ripple effect on major cost figures for total patient care. Once a single pulse has been found and appropriate computerized control mechanisms

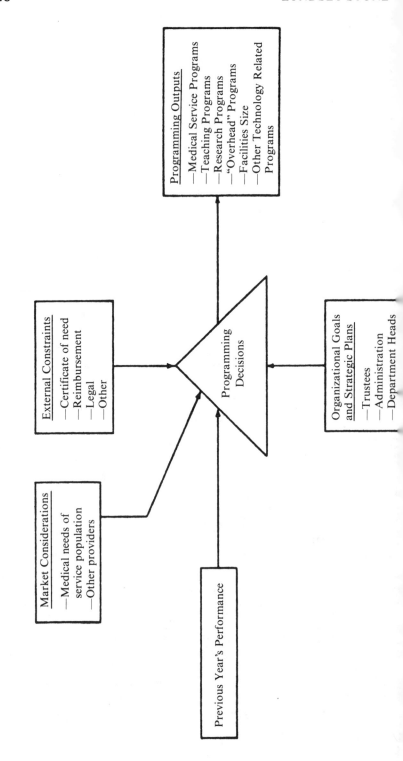

**FIGURE I**

**Schematic Diagram of Programming Phase**

set in place (e.g., a system to detect massive shifts in diagnoses), it is necessary to try to keep hospitals and practitioners from raising costs to a comfortable margin, spinoff concerns will be addressed at a later point, for example, DRG's for outpatient care by physicians is a spinoff.

To summarize, health care systems have developed in most Atlantic nations with idiosyncratic relationships between public and private institutions, and with differences in the extent to which policy, planning, and resources are integrated through strategic management. An integrating strategic approach would require the application of appropriate qualitative and quantitative methods of describing the planning process based on policy priorities. Resource availability would interact with priorities to determine allocations. Quantitative and qualitative methods could be used by nations to measure the accomplishment of strategic health care planning; these must be flexible enough for adaptation to political, economic, and social changes. Furthermore, computation must be simple and planning evaluation formulas readily usable by managers on a daily basis.

Quantitative and qualitative approaches are currently available for health care system strategic planning and they can integrate a variety of techniques to spin out future scenarios and contingencies. The structuring of management information systems can simplify data presentation and samplings of computerized data can be used to initially structure the norms and standards of health system controls. Minimal computer literacy is, of course, necessary for the interface of policymakers with MIS specialists.

A larger problem exists, however, in making public sector policy decisions, and that is the specification, implementation, and monitoring of policies after legislation or administrative reorganization. Public decision systems live with different constraints and without the profit motive of private industry. Strategic planning systems must simultaneously parallel appropriate program budgeting procedures or else they become a mockery of the policymaker's intent. In the public there are multiple clients, but the crucial client is the citizen, who must be able to determine the accomplishments of government. The late Robert Mowitz stated that [1980, pp. ix–x]:

> ". . . the deluge of detailed reports and statistics produced by contemporary bureaucracies and smothered in public relations creates an aura of incomprehensibility. If the executive and the legislature cannot observe and report the status of the governmental system as a whole, i.e., if they have no scorekeeping capability, then certainly their decision–making capacity is seriously restricted. If such ignorance is self–imposed, the citizen can challenge the implied hypothesis that ignorance is bliss."

It is necessary to tie the management information system and the strategic planning effort into a decision cycle which recognizes the nature of government in a democracy. Mowitz has described such a model (see Figures II and III). Policymaking, from this perspective [Mowitz, 1980, p. 42]:

**FIGURE II**
**Decision Logic and Structure**

| | A | B | C | Program Decision Taxonomy | |
|---|---|---|---|---|---|
| | | | | D | E |
| 1 | Values | Preferred States | Subjective/Words | Goals | Programs/Program Categories |
| 2 | Facts | Physical/Behavioral States | Observable/Quantifiable Impact/Outcome Measures | Objectives | Subcategories |
| 3 | Work | Clusters of Activities Knowledge/Skills | Resources Men/Materials/$ | $\dfrac{\text{Outputs}}{\text{Need/Demand}}$ Estimators | Elements |

The program hypothesis: that the outputs produced by work will bring about the physical and behavioral states that satisfy the values of the system. Program analysis tests this hypothesis and searches for work alternatives. Confirmed program hypothesis yield verified program doctrine.

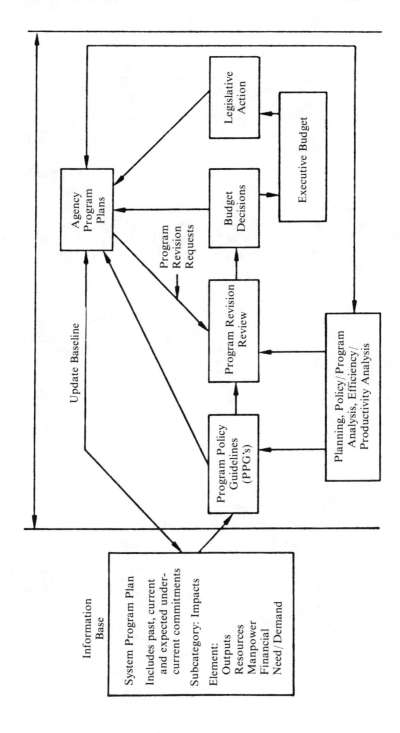

". . . is . . . the process of deciding what the goals of government should be and what specific behavioral and environmental states should be maintained or achieved in order to satisfy those goals. Employing the decision logic, policy-making involves value selection and the translation of values into facts through selection of desired impacts (behavioral and environmental states). This is not simply a process of selecting a value and a condition to satisfy it, but also a consideration of what is attainable given the existing scientific knowledge, technology and program doctrine."

The eight essential conditions listed below [Mowitz, 1980, pp. 59–60] identify what the system does:

1. Identify the major substantive values of the system (Figure II).

2. Convert the values into observable and quantifiable physical and behavioral states acceptable as satisfying the values. These states become the performance objectives of the system (Figure II).

3. Identify work and resources that will produce outputs that have some known capacity to bring about or to maintain the performance objectives (Figure II).

4. Periodically review the relationship between values and objectives and establish boundaries and priorities for decision–making that reflect political values (Program Policy Guidelines, Figure II).

5. Establish an annual decision cycle that forces a review of past experience and projects the likelihood of future success through the review of alternatives (Figure III).

6. Base the scanning of alternatives upon available knowledge reflecting current science and technology by institutionalizing the requirement of analysis as a condition for entering the decision stream (Program Revision Request and Review Process, Figure III).

7. Establish a reporting system that includes information about the external effects or impacts of the organization; about the outputs of work; for monitoring results; and for providing a historical base for future decisions against which management can be judged (Maintaining the System Program Plan, Figure III).

8. Finally, institutionalize the decision process and assume that any set of organizational arrangements is functional as long as the decision requirements are being met, that is, outputs are being produced that satisfy the performance objectives of the system with an acceptable degree of efficiency. Organizational adjustments should be justified in terms of enhancing effectiveness and efficiency, as determined by effects upon impacts and the cost of producing outputs.

The basic issue being raised as one examines health care system–wide strategic planning is the workability of democracy. A viable, adaptive, pluralistic control system of multi–level government necessitates decision analysis and control systems. Such systems must respond to their environments and still retain their integrity. Most importantly, they must be accountable, responsible, and understandable. One has at his disposal quantitative and qualitative analytic tools which are adequate for the task.

Now, it is a question of larger–scale use and conveying to the public, to interest groups, to legislators, and to executives which tools are most appropriate in specific situations and the advantages and constraints of each. The success of system–wide strategic planning may rest with the ability of decision makers to fully use computerized management information systems to enlarge their appreciation of alternative strategies and their outcomes for citizens and their health.

## REFERENCES

R. N. Anthony and J. S. Reece, *Management Accounting: Text and Cases,* 5th Ed., Homewood, Illinois: Richard D. Irwin, Inc., 1975.

Bernard S. Bloom and S. E. Berki, eds., *Cost Benefit, Cost Effectiveness and Other Decision–Making Techniques in Health Care Resource Allocation,* Proceedings of a Regional Symposium, May 19–21, 1983, Chicago, Illinois.

Bernard S. Bloom and Harold S. Luft, *Cost Benefit, Cost Effectiveness, and Other Decision–Making Techniques in Health Care Resource Allocation,* Proceedings of a Regional Symposium, November 4–6, 1982, Phoenix, Arizona, Biomedical Information Corporation, 1983.

"Business: The Big Business of Medicine," *Newsweek,* October 31, 1983.

Lewis Freeberg, "Hospital Utilization: Estimation and Simulation Tools for the Development of Systematic Plans and Marketing Strategies," *Journal of Health Care Marketing,* 1, No. 4, Fall 1981.

Kenneth M. Jones, Jr., "Long-Range Strategic Financial Planning," *Topics in Health Care Financing,* Summer 1981.

Ronald T. La Conte, "Learning Skills for the Emerging Technology," *Public Management,* December 1982.

Barry L. Meiselman, "Strategic Planning and the Design of a Hospital Ambulatory Care Financial Strategy," *Topics in Health Care Financing,* Fall 1982.

Robert J. Mowitz, *The Design of Public Decision Systems,* Baltimore: University Park Press, 1980.

Michael Nathanson, "Tax Act Speeds Automated Merging of Clinical and Financial Information," *Modern Healthcare,* March 1983.

Arnold P. Silver, "A Futuristic Look at Cost and Rate Controls," *Topics in Health Care Financing,* Summer 1981.

John D. Thompson, Richard F. Averill, and Robert B. Felter, "Planning, Budgeting, and Controlling—One Look at the Future: Case Mix Cost Accounting," *Health Services Research,* 14, No. 2, Summer 1979.

Alvin Toffler, *The Third Wave,* New York: Morrow & Co., 1980.

Robert A. Vraciu, "Programming, Budgeting, and Control in Health Care Organizations: The State of the Art," *Health Serices Research,* Summer 1979.

G. Rodney Wolford, "Is Diversification for You?" *Topics in Health Care Financing,* Summer 1981.

# Chapter Fifteen

## Hospital Cost-Shifting Under Prospective Payment

**MICHAEL D. ROSKO**

### Introduction

In response to the alarming increase in hospital expenditures, governmental authorities and other third party payors have experimented with prospective payment (PP) mechanisms. As of May 1982, eight states were using PP to regulate hospital cost increases [Esposito, et al, 1982]. On October 1, 1983, the Health Care Financing Administration began to replace a retrospective method of financing inpatient hospital care for Medicare beneficiaries with a PP system in which Diagnosis Related Groups (DRG's) are employed to establish hospital payment rates.

A number of recent studies have concluded that state-mandated PP systems have controlled the rate of increase of hospital expenditures [Biles, et al, 1980; Coelen and Sullivan, 1981; Comptroller General, 1980; Melnick, et al, 1981; Rosko, 1982(a); Sloan, 1981, 1983]. However, PP may create some perverse incentives. Cleverly [1979] argued that PP, irrespective of whether payment is based on patient days or DRG's, creates a strong incentive to shift costs from regulated patients to non-regulated patients. This may reduce the rigor of PP because the extent to which fiscal restraints imposed by PP result in cost control may depend upon the ability of the institution to subsidize losses in regulated areas by transferring costs to unregulated areas of activity, or by charging unregulated patients or payors differential prices.

Several studies have examined the influence of insurance mix on these dimensions of hospital behavior and, although contradictory findings have been reported [Fitzmaurice, 1981], available evidence seems to suggest that costs, charges, and profitability differ among multiple payors [Danzon, 1982; Sloan and Becker, 1982]. Although the effects of PP on hospital expenditures have been studied extensively, there is a paucity of published empirical data on the impact of PP on hospital cost-shifting. This study attempts to fill part of the void.

Results are presented from an analysis of the Standard Hospital Accounting and Rate Evaluation (SHARE) program, a mandatory, formula-based PP system which was implemented by the New Jersey Department of Health in 1975. A detailed description of this program is available elsewhere [Worthington, et al, 1979(a)]. The next section pro-

155

vides a simple conceptual model which illustrates cost–shifting incentives that may be created by PP. This is followed by a description of the data and methods used in this study. Results are presented in the fourth section. Finally, the implications of the results for national policy are discussed in the concluding section.

### Model of Cost–Shifting Behavior

The model of the impact of PP on hospital cost–shifting is based upon the utility maximizing model of the behavior of the firm. This is a model of non–profit maximizing behavior that is frequently found in economic literature [Miller, 1978].

Martin Feldstein developed a utility maximizing model of hospital behavior as part of a 12 equation model of non–profit hospital price dynamics [Feldstein, 1971]. This model is depicted in Figure I. Feldstein's model is based on the simplifying assumption that, given a fixed budget, a hospital faces the opportunity locus (or product transformation curve), $AB$. This opportunity locus depicts a situation in which the hospital faces a trade–off between patient days ($PDS$) provided and the quality of hospital care ($QH$). This model can be extended to include more outputs. However, more than two outputs cannot be shown on a graph.

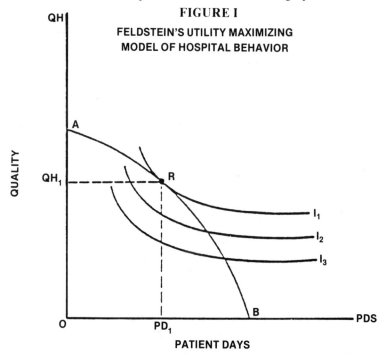

**FIGURE I**

**FELDSTEIN'S UTILITY MAXIMIZING MODEL OF HOSPITAL BEHAVIOR**

Source: Martin Felstein, *Hospital Costs and Health Insurance* (Cambridge: Harvard University Press, 1981), p. 112, Figure 3-2.

Quality is defined in Feldstein's model as the intensity of services provided (i.e, the number of inputs per patient day). This may not be a well-chosen measure of quality for an empirical model. Dowling reported serious difficulties in acquiring valid and reliable measures of intensity [Dowling, 1976]. Therefore, the reader is asked to assume that quality, as used in the Feldstein model, pertains to something that can be conceptualized but cannot be measured.

The opportunity locus in Feldstein's model is drawn concave with respect to the origin. This indicates that as the hospital moves from point $B$ toward point $A$ on the product transformation curve, an increasing amount of $PDS$ must be sacrificed to obtain each extra unit of $QH$. This reflects rising marginal costs as $QH$ is increased. The model also includes indifference curves $I_1$, $I_2$, and $I_3$, which indicate that the utility of the hospital administrator is a function of patient days and quality. The indifference curves are drawn convex with respect to the origin. This reflects the assumption that the administrator's marginal evaluation of quality decreases as the level of quality increases. The higher the indifference curve, the greater the level of satisfaction. Utility of the hospital's chief executive officer is maximized at point $R$ in Figure I. At this point, the marginal rate of product transformation equals the marginal rate of substitution.

Feldstein's model must be altered in order to show the effects of PP on hospital behavior (see Figure II). The revenue constraint imposed by PP can be entered into the model as a price ceiling for each patient day. Cromwell depicted this as a kink in the product transformation curve [Cromwell, et al, 1976]. This is shown as $QH_2GF$ in Figure II. The hospital's opportunity locus becomes $QH_2GFB$ because the revenue ceiling imposed by PP does not allow the hospital to provide care that is more expensive than the value of the inputs needed to provide $QH_2$ amount of $QH$ per patient day. At the new equilibrium position, point $F$, the hospital will provide more patient days but at a lower level of quality than prior to the imposition of PP controls. The net result of PP will be lower per diem costs.

It is possible for the hospital to operate at the initial equilibrium position at point $E$, even with the price ceiling in effect. This can be done if the hospital is willing to suffer a loss per patient day equal to the vertical distance $EG$. $PD_1E$ is equal to the cost per patient day, when $QH_1$ quality and $PD_1$ patient days are provided. $PD_1G$ is the per diem prospective rate set for this hospital. Alternatively, the hospital can avoid suffering a loss if it is able to subsidize the losses associated with the care provided to the regulated patients by raising charges to non-regulated patients or by increasing its level of endowment. Cross-subsidization may be preferred over debt financing as a response to PP because it does not threaten the solvency of hospitals if this strategy is successfully carried out.

158　　　　　　　　　　　　　　　　　　　MICHAEL D. ROSKO

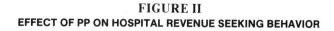

**FIGURE II**
**EFFECT OF PP ON HOSPITAL REVENUE SEEKING BEHAVIOR**

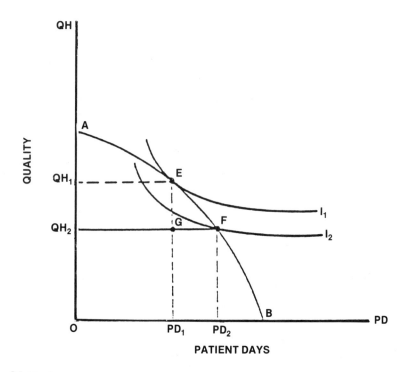

## Methods

The experience of the New Jersey PP program was used in this study for a number of reasons. First, the ability of the New Jersey program to contain hospital expenditures has been documented in two separate multivariate studies which used different research methods [Coelen and Sullivan, 1981; Rosko, 1982(a)]. Second, this program did not regulate reimbursement to all payors [Worthington, et al, 1979(b)]. The absence of universal rate regulation allows one to test the cost–shifting hypothesis. Third, the use of a single state allows for a more reliable identification of hospitals which are likely to successfully shift costs to non–regulated patients.

Data were drawn primarily from audited *Medicare Cost Reports*. These are a more reliable source of data than the self–reported American Hospital Association, *Survey of Hospitals* which has been used in most previous PP evaluations.

The observational unit for the empirical analysis was the individual hospital. A multiple time series, quasi–experimental design was used in this study [Cambell and Stanley, 1963]. The evaluation period included the years 1971 to 1978. This allowed for a four year pre-test period (1971 through 1974) and a four year post–test period (1975 through 1978).

The study population ($n$ = 86) included all New Jersey short–term general not–for–profit hospitals (hereafter called New Jersey hospitals) which had been in operation during the evaluation period. Sixty–six hospitals, located in eastern Pennsylvania, served as comparison hospitals. The comparison group had the same ownership and service characteristics as the study group (i.e., they were short–term, general, not–for–profit, non-governmental hospitals).

Analysis of data for available hospital market characteristics and sample hospital characteristics suggested that eastern Pennsylvania was a suitable comparison region for New Jersey [Rosko, 1982(a)]. The statistical significance of differences between the study and comparison regions, for changes in levels of available market supply and demand variables (i.e., per capita income, mortality rate per 1,000 population, non–federal physicians per 100,000 population, specialist physicians per 1,000 population 65 years of age or older, and non–federal hospital beds) which occurred during the evaluation period, was evaluated by the Student $t$-test. With the exception of change in non–federal hospital beds ($p < 0.04$), none of the $t$-values for regional differences were statistically significant at conventional levels ($p < 0.10$).

Differences between study and control hospitals were assessed for eight variables pertaining to size, volume, case–mix, and teaching activity. Hospitals in the two regions were remarkably similar in terms of the above types of variables. The largest value of $t$ for the difference in the mean value of the above variables, between New Jersey and eastern Pennsylvania hospitals, was less than 1.37.

Cost function analysis was used to isolate and estimate the effects of prospective reimbursement on inpatient hospital expenditures per admission. The cost function model is expressed in Equation 1. A description of the variables used in this model is presented in Table 1.

$$EXP/ADMIT_{it} = a_0 + B_1 (PP_{it}) + B_2 (YR_{it}) + B_3 (STATE_{it}) +$$

$$B_4 (OCCUP_{it}) + B_5 (NCS_{it}) + B_6 (RESBED_{it}) + e_{it} \qquad (1)$$

The dependent variable includes only inpatient expenditures because most outpatient charges were not regulated by the rate–setting program. The last three independent variables—$OCCUP$, $NCS$, and $RESDBED$—have been used frequently in empirical research and their inclusion has theoretical justification [Feldstein, 1979; Watts and Klastorin, 1980]. These variables were used in this analysis to control for inter–hospital

**TABLE 1**

Variable Definitions, Mean Values and
Standard Deviations

| VARIABLE | Definition | All Hospitals MEAN (Std.Dev.) | Inner-City Hospitals MEAN (Std.Dev.) | All Other Hospitals MEAN (Std.Dev.) |
|---|---|---|---|---|
| Dependent Variable | | | | |
| EXP/ADMIT | Total inpatient expenses/admissions, expressed in 1975 constant dollars. | $1011.03 (303.89) | $1214.77 (435.71) | $957.71 (230.87) |
| Independent Variables | | | | |
| OCCUP | Occupancy rate (%) | 80.55 (9.10) | 80.26 (7.34) | 80.62 (9.51) |
| NCS | Number of AHA listed complex services | 6.23 (2.65) | 7.09 (2.53) | 6.01 (2.63) |
| RESDBED | Number of residents/100 beds | 2.95 (5.18) | 5.32 (6.73) | 2.33 (4.49) |
| YR | Linear time trend variable set equal to last digit of year, i | — | — | — |
| PP | Binary rate-setting variable set equal to 1 if observation occurred in a New Jersey hospital during the period 1975-1978 | — | — | — |
| STATE | Binary variable: equals 1 if observation occurred in New Jersey | — | — | — |
| HOSPOO2, ·· ·· HOSP152 | Binary variables: equal 1 in hospital identified by the three digits | — | — | — |

differences which effect expense per admission.[1]

Occupancy rate ($OCCUP$) measures the intensity with which the hospital and its fixed resources are used. Accordingly, this variable is expected to be inversely related with $EXP/ADMIT$. The number of complex services ($NCS$) is a scope of service measure. As a hospital's scope of services increases, a more complex case–mix is likely to be attracted. Thus, this variable should have a positive regression coefficient. Other scope of services variables (i.e., number of basic services, number of quality enhancing services, and number of community services) were not used in order to avoid multi–collinearity problems [Berry, 1973]. $RESDBED$ (medical residents per 100 beds) measures the intensity of medical teaching activities. This variable should be positively related with $EXP/ADMIT$ because teaching programs are expensive to operate. They also tend to attract a more complex case–mix.

It was necessary to account for unmeasured changes which occurred over time—e.g., technological change, physician practices, and so forth—by using a linear time trend variable, $YR$. The binary variable, $STATE$, controls for initial differences in unmeasured variables between study and comparison hospitals. The intercept and error terms are represented by $a$ and $e$, respectively.

$PP$ is a binary variable which measures the differences in average increases in inpatient expenses per admission (while holding the effects of all other independent variables constant), between the study and the comparison hospitals, that occurred annually during the period (1975–1978) in which the rate–setting program was in effect. If the rate–setting program was successful in constraining the growth of inpatient expenditures per admission, the estimated coefficient of $PP$ will have a negative sign.

The regression model shown in Equation 1 is based on the assumption that the error terms are independent. However, some serial correlation was detected. Thus, it was necessary to estimate cost functions by using a fixed–effects model. This was accomplished by entering a binary variable for each hospital into the regression equation. The fixed–effects model controls for omitted hospital specific variables, such as location or physical layout of facilities, which are invariant with respect to time. A detailed discussion of fixed–effects models is available elsewhere [Hausman, 1979].

It has been hypothesized that, *ceteris paribus,* the incentive for hospital administrators to contain costs is directly related to the percentage of

---

[1] It might be argued that it is inappropriate to use hospital–specific explanatory variables in the regression equation because they may be affected by the PP program. However, this was not the case. Regression analysis was performed on each of the hospital characteristics variables and no significant ($p < 0.05$) interstate difference was detected in the change in the level of these variables during the period in which the PP program was in operation. Corroborating evidence is provided by the *National Hospital Rate Setting Study,* which found that the New Jersey PP program did not have a statistically significant ($p < 0.10$) effect on occupancy rate or scope of service. Teaching activities were not investigated in the national study [Worthington and Piro, 1982; Cromwell and Kanak, 1982].

revenues regulated by the PP program [Dowling, 1976]. As the percentage of regulated revenues increases, it becomes more difficult for the hospital to use non–regulated payors to subsidize operating losses suffered in the provision of services to regulated patients. Thus, one would predict that, *ceteris paribus,* the impact of PP on hospital expenditures will increase as the percentage of revenue regulated by the PP program is increased. Unavailability of revenue data precluded a direct test of this hypothesis.

However, it was possible to test this hypothesis indirectly. The program under evaluation regulated only Medicaid and Blue Cross patients. Revenues from these sources were about 45 percent of total inpatient revenues in the typical New Jersey hospital. However, the percent of hospital revenue that was regulated varied substantially by location. Compared to hospitals located in other catchment areas, New Jersey inner–city hospitals had a greater percentage of Medicaid patients, whose payments were regulated, and Medicare patients, whose payments were not regulated [Worthington, *et al,* 1979(b)]. However, the cost–based Medicare reimbursement formula made it difficult for hospitals to use this group of patients for cross–subsidization purposes. In contrast, hospitals located in other catchment areas typically have a greater proportion of charge–based commercially insured patients whose charges can be increased more easily.

Thus, it is hypothesized that if cost–shifting was practiced in New Jersey hospitals, the rate regulation program would have a more pronounced effect upon inpatient expenditures per admission in hospitals located in inner–city areas than in hospitals located in other catchment areas. This hypothesis was tested by estimating separate cost functions for hospitals located in inner–city catchment areas ($n$ = 36) and hospitals located in all other catchment areas ($n$ = 116). Catchment area criteria developed by the New Jersey Department of Health are used in this study. Classification criteria included: total population, population density, and percent population with income less than the poverty level [Worthington, *et al,* 1979(b)].

### Results

Table 2 presents estimated cost functions for: all hospitals (Model 1), inner–city hospitals (Model 2), and hospitals located in all other areas (Model 3). The adjusted $R$–square exceeded 0.88 in all models. The highest correlation coefficient between any two independent variables was only 0.58. This suggests that multi–collinearity did not cause the parameter estimates to be unreliable. All of the coefficients in Model 1 and Model 3 were statistically significant ($p < 0.05$) and of the expected sign. In model 2, *NCS* and *RESDBED* had insignificant ($p < 0.05$) regression coefficients. This may be due to the fact that most inner–city hospitals in New Jersey and eastern Pennsylvania have had extensive teaching programs and a large number of complex services throughout the evaluation period. Therefore, it is likely that the effects of these factors were captured by the

individual hospital variables of the fixed–effects model. In contrast, suburban and rural hospitals added these programs over time and thus, they
were not reflected by the individual hospital variables.

### TABLE 2

### Average Cost Regression Results

|  | Model 1*<br>All Hospitals<br>(Std.Error) | Model 2*<br>Inner City Hospitals<br>(Std. Error) | Model 3*<br>All Other Hospitals<br>(Std.Error) |
|---|---|---|---|
| PP | −40.734**<br>(9.96) | −61.483***<br>(28.72) | −25.194**<br>(9.37) |
| YR | 51.601**<br>(1.65) | 65.577**<br>(4.86) | 45.710**<br>(1.55) |
| STATE | 59.628**<br>(13.90) | 175.234**<br>(56.06) | 36.531**<br>(12.73) |
| OCCUP | −3.507**<br>(0.433) | −7.917**<br>(1.61) | −2.912**<br>(0.39) |
| NCS | 7.546**<br>(2.14) | 8.007<br>(5.97) | 5.386**<br>(2.09) |
| RESDBED | 9.937**<br>(1.13) | 2.506<br>(3.65) | 11.078**<br>(1.06) |
| INTERCEPT | 53.164 | 125.332 | 79.72 |
| Adjusted<br>R-Square | 0.907 | 0.924 | 0.887 |

*Estimated coefficients for the individual hospital binary variables are not reported.
**Significant at $p < 0.01$.
***Significant at $p < 0.05$.

The coefficient of the rate regulation variable, $PP$, was negative and
statistically significant ($p < 0.05$) in each equation. However, the coefficient of $PP$ was much larger in the equation (Model 2) for inner–city
hospitals than in the equation (Model 3) which used the data set for hospitals located in all other areas. The results suggest that from 1975 to 1978
annual savings attributed to the rate regulation program, in terms of inpatient expenditures per admission, amounted to $61.48 in inner–city hospi-
tals and $25.19 in hospitals located in other catchment areas. These sav-
ings represent 5.1 percent and 2.6 percent of mean base year (1974)
expenditures of inner–city hospitals and other catchment area hospitals,
respectively.

**Implications**

The most appealing explanation for the disparate performance between inner–city hospitals and hospitals located in other areas is that the inner–city hospitals felt greater pressures to contain costs. A brief review of the PP mechanism is necessary to develop this explanation. A tight prospective rate creates a strong possibility that a hospital might suffer financial operating losses during the forthcoming year. The threat to a hospital's solvency may cause a change in behavior of hospital administrators. More specifically, in order to avoid a forecasted deficit, hospital administrators are likely to take action to increase revenue or to reduce costs. It is likely that hospital administrators will prefer to respond to the revenue constraints of PP by taking revenue–increasing actions, because these measures are less traumatic to the organization than cost–cutting actions. If the hospital is able to increase revenue by a sufficient amount, then it will be able to maintain its current level of goal–attainment without making difficult and unpopular decisions about eliminating or reducing personnel or programs within the hospital.

This conclusion follows Schultz and Rose's observation that the effectiveness of hospital administrators is evaluated by hospital trustees on the basis of: (1) solvency; (2) quality of services; (3) institutional harmony, which may be defined as the level of employee and medical staff satisfaction and which, for employees, is undoubtedly related to compensation, job security, and working conditions; and (4) institutional growth [Schultz and Rose, 1973]. All of these criteria of managerial success can be influenced by revenue–increasing behavior, while only the first criterion, solvency, is directly related to cost–containing behavior.

One conclusion that can be drawn from the above model is that inner–city hospitals faced a stronger incentive to contain cost, because they were less successful in generating additional revenue than hospitals located in other areas. However, this conclusion is based upon the following indirect evidence: inner–city hospitals have a smaller proportion of charge–based patients, whose charges can be increased with relative ease, than hospitals located in other catchment areas [Worthington, et al, 1979(b)]; and, an analysis of tabular data which concluded that the financial position (e.g., profitability, liquidity, and capital structure) of inner–city hospitals declined more than that of other hospitals during the period (1975-1979) in which the rates for New Jersey hospitals were regulated [Rosko and Broyles, forthcoming]. The latter finding was based upon rather unsophisticated analysis and further research in this area is needed. Anecdotal evidence from a survey of hospital administrators and hospital chief financial officers also supports the cost–shifting hypothesis [Rosko, 1982(b)].

The results of the evaluation of the New Jersey rate regulation program have some important implications for the recent changes in the Medicare program which alter the reimbursement mechanism from retrospective, cost–based to prospective, DRG–based. Both the New Jersey SHARE program and the recently implemented Medicare program use prospective payments to motivate hospitals to contain costs. However, both programs do not regulate the charges paid by all payors and this may create a strong incentive to shift costs to the non–regulated payors.

Thus, the Medicare DRG–based payment system may result in the following consequences. First, hospitals may shift costs to non–regulated patients. Thus, the gains in Medicare program cost savings will be offset, to some extent, by increased charges borne by other groups. Second, hospitals that are more successful in cost–shifting will have less incentive to initiate cost–containment programs. Thus, cost–savings in the DRG–based Medicare payment system may be less than estimated in previous evaluations of PP programs, which regulated a greater percentage of hospital revenues than Medicare revenues represent for the typical hospital. Third, DRG–driven PP systems reward hospitals with a lower average length of stay within a DRG and punish those with a higher average length of stay within a DRG. It is desirable to reward hospitals for efficient clinical management which results in the timely discharge of patients. However, it is undesirable to punish hospitals for external factors, such as complexity of case–mix and availability of nursing home beds, which lengthen a patient's stay. Results from several exploratory studies of DRG's suggest that this type of patient classification scheme is not sufficiently refined to account for variations in average length of stay within a DRG which are due to complexity and severity of illness [Grimaldi and Micheletti, 1980; Young, et al, 1980; Berki, et al, 1981].

For example, multivariate analysis found that, within seven of eight DRG's studied, the number of recorded diagnoses had a direct and significant ($p < 0.10$) relationship with average length of stay of patients grouped in the same DRG [Berki, et al, 1981]. Additionally, average length of stay may be affected by discharge disposition problems. Patients in inner–city hospitals are more likely to have multiple diagnoses and disposition problems, because of their low income status, than other patients. In the combined New Jersey and eastern Pennsylvania sample, the average length of stay ranged from 9.1 days in inner–city hospitals to 8.3 days in hospitals located in other catchment areas.

Thus, a DRG system which does not account for differences in average length of stay, which are due to factors correlated with location, may result in windfall profits to suburban hospitals and harsh penalties to inner–city hospitals. This may lead to the deterioration of service capability of inner–city hospitals.

Finally, it is appropriate to note that during the years 1980 to 1982 the State of New Jersey began to phase out the SHARE program which was replaced by a DRG–based system which regulated all payers. Many of the provisions of the enabling legislation, S–446, for the New Jersey DRG system were made in response to the problems encountered in the

SHARE program that were discussed in this paper, i.e., cost–shifting and deteriorating financial status of inner–city hospitals. It is interesting to note that although the New Jersey DRG system is recognized as the prototype for the Medicare PP system, these particular problems were not addressed in the federal legislation.

## REFERENCES

Sylvester E. Berki, Marie Ashcraft, and William Newbrander, "Length–of–Stay Within DRG's," Paper presented at the American Public Health Association Meetings, Los Angeles, November 1981.

Ralph Berry, Jr., "On Grouping Hospitals for Economic Analysis," *Inquiry*, 10, Spring 1973.

Brian Biles, Carl Schramm, and J. Graham Atkinson, "Hospital Cost Inflation Under State Rate–Setting Programs," *New England Journal of Medicine*, 303, September 1980.

Donald Cambell and Julian Stanley, *Experimental and Quasi–Experimental Designs for Research*, Chicago: Rand McNally College Publishing Company, 1963.

William Cleverly, "Evaluation of Alternative Payment Strategies for Hospitals: A Conceptual Approach," *Inquiry*, 16, Summer 1979.

Craig Coelen and Daniel Sullivan, "An Analysis of the Effects of Prospective Reimbursement Programs on Hospital Expenditures," *Health Care Financing Review*, 2, Winter 1981.

Comptroller General, *Report to the Congress of the United States*, "Rising Hospital Costs Can be Restrained by Regulating Payments and Improving Management," HRD–80–72, Gaithersberg: General Accounting Office, 1980.

Jerry Cromwell, Craig Coelen, Lee Edlefsen, Diane Hamilton, and Jan Mitchell, "Analysis of Prospective Payment Systems for Upstate New York: Summary," Final report prepared for Department of Health, Education and Welfare under SSA/ORA contract HEW/OS–74–261, Cambridge: Abt Associates, 1976.

Jerry Cromwell and James Kanak, "The Effects of Prospective Reimbursement Programs on Hospital Adoption and Service Sharing," *Health Care Financing Review*, 4, December 1982.

P. M. Danzon, "Hospital Profits: The Effects of Reimbursement Policies," *Journal of Health Economics*, 1, Winter 1982.

William Dowling, "Prospective Rate Setting: Concept and Practice," *Topics in Health Care Financing*, 3, Winter 1976.

Alfonso Esposito, Michael Hupfer, Cynthia Mason, and Diane Rogler, "Abstracts of State Legislated Hospital Cost Containment Programs," *Health Care Financing Review*, 4, December 1982.

Martin Feldstein, "Hospital Cost Inflation: A Study of Nonprofit Price Dynamics," *American Economic Review*, 51, December 1971.

Paul Feldstein, *Health Care Economics*, New York: John Wiley and Sons, 1979.

Michael J. Fitzmaurice, "A Statistical Analysis of the Medicare Hospital Routine Cost Differential," Health Care Financing Administration, August 1981 (unpublished).

Paul Grimaldi and Julie Micheletti, "On the Homogeneity of Diagnostic Related Groups," *Journal of the American Medical Record Association*, 10, January 1980.

J. A. Hausman, "Specification Tests in Econometrics," *Econometrics*, 46, November 1979.

Glenn Melnick, John Wheeler, and Paul Feldstein, "Effects of Rate Regulation on Selected Components of Hospital Expenses," *Inquiry*, 18, Fall 1981.

Roger Miller, *Intermediate Microeconomics*, New York: McGraw–Hill, 1978.

Michael Rosko, "Impact of Prospective Rate–Setting: Cost Containment or Cost Shifting?," Paper presented to American Economic Association Annual Meeting, New York, December 1982(a).

_____, *Hospital Responses to Prospective Rate Setting*, unpublished Ph.D. dissertation, Temple University, 1982(b).

_____ and Robert Broyles, "Unintended Consequences of Prospective Reimbursement: Cost–Shifting and Erosion of Hospital Financial Position," *Health Care Management Review*, forthcoming.

Rockwell Schultz and Jerry Rose, "Can Hospitals be Expected to Control Costs?," *Inquiry*, 10, June 1973.

Frank Sloan, "Regulation and the Rising Costs of Hospital Care," *Review of Economics and Statistics*, 63, November 1981.

―――― , "Rate Regulation as a Strategy for Hospital Cost Control: Evidence From the Last Decade," *Health and Society*, 61, Summer 1983.

―――― and Edmund Becker, "Cross Subsidies and Payment for Hospital Care," Report submitted to the National Center for Health Services Research, August 1982.

Carolyn A. Watts and T. D. Klastorin, "The Impact of Case Mix on Hospital Cost: A Comparative Analysis," *Inquiry*, 17, Winter 1980.

Nancy Worthington, Jerry Cromwell, and Gilby Kamens, "Prospective Reimbursement in New Jersey," *Topics in Health Care Financing*, 17, Fall 1979(a).

―――― , "Case Study of Prospective Reimbursement in New Jersey," *National Hospital Rate Setting Study*, Baltimore: Health Care Financing Administration, 1979(b).

Nancy Worthington and Paula Piro, "The Effects of Hospital Rate Setting Programs on Volumes of Hospital Services: A Preliminary Analysis," *Health Care Financing Review*, 4, December 1982.

Wanda Young, Roger Swinkola, and Martha Hutton, "Assessment of the Autogrp Patient Classification System," *Medical Care*, 18, February 1980.

# Chapter Sixteen

## Changing Health Care Payment Mechanisms

### RICHARD C. McKIBBIN[1]

## Introduction

Sweeping changes in the way in which hospitals are paid for the care of individuals covered by Medicare have been introduced in the past two years. Cost-based retrospective reimbursement has been eliminated, replaced initially by a system of target rates and Section 223 limits introduced as part of the 1982 Tax Equity and Fiscal Responsibility Act (TEFRA). Even more importantly, prospectively–set, diagnosis related group (DRG) based payment rates began to be phased in over a three–year period on October 1, 1983. A number of conceptual and operational issues associated with the new hospital payment mechanisms have been addressed in numerous other studies.

The emphasis here is not to review the characteristics of the new payment mechanisms because these have already been described. Rather, this study identifies some of the likely future impacts of changing payment mechanisms for health services generally, as opposed to hospital care specifically. It explores some of their potential consequences for professional relationships, which will affect both health professionals and others employed in health care, and the structure of the health care delivery system itself. Professional relationships will be subject to potential changes of great significance, altering traditional roles and relationships for all types of health care employees, as a result of recent and likely future changes in the payment mechanisms for health care services in the United States.

## Payment by DRG: Incentives and Implications

The shift to prospective payment by Medicare will have a significant impact on community hospitals; the Medicare program is the source of 31.7 percent of their revenues [Davis, 1982, p. 36]. Even though the three-year phased introduction of DRG–based payments for Medicare beneficiaries began last year, the new system involves a number of unresolved issues and uncertain consequences. For example, no procedures have been developed for the way in which hospital's capital costs (expenditures for

---

[1] The views expressed are the author's and do not necessarily reflect the views of the American Nurses' Association.

new construction, purchases of additional facilities and durable equipment, and their associated interest and depreciation expenses) will be treated. For now, a "window" exists and such costs are allowed to "pass through." That is, a hospital is reimbursed by Medicare for capital costs to the extent that the facility provides services to Medicare beneficiaries.

In the current absence of controls on the payment for capital costs, capital expenditures by hospitals have increased at dramatic rates and can be expected to continue at high levels until 1986, when the government is expected to establish a methodology for incorporating allowable capital costs in the DRG–based payment mechanism ["National Hospital 'Cap'. . . ," 1983]. An intense debate involving a variety of complex alternative possible capital cost methods is underway, the results of which could have a major and differing financial impact on hospitals, depending on whether they undergo significant expansion or modernization during this period of time.

A more immediate consequence of the new Medicare inpatient hospital payment mechanism flows from the new system's incentives for increased operational data by DRG and by physician, for reduced lengths of stay, and for enhanced discharge planning. These involve more careful identification of essential and cost–effective activities to assist the hospitals in providing care, by diagnosis, at costs below the payment rates. These incentives are the result of several characteristics of the new payment mechanism, which are described in Table 1.

As a result, hospital decision makers are working more closely with representatives from the medical staff, accounting, medical records, and nursing to identify and examine care patterns, particularly for those DRG's in which hospitals experience a high volume of admissions. Computerized hospital information systems, often incorporating patient classification measures as indicators of the severity of illness and extent of intervention required, as well as medical, financial, and DRG-based operational information, are being introduced into the nation's hospitals at unprecedented rates. In a recent survey, more than 150 companies were identified that provide computerized management information systems to hospitals [Dorenfest, 1983, p. 129]. Because of these developing information–based hospital management systems, it is essential for health professionals to develop familiarity with computerized information systems and to insure that the essential and cost–effective characteristics of hospital care are identified and incorporated in the hospital's decision–making processes.

As a part of the changes brought about by the new payment mechanisms and their associated incentives, professional and staffing relationships in the hospital are being reexamined. Physicians have long viewed hospitals as their workshops, but have traditionally not been financially responsible or accountable to the hospital as a result of their actions. Individual hospitals, utilizing per–physician DRG length of stay and ancil-

| | TRADITIONAL | DRG |
|---|---|---|
| Payment mechanism is: | Per diem, or total hospital costs divided by patient days. | By the case, or costs related to treatment of specific DRG. |
| Payment unit is: | The patient day. | The diagnosis. |
| Calculation of rates: | Rates reflect hospital's own costs. | Rates are derived from a blending of hospital-specific amounts based on each hospital's cost experience. National and regional (for nine census divisions) DRG amounts for both urban and rural hospitals. Transitional period—by October 1, 1986, payment will be 100 percent of the national urban or rural DRG rate. |
| Timeframe: | Retrospective. | Prospective. |
| System incentives: | Hospital has limited incentive to contain costs, since expenses are reimbursed retrospectively. | Hospital profits from cost containment through receipt of incentive payments when length of stay is lower than average, and experiences disincentives when costs exceed the standard. |
| Payers: | Commercial Payers are billed for costs disallowed by noncommercial payers. | The system will apply to all Medicare participating hospitals, except psychiatric, long-term care, rehabilitation, and children's hospitals, and hospitals outside the 50 states and Washington, D.C. |

*Source:* Shaffer [1983, p. 393].

lary service utilization analyses, can now identify medical staff members
whose clients appear to stay, on average, for excessive periods of time,
receive unnecessary tests, or undergo unnecessary procedures. Such
information clearly presents potential confrontational situations, in which
the physician's position as an autonomous decision maker is subject to
challenge by hospital administrators. In the extreme, a physician's staff
privileges at a particular institution, theoretically, could be terminated for
economic reasons.

The potential for conflict between the medical staff and hospital administration stems from obviously divergent incentives. Given a fixed payment rate per Medicare DRG, the administrator's incentive is to encourage activities that enhance discharge planning, thereby reducing length of
stay. Physicians, however, are potentially liable for any problems resulting
from early discharges, and their Medicare payment is still on a fee-for-
service basis, so that reduced stay lengths tend to reduce the number of
physician contacts, and thus income.

On the other hand, conflict between physicians and administrators may
be reduced if physicians themselves police their own ranks. Physicians do
appear to be, in the aggregate, cooperating with the hospitals' desires to
reduce lengths of stay as a result of prospective payment for Medicare;
hospital lengths of stay have recently declined, particularly for those
patients covered by Medicare. Comparing the third quarters of 1982 and
1983, it is notable that average length of stay fell 1.7 percent for inpatients
under 65, but fell by 4.6 percent for inpatients 65 and over [AHA, 1983, p.
2].

While such data cannot be unequivocably or fully identified as a result
of cooperative physician responses to prospective payment incentives, it is
almost certainly related to them. Anecdotal evidence also seems supportive of such a view: Jeff Goldsmith, author of *Can Hospitals Survive?* and
a consultant for Ernst and Whinney, believes that "doctors seem amaz-
ingly willing to take the long view of this thing," and Paul Cooper, administrator of a hospital in New Jersey, subject to a DRG–based—all payers
payment system since 1980, indicates that, during efforts to get physicians
to reduce lengths of stay, "we've had resistance, but when push comes to
shove they come around." ["Hospitals and Doctors Clash . . . ," January
19, 1984, p. 31].

However, the initial apparently cooperative physician response to prospective payment may erode as pressures to control hospital costs become
more intense as the phase–in continues, and as related factors exacerbate
the situation. These include an emerging surplus of physicians
[GEMENAC, 1981], and a resultant difficulty for physicians to maintain
their incomes. Yet another factor may come into play: physicians and
health administrators tend to think differently. Physicians [Reece, p. 674]

". . . are educated to concentrate on the *individual transaction*—the one-
on-one encounter with a specific problem or a specific patient. For the most

part, (physicians) do not stop to think how the impact of each transaction ripples through a system. The professional manager, on the other hand, is taught to think in terms of events as a *process with a series of transactions.* Each transaction has a cost and a profit—and each is to be minimized or maximized by a *systematic, organized, and purposeful team approach.*

"Because of these differences in education, tension inevitably exists between physicians, who wish to maximize what they can do for the individual patient no matter what the cost, and professional health care manager, who desires to moderate costs by routinizing the transaction or reducing the number of transactions, or minimizing deviations from routine transactions."

Stated differently, there appear to be inherent potential conflicts between organizational and professional needs. These are not limited to the hospital administrator–physician relationship, but to general relationships between practicing health professionals of all types and administrative decision makers. These strains have been summarized in Table 2.

**TABLE 2**

**Strains Between Administrative and Professional Needs**

| ADMINISTRATIVE NEEDS | PROFESSIONAL NEEDS |
|---|---|
| 1. Predictability. | 1. Freedom to operate in the face of uncertainty; the exceptional case syndrome. |
| 2. Commitment to organizational goals—organizational maintenance. | 2. Commitment to the goals of one's profession and peers; more narrowly focused than the organization's goals. |
| 3. Coordination and integration across tasks, services, and departments. | 3. Freedom to function within specialized interest areas; loose coordination that does not interfere with one's professional work. |
| 4. Control and feedback to ensure public accountability. | 4. Emphasis on individual accountability to patients and professional peers. |
| 5. Specialization of labor to accomplish organizational-relevant tasks. | 5. Specialization of labor to accomplish individual-specific tasks. |

*Source:* Adapted from Shortell [1982, p. 11].

To the extent that these differences are indeed real, then the long–term ability of physicians, other health professionals, and administrators to respond cooperatively to the incentives brought about by prospective payment may be constrained. Younger physicians who, for example, may face difficulties in establishing their practices and attaining a secure income, could be expected to be more cooperative than established physicians, creating the possibility of the future intra–professional conflict as well.

### Prospective Payment for Other Health Services

The interest of government health policymakers in revising payment mechanisms and their associated incentives is not limited to the payment for the hospital care of inpatient Medicare beneficiaries. Rather, an interest exists in developing prospective payment systems for other health services. Physician payment, payment for nursing homes and other extended care facilities, for home health services, and for various health care services rendered in ambulatory care settings are all being studied.

It is beyond the scope of this analysis to describe the potential prospective payment mechanisms for these services and care settings. However, it is important to note that the rapidly rising cost of health care programs financed with federal funds makes these efforts likely to be implemented in the future; it appears that prospective payment for the hospital care of the elderly under Medicare was introduced first, primarily because this program involves the greatest expenditure of all federal health programs. It was, therefore, identified as the first area to be reformed. Reforms in payment mechanisms for other health services will create both challenges and opportunities for health care workers involved with these settings.

The possible introduction of prospective payment for long–term care, both in institutional settings and in the home, will challenge providers to render even more cost–effective care than at present in these settings. It will also become increasingly necessary to demonstrate the cost–effectiveness of certain services compared to others in order to retain reimbursement for them. Providers may find themselves more directly competing for clients and dollars. Which providers will be paid? Probably those that are least costly but competent to perform the necessary range of services. For example, reimbursement for an expanded range of nursing services may be achieved, but this is likely to occur only if the beneficial cost consequences of such services are rigorously demonstrated. While some studies have begun to document the cost–effectiveness of various health professionals, further cost–effectiveness research is necessary [McKibbin, 1978, pp. 110–15; Fagin, 1982, pp. 459–73].

New organizational arrangements for responding to incentives associated with prospective payment will also emerge. One interesting example of such an arrangement is the continuing care program recently developed by a health maintenance organization in Kansas City [Prime Health, 1983, pp. 2–3]. This program utilizes highly skilled nurse practitioners to reduce hospital lengths of stay. The organization markets a program to community hospitals to reduce length of stay, a prime incentive for hospitals as a result of the new DRG payment system, by arranging for the patient care services at home that would otherwise require hospital care. It also develops procedures for pre–hospitalization patient education which may reduce the length of stay or the likelihood that hospitalization will be required. In addition, management contracts may be secured to manage discharge planning, home health care, extended care facilities services, hospice care, and pre–authorization reviews of elective hospital admissions as alternatives to costly hospital services, which may not be necessary. Thus, the probable extension of prospective payment for other health services can be expected to offer additional new and innovative business and employment opportunities for health professionals.

These new arrangements will contribute to an increasingly competitive health care environment. As an example, consider the fact that some services which are usually rendered by physicians can also be provided by nurse practitioners. The extent of such overlap varies among states and situations, but does exist. In terms of the two professionals range or scope of practice, perhaps 50 percent of the services rendered by nurse practitioners are also commonly provided by physicians, but nurse practitioners' scope of practice overlaps with perhaps only 10 percent of the range of services provided by primary care physicians. To enhance their professional status, demand for services, possibilities for reimbursement, and autonomy as practitioners,' nurse practitioners have an interest in expanding their scope of practice. Typically, this would occur in areas in which physicians are also active, unless encroachment onto their professional turf were prevented by legal or other means.

In an era of increasing demand for health services and ready availability of funding for such services, a situation such as that described for nurse practitioners and physicians may be of limited concern to both groups. Physicians may abandon the performance of some services to the competing professionals; the professional and economic rewards available to each group expand, even though for one group it is partly at the expense of a reduced rate of growth. However, in an era of restrictive financing and emerging manpower surpluses, confrontations between the two groups over the extent of and rate of change in—indeed, possibly in the continued existence of—such overlapping professional services are likely to be challenged.

For example, in the State of Missouri, a supreme court decision was reached on November 22, 1983, in the case of *Sermchief v. Gonzales*. This decision overturned an earlier circuit court ruling which had enjoined nurse practitioners from performing certain examinations and dispensing medications unless prescribed by a physician. Suit had been brought by the state's healing arts board, but the court found that the state's legislature had adopted an open–ended definition of nursing and that changes in the nursing practice act revealed "a manifest legislative desire to expand the scope of authorized nursing practices" and "to avoid statutory constraints on the evolution of new functions for nurses . . ." ["Missouri NPs Win Appeal . . . ," 1984, p. 132]. Prospective payment appears likely to usher in an era of increasing numbers of challenges of this type.

**All Payers Systems and Generalized Prospective Payment Mechanisms**

Unlike the system established nationally for Medicare, New Jersey has developed a DRG-based prospective payment system which encompasses the payment rates for all persons hospitalized in that state. All payers, not just Medicare, pay the hospitals the rates established by the New Jersey Hospital Rate Setting Commission. Such a system has the advantage that cost shifting cannot occur; that is, costs not paid by one third party, such as Medicare, cannot be added to the rate base for determination of the level of charges to other third parties and private payers. Thus, an all payers system can restrain the level of *total* hospital payments, while a system such as the national DRG-based prospective payment system is capable only of restricting the level of hospital payments made by Medicare. While there is contention about whether or not hospitals are, in fact, able to completely shift costs not fully compensated by one payer to other payers, this issue is of concern to Blue Cross and Blue Shield, private insurance carriers, employers with self-insurance arrangements, as well as to employers generally because of its potential adverse effects on health insurance premiums.

Three states in addition to New Jersey—Maryland, Massachusetts, and New York—hold waivers which permit them to use their own state hospital payment system in lieu of the federal DRG-based Medicare payment mechanisms. These state plans also address hospital rates for all payers, but are not based on DRG's. Other states have applied or plan to apply for waivers, but it has been argued that individual state programs may be more expensive than the Medicare plan, so it is uncertain whether or not more waivers will be granted. At the same time, it appears unlikely that the Reagan Administration would support a plan to control hospital rates which would incorporate rate setting for non-federal payers. Thus, the most likely outcome would appear to be efforts on the part of non-Medicare payers of hospital bills to attempt to make contractual arrangements with hospitals to keep rates they are charged in line with federal DRG-based rates. The current trend toward the emergence of Preferred Provider Organizations (PPO's), which contract with hospitals, physicians, and other providers for coverage at specified discounts from standard charges for services, appears to be such an effort.

Future initiatives to moderate the rate of cost increases for the Medicare program and other sources of payment for health services may lead to even more profound changes in payment mechanisms than those which have so far occurred. The present federal administration came into office in 1981, amid much discussion of and many proposals for establishing competitive incentives in health care delivery. The voucher proposal for Medicare represented one effort in this direction. Current discussions on health policy focus on the evolution of prospective payment into a more generalized format, not specifically linked to any particular providers or institutions. Such a concept could take the form of proposals to contract with organizations which would, for a prospectively-determined fee, agree to assume the risk for any and all health services required by a specific enrolled group, such as a subgroup of the entire Medicare population. An organization would then arrange for the total health service requirements—hospital care, physician visits, long-term home or institutionally-based nursing care, and so forth—of the enrolled population. Such organizations would compete for enrollees, who would be entitled to a defined federal annual contribution, or voucher amount, for their health services requirements.

A generalized prospective payment system could replace not only the new Medicare DRG-based hospital payment arrangements but also the developing prospective payment systems for other health services. From an administrative perspective, this kind of a plan would be attractive because it is relatively simple. However, some health groups have expressed reservations about the development of a generalized umbrella prospective payment arrangement, as a result of unanswered questions regarding the range of services covered and possible detrimental quality assurance effects that may be associated with it.

However, any sweeping change in the organizational and institutional arrangements for health delivery will take time. Regulations, fee structures, and administrative rules for HMO's to enroll Medicare beneficiaries have been developed over the past several years, but these are still in an experimental stage. A vast program of contracting with millions of Medicare beneficiaries through HMO-like, voucher financed plans will not be forthcoming in the near future, athough they could conceivably be implemented by 1990.

It is not possible to predict what precise form will develop for the future structure of payment mechanisms for health services. It is certain, however, that change will continue. Economic incentives will increasingly influence clinical decisions [Luft, 1983, pp. 103–23]. In such a changing health care environment, health professionals need to be able to respond and adapt rapidly to the evolution of payment mechanisms for health services.

## Impact on Health Professionals

Developments associated with the new incentives that are part of prospective payment have a number of consequences for health professionals. They include:

1. Increased direct competition among providers for patients and health care dollars.

2. Increased responsibility for cost control.

3. Increased emphasis on discharge planning.

4. Greater expectations regarding productivity.

5. Enhanced opportunities for direct business involvement in health services delivery.

6. Expanded requirements for computer-based information systems, integrating medical, nursing, financial, and operational information.

7. Increased reliance on highly-technical diagnostic and therapeutic equipment.

8. Enlarged requirements for employment in home-based and elderly care settings.

9. Increased expectations regarding the demonstrated cost-effectiveness of health care services of all types.

These consequences will have far reaching economic and employment effects for health professionals. An individual health professional's career over the next decade will be far from static. It will change dramatically. Patient care will, of course, remain as the focus but the nature of health related interventions, the settings in which they occur, the technical complexity with which they are conducted, the documentation required to accompany them, the source and basis of payments for services rendered, and the individual range of service and degree of autonomy as a provider are all likely to change remarkably. Some of these changes will flow from social and demographic factors associated with an increasingly aged population. Other changes will result more directly from the evolution of payment mechanisms and their associated organizational and operational incentives. Taken together, these changes and their effects represent dramatic challenges and opportunities for health professionals.

## REFERENCES

American Hospital Association, *Trends,* Office of Public Policy Analysis, 73, Chicago, December 1983.

C. Davis, "Effects of Medicare, Medicaid on Community Hospitals," *Healthcare Financial Management,* July 1982.

S. Dorenfest, "More Computer Firms Entering Already Crowded Hospital Market," *Modern Healthcare,* 1983.

C. Fagin, "Nursing's Pivotal Role in American Health Care," L. Aiken, ed., *Nursing in the 1980's: Crises, Opportunities, Challenges,* Philadelphia: J.B. Lippincott, 1982.

Graduate Medical Education National Advisory Committee, *Report,* U.S. Department of Health and Human Services, Pub. No. (HRA) 81-652.

"Hospitals and Doctors Clash Over Efforts by Administrators to Cut Medicare Costs," *The Wall Street Journal,* January 19, 1984.

H. Luft, "Economic Incentives and Clinical Decisions," in B. Gray, ed., *The New Health Care for Profit,* Washington, D.C.: Institute of Medicine, National Academy Press, 1983.

R. McKibbin, "Cost-Effectiveness of Physicians' Assistants: A Review of Recent Evidence," *The Physicians' Assistants Journal,* 8, 1978.

"Missouri NPs Win Appeal in Medical Practice Suit," *American Journal of Nursing,* 84, 1984.

"National Hospital 'Cap' Seen as One Option by Commission," *Health Services Information,* Washington, D.C.: Healthcare Publications, December 26, 1983.

Prime Health, "Continuing Care Plan—Policy Proposal," unpublished, Kansas City: September 28, 1983.

R. I. Reece, "The Corporate Transformation of Medicine in Minnesota: First of a Series:

The Accelerating Industrialization of Health Care in The Twin Cities," *Minnesota Medicine,* November 1983.

Shaffer, *Nursing and Health Care,* adapted from the *1982 Annual Report,* New Jersey Rate Setting Commission, September 1983.

S. Shortell, "Theory Z: Implications and Relevance for Health Care Management," *Health Care Management Review,* 7, Fall 1982.

# Chapter Seventeen

## Networking Hospitals for Cost Identification, Productivity, and Resource Utilization

### CHARLES T. WOOD

## Introduction

Society is currently witnessing the most dramatic and far-reaching change in the history of health care management. With the advent of the Prospective Payment System (PPS), health care providers, as well as regulators and third-party payors, have thrust themselves, or have been pushed, into an environment which is foreign to the mind set they have cultivated for many years.

Most hospital managers are very comfortable with retrospective cost reimbursement and per diem averaging. But, PPS will change hospital management systems, including budgeting, financing, accounting, costing, pricing, marketing, and planning. PPS will also alter the medical staff-management-trustee relationship. It will affect hospital-doctor-patient interactions, as well as hospital and community communications.

This paper will outline some of the changes brought about by PPS and the necessities for drastically altering hospital management systems of cost identification, productivity, and resource utilization control. It will introduce the concept of cost identification by specific diagnosis, by day of hospitalization, and networking for optimum efficiency of resource management and profitability.

## Management Incentives Under DRG and PPS Programs

Hospital prospective payment presently comes in two forms. One system is fixed payment per Diagnosis Related Group (DRG) as payment for the care of the hospitalized patient, such as in the Medicare system. The second is a cost and income ceiling on the aggregate annual cost and income of the hospital, as in Massachusetts Chapter 372. All states in the U.S. either have or will have a PPS program similar to one of these systems. Most countries, other than the U.S., either have or are looking toward very similar systems.

The Massachusetts Chapter 372 places a ceiling on maximum allowable cost and, also, on aggregate income allowed from hospital operations. As in PPS, increases are allowed each year, based on certain inflation factors. There are also allowances for increased volume, but actually the incentives are greater for a hospital to decrease rather than increase volume.

The following are some of the more obvious management incentives for hospitals under both PPS systems. These points will generally apply to either the DRG program or the cost–income ceiling. The initiatives required by a hospital may be slightly different but the end result will be the same.

1. *Minimum Acceptable Care.* Except for conscience, criminal law, or regulatory authority, hospital managers could encourage physicians and other staff to give only minimal care to patients.

2. *Internal Price Shifting.* Since there are no controls on pricing, hospitals could inflate the price of treatments or services where there is little or no competition or, in the case of a DRG system, raise the price to the maximum allowable payment. The same price inflation could be practiced where the hospital, by policy, does not want to encourage a particular type of patient admission.

Conversely, hospitals could encourage patient admissions by underpricing certain types of treatments or services. Additionally, a hospital under PPS could manage prices to encourage admissions of certain patients that will tend to bring in other business of a more profitable nature.

3. *Internal and External Cost Shifting.* A hospital could take advantage of allowable volume increases, shifting as much of the cost as possible to those growth areas. There is a new form of external cost shifting emerging now in Massachusetts. External cost shifting was to have ended with income–cost controlled prospective payment for all payors under a Medicare waiver for Massachusetts. Because of per diem averaging, it is still possible for third–party payors to cost shift by using private utilization review programs to shorten the length of stay.

Not as much money is saved for the total health care system by cutting off the last day of hospitalization as some people think. At the Massachusetts Eye and Ear Infirmary, the last day cost of semi–private hospitalization is only about 20 percent of the average per diem all–inclusive cost, or roughly 43 percent of the average routine daily service cost excluding all ancillaries. The last day cost is 5 percent of the average per case cost. Cutting off the last day actually saves approximately 20 percent of a hospital's average daily cost. A single payor, however, could save 100 percent of the average per diem charges. The 80 percent would be shifted to other payors when the average daily cost is recalculated. This is a result of the per diem averaging method of cost identification which the PPS programs still recognize.

4. *PPS Recognizes Traditional Cost Identification.* Per diem averaging of the cost of all expenses, regardless of the effort expended on the specific treatment, is like a business averaging the costs of its entire product line. For example, the health care system's practice of per diem averaging is comparable to a shoe manufacturer costing and pricing all styles of shoes the same and selling all products at the average price. DRG's on the other hand, have only changed *total* product line averaging to *partial* pro-

duct line averaging. DRG's have *changed* costing methods but have *not improved* them. The PPS, using DRG's, is diagnostic related—not cost related.

In terms of a non-health care business, DRG costing and pricing is like taking a few related products and averaging the cost of that partial product line. It would be like averaging the price of all women's shoes, regardless of the style or production effort that went into the individual shoes in that production group. Based on this thinking, there would be a different average price per shoe for all men's shoes and children's shoes as well.

The continuation of this industry-wide practice of total or partial product line averaging of the PPS will give hospitals which identify definitive product costs an opportunity to engage in marketing practices not available to hospitals in the past. Hospitals simply *must* adopt definitive product cost identification, budgeting, and management techniques by definitive product cost identification. This means the costing of specific diagnosis by day of hospitalization.

Definitive product management is a well-established practice in health care, though it may not have been recognized by that label. For instance, a decision by a for-profit chain of hospitals not to move into a geographical area heavily populated by the poor and underprivileged is definitive product management (DPM).

Another example of DPM is a decision by an HMO to operate its own hospital for the treatment of less severe patients. That practice, in today's per diem averaging mode, will leave the more complicated and expensive cases to the care of other hospitals. Woe be to the manager of an independent hospital affiliated with an HMO who doesn't understand that in these days of prospective payments, still coupled with per diem averaging, the profitability of the independent hospital would suffer. Once DPM is understood, the possibilities are endless.

Still another example of DPM would be a decision by a hospital to operate its own preferred provider organization exclusively for its employees, with catastrophic coverage by a third party. Product management has been possible in the past for selected hospitals and provider organizations. With PPS and DPM there is an opportunity for all to now manage by product costing and marketing.

5. *Marketing by Controlling the Medical Staff.* Hospitals have as much right as other businesses to choose their product lines in order to avoid unprofitable products. Using this theory, a hospital could control, to a certain extent, the diagnoses it wishes to encourage or discourage by accepting or denying medical staff privileges, or by limiting admissions by diagnoses or by physician.

There is a way to build an equitable and cost-effective PPS. This author recommends a system more relative to definitive product costing. Even *cost related groups* would be better than diagnosis related groups and, in this computer age, identifying cost by diagnosis by day of hospital-ization is easy to accomplish.

It is believed that in the future there will be costing by diagnosis by day as a component of the PPS. There will be a gradual adjustment of DRG's to more closely reflect individual diagnostic costs and come closer and closer to CRG's—cost related groups.

One will probably go on calling them DRG's because that seems to be the way the health care industry relates to hospital statistics. For example, for centuries nursing care has been called "room and board." In 1966, the combined services of nursing and room and board was changed to "rou-tine daily services" and it has been called that ever since. Modern nursing care is not just routine daily services but it continues to be called by that misnomer. So, one is probably stuck with DRG's whether or not they reflect a diagnosis related group or a cost related group.

### An Integrative Management System

Hospitals need to establish an integrative management response by set-ting up a *networking system* of two or more hospitals for *definitive cost identification, productivity management, and resource utilization controls.* It is imperative that hospitals look at the real cost of each of their products.

The health care management team must get the correct mind set because there are some hospital managers who believe that costing by DRG's is cost identification by product. It should be made clear that neither DRG cost identification, nor per diem cost identification, gives adequate tools for management. Currently, when hospital cost accoun-tants average routine daily cost they include nursing and other cost cen-ters unrelated to providing relatively similar services to each patient each day—regardless of the diagnosis. This system is not definitive enough for accurate product costing. Examples of similar services for all cases that *can* be averaged per diem are the room cost, the cost of linen and laundry, and routine food service—almost nothing else. If the state of federal governments mandate that an institution be paid on a per diem calcula-tion, a DRG, or whatever, little can be done. However, an individual hospital needs to know its true cost in order to survive.

Identification of unit cost can be obtained through the following formula:

Cost by day for each diagnosis, subdiagnosis or, common mul-tiple diagnoses

equals

Cost of medical records, cashier, admitting, scheduling, and other areas that should be included one time on the day of admission

plus

Cost of average daily room and board for each day of stay

plus

Cost of average daily routine medications and dressings for each day of stay

plus

Cost of nursing and physician care by relative value units for that diagnosis for each day of stay

plus

Cost of non–routine drugs, equipment, and services on the day they are given

plus

Cost of operating room, anesthesia, radiology, laboratory services, and other diagnostic or therapeutic services on the day each is given

plus

Direct and indirect overhead as apportioned through each cost center above

The total cost for that diagnosis then is the sum of each day's cost. Once the cost by diagnosis by day is established it is possible to average the cost of each diagnosis by day. That is, for example, the average cost on the day of admission, the second day, the third day, and so on for a patient with carcinoma of the larynx with radical neck dissection. The total of these days will become the average cost for a patient with a certain diagnosis. A hospital should do this for all its diagnoses, whether it's an appendectomy, a leg fracture, or whatever.

In order to practice productivity management, the ancillary services and other cost centers must be costed by their own individual product so that they reflect their true costs—*not price but true cost*. It is not important that a hospital have routine chest X–rays or a CT scan overpriced and a barium swallow underpriced; the *cost* is the *important* element when making internal management decisions. A system must be established to measure productivity by product.

There are even some national, full–scale management information systems which refer only to prices charged by hospitals! And even they often refer to per diem average charges.

Finally, a system to measure resource utilization is needed to control the use of resources. It is no use under PPS to have the most efficient ancillary departments in the world if the utilization of ancillaries or other services for each diagnosis is excessive, or unexplainably out of the ordinary mode of treatment.

A recent *Wall Street Journal* article [January 18, 1984], quotes Alex McMahon, President of the American Hospital Association, "we all know there has been extra testing going on because under cost reimbursement, the idea was if you can do it, do it." John Koury, Jr., Chairman of the American Medical Association, is quoted in that same article, "most physicians feel that the ratchet will be turned so tight that quality of care will suffer."

To this author's knowledge, there does not as yet exist a system which supplies resource utilization data in any useful way. The reason one cannot compare is that no uniform system of definitive product cost identification exists. A system that has more than 10 to 12 percent of inpatient cost expressed in terms of patient days is nearing invalidity.

One needs to concentrate on developing networks of hospitals for the sole purpose of truly identifying cost, for measuring productivity, and controlling resource utilization. Two or more hospitals can form a network. However, the more hospitals comprising a network, the more precise the comparative statistics.

In order to have an effective network, the following management systems will be necessary.

1. An accurate product related and unit related cost identification and data management system is needed. There are two kinds of product costing. One is by diagnosis by day, which is a daily total of each treatment, modality, or clinical relative value unit. The other is unit related. By unit is meant the actual cost of the individual products in a hospital department or service, such as the cost of each different lab test or each different radiological exam. Another example of a unit cost would be the cost of a nursing clinical care unit or some other relative value unit for nursing or other clinical department. In other words, one needs to know the true cost of the shoe laces, the leather, the beads, buttons and bows, as well as the labor hours.

2. A system should be established for measuring unit outputs by diagnosis, subdiagnosis, and common multidiagnoses cases by day. The sum of the cost of the buttons and bows, labor, shoe laces, and all the other products that go into a specific style shoe will be the cost of that product—exactly like the cost for a specific diagnosis. The sum cost of the ingredients, plus labor and overhead, will be the cost of a case by diagnosis.

3. A system should be implemented for monitoring resource utilization by physician, clinical units, and hospital. As the *Wall Street Journal* article, quoted earlier stated, one needs to know if production products are being wasted and, if so, by whom.

4. A system to measure productivity is needed. Are there efficient operating rooms, anesthesia departments, laboratories, nursing services, and housekeeping departments? After there is definitive product related costing, one can then measure efficiency.

5. Standardized methodology among hospitals can aid in comparing productivity. Without a standardized methodology and a way to measure utilization and efficiencies among hospitals and units of hospitals, they

simply will not know whether the hospital is productive or not. That is why there is a need for networking.

6. A system for data sharing is needed. There has been a reluctance by hospitals to share data; especially within the same market area. Networks can be organized in such a way that data sharing need not be either burdensome or run afoul of antitrust laws—networking can occur among hospitals in widely separated market areas. A multihospital system obviously has a very effective network already. For-profit hospital chains have a network. Another network could be a state association or council of affiliated hospitals. Individual hospitals and multihospital systems, alike, may wish to network along other lines.

Any group of hospitals can form a network anywhere, of any size. In order for networks to be effective, however, they must follow the management systems just outlined: an accurate product related production unit, relative cost identification, and data management system; a system for measuring outputs by diagnosis by day; a system for monitoring and controlling resource utilization by physician, clinical unit, and hospital; a system to measure productivity; standardized methodologies; and a network for data sharing.

## Conclusion

There will be a prospective payment system of one form or another for the foreseeable future. Presently, the existing cost identification systems are inaccurate and are not likely to change very rapidly. Individual hospitals and multihospital systems alike, however, have an excellent opportunity to manage effectively by identifying the true cost of their products and by networking, or organizing in such a way as to engage in productivity measurements and resource utilization control.

# Part Six

**Management Systems**

# Chapter Eighteen

## A Method for Analysis of Health Care Delivery Systems

### RONALD E. BELLER

## Introduction

The divergent ways that the label health care delivery system is used make it difficult to find definitions or analytical models which aid significantly in the understanding of these complex systems. Yet health care is a topic of uppermost concern in most societies. Each year, increasing amounts of nations' resources are committed to facilities, to the education of care providers, and to assist in payment for health care services, reflecting the high priority given human health. Coincident with this concern has been the development of the attitude that access to health services is an inescapable result of progress and irrefutable right.

Anxiety grows about the limited availability of primary care, about the lack of emphasis on the promotion of health and prevention of disease and injury, about the growing array of organizational forms emerging for the delivery of care, about new concepts of third party payment for care, and about the impact of technology on care and support services. When these issues are juxtaposed to the inadequate notions of the systems that are supposed to deliver health care, one finds a disconcerting lack of focus and rigor in the analysis of such systems, and, not surprisingly, uncoordinated and contradictory efforts at changing them.

This paper will attempt to advance the understanding of health care systems and the ability to cope with them in the real world. Not all of the many health issues or the full complexity of delivery systems could be incorporated in this effort. What is here, hopefully, is a beginning which can support continuing efforts in the future.

## General Systems

Before considering health care delivery systems, it is necessary to review optional systems' concepts, ways of thinking about systems, and models of systems. The general categories to be described are representative of those presented in the literature. The combined thrust of the categories defines a span of concepts and models from broad to relatively narrow notions of the nature of systems.

All of the examples assume that the analyst is dealing with open systems. Open systems, health care delivery systems being a particular type,

191

interact or exchange energy with their environments. These systems seek to achieve a steady state through dynamic exchange with the nonsystem portion of the defined operating milieu.

A reasonable understanding of the properties of open systems adds to the appreciation of the complexity of health care delivery and of the difficulty of describing its multivariate nature. Models for analysis of health care must necessarily include elements from the full range of categories of systems that will be reviewed, if they are to have sufficient power in analysis and description.

### Behavioral Approaches

The behavioral approach to the nature of systems provides relatively broad systems concepts and models. This approach is concerned with the general properties of social systems, and in viewing and describing such systems, the analyst addresses social interaction, patterns of relationships which can be characterized as to their qualitative and quantitative nature. Loomis states [1960, p. 1] that the frame of reference of sociology is:

> ". . . *interaction,* characterized by patterned *social relations* that display in their uniformities social *elements,* articulated by social *processes,* the dynamics of which account for the emergence, maintenance, and change of *social systems.*"

Whatever the system or its relative complexity [Loomis, 1960, p. 5] *"the elements that constitute it as a social system and the processes that articulate it remain the same."*

Loomis also provides a useful means of differentiating social systems in terms of their *gemeinschaft* as opposed to *gesellschaft* qualities. The addition of this qualitative dimension to the elements and processes of the model aids greatly the analysis and understanding of on-going social systems. Further, in discussing conditions of social action, Loomis mentions territoriality, time, and size of the social system as being both system and environment and having significant impact on the system and its features.

Loomis' model contributes to an understanding of complex social systems via his proposition that their structures are definable in terms of a limited number of elements, and his designation of elemental and master processes which not only further define structure, but describe the type and nature of elemental interplay. Though the Loomis model parallels those presented below as input-output models, it is broader in the range of systems thinking and analysis it supports. The inclusion of territory and time in Loomis' model also provides linkage to the holistic approaches to systems.

### Holistic Approaches

Proponents of holistic approaches downplay the importance of relationships in portrayal of systems and seek what they believe are more encompassing and meaningful connections of members of wholes. As Angyal states [1941, p. 247]:

> "The term 'system,' as used in this discussion, is . . . at variance with the common usage . . . the type of connexions in a whole is very different from (those) which exist in an aggregate. The term 'system' is used here to denote a *holistic system.*"

The components or objects of a system, according to Angyal, do not participate solely through relationships, but more generally through their spatial arrangement in what he calls dimensional domains such as space and time. Holistic approaches such as Angyal's allow space and time to become determinants of the system itself. Structure and process, as they exist in relationships, take on unique systems meaning through their spatial arrangement in a dimensional domain.

Holistic approaches move system definition beyond the common relations-based versions; input-output models, though useful in some contexts, provide little insight in others. Holistic approaches enrich the understanding of health care delivery systems by making it possible to include important aspects of health care frequently omitted from analyses, such as health education and environmental health, for which current relationships to curative health services are either sketchy or non-existent.

*Input-Output Approaches*

Another approach to systems moves to the endpoint of systems thinking to the generation of tight, relational models. These models simplify human behavior and system performance to deterministic states and take the form of open input-output systems as portrayed in Figure I.[1] Each system is [Churchman, 1968, p. 11] "made up of sets of components that work together for the overall objective of the whole." A more mechanistic concept of systems is used by Optner in describing three basic types: machine-like, man-dominated, and man-machine systems. Any of these types of systems can be networks of input-output processes of greater or lesser complexity [Optner, 1960, pp. 3-15].

Feedback is defined as system output returned as input for the purpose of controlling or correcting the system's performance relative to its environment. Hare [1967, pp. 111-13, 125-29] discusses simple feedback and higher order feedback loops featuring memory, learning, and goal changing as depicted in Figure I. Extension of the simple input-output model to the higher order forms defines open systems which can resist entropic decay.

Input-output models of health care systems have obvious value where relationships can be specified and usefully described in input-output terms. The ability to create networks through linkage of input-output subsystems and to perceive higher order system properties strengthens analysis of increasingly complex health care delivery systems.

---

[1] In addition to the basic input-output model, the figure incorporates feedback loops discussed a bit further in the text.

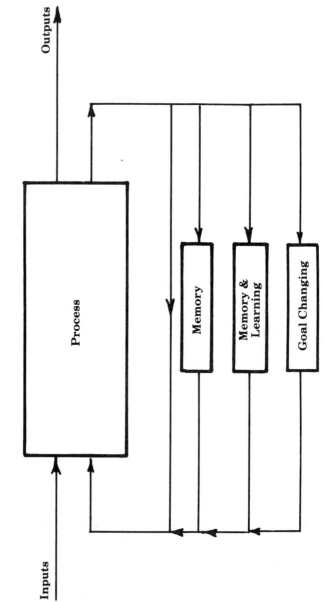

Figure I
Open Input/Output System With First, Second, Third and Fourth Degree Feedback Loops

*Bridging Approaches*

There are approaches to systems which combine two or more of the features of the behavioral, holistic, and input-output approaches. In doing so, bridging approaches show that the various ways of thinking about systems can be combined to form enhanced models for particular use.

Katz and Kahn link concepts from all of the other approaches. They point to the primacy of input-output relationships and structure in systems theory, but they also state that structure can be observed in physical arrangements. In addition, they argue that structure is to be found in cyclic, interrelated events, that it [Katz and Kahn, 1966, p. 21] "is events rather than things which are structured." These authors also discuss the effects of entropy on systems and the need for its control if systems are to persist by reaching and maintaining a steady state in dynamic exchange with their environments [pp. 21-4].

Tichy reports on the application of a diagnostic model to a chain of non-profit hospital and primary care clinics. His model includes as components: mission, strategy, and objectives; sociotechnical arrangements; organizational processes; people; and emergent networks. Since system performance relates to the nature of these components and their interrelationships, diagnosis of functioning systems must encompass both [Tichy, 1978, pp. 306-07]. Tichy's use of his model in a case study shows strong ties to the behavioral and input-output approaches, but his components provide a means of characterizing mission, elements, structure, and processes not found in preceding models.

*Systems Thinking*

The specific approaches to systems each embody what has been termed systems thinking. Whether it is social interaction, holism, or patterns of relationships, each approach gives clear evidence of looking at phenomena in different ways yielding a variety of portrayals of essentially the same objects of study.

In a more fundamental sense, there is a form of thinking which yields systems rather than some other concept of phenomena. Such thinking moves the analyst from relatively unstructured descriptions of observations, to the delineation of specific systems models [Beller and White, 1972, pp. 855-61]. The variety of systems thinking in the various approaches increases the possibility of finding concepts of systems which might provide special ways of looking at and connecting the phenomena being studied.

## Health Care Systems

Analysis of health care delivery systems would be aided measurably if a commonly used, analytically useful definition of health could be elicited from the literature. Several authors mention the Preamble to the Constitution of the World Health Organization (WHO):

"Health means more than freedom from disease, freedom from pain, freedom
from untimely death. It means optimum physical, mental, and social efficiency
and well-being."

Klarman, upon noting this definition, states that it [1965, p. 3] "is probably too broad to furnish guidance regarding a society's real aims in the
health field and too vague for the purpose of evaluating existing programs." Callahan [1977, pp. 2-6] finds the WHO definition to be danger-
ous, needing to be supplanted by something less ambitious: "its emphasis
on 'complete physical, mental, and social well-being' puts both medicine
and society in the untenable position of being required to attain unattai-
nable goals." Though the terms health and medical care are used in tan-
dem throughout Klarman's treatise, the data used are drawn predomi-
nantly from medical care.

Many modern societies seem increasingly preoccupied with health, yet
it has been observed that illness is the prevalent human state [Zola, 1966,
pp. 615-16]. Wildavsky, in noting the popular practice of equating health
and medical care talks about goal displacement. Since one cannot find
useful definitions of health and, therefore, cannot set goals and measure
progress, one can shift to something for which goals can be set. He notes
[1977, p. 106]: ". . . In this case 'health' has become equivalent to 'equal
access to medicine'."

On the other hand, most of what is measured in human health in morbidity and mortality statistics is beyond the reach of medical care, being
primarily influenced by individuals' personal habits and their physical
environment [Knowles, 1977, p. 58; Duval, 1977, p. 185]. These observations lead to the advocacy of health education, preventive medicine,
environmental quality, and other non-curative approaches.

If studies show that clinically-defined illness is a fairly prevalent state,
then health and illness as commonly used may be nearly equiprobable
states of being in humans. As such, a minimum entropic decay of health,
as an organized condition, yields illness. Should this premise be accurate,
a society's preoccupation with curative medicine need not involve goal
displacement or typify misplaced emphasis. Rather, regular seeking of
care can be seen as a rational effort to return to health, the steady state
humans perceive to be the way they want to be "organized" as biological
organisms.

Illness, real or imagined, and attempts to "return to health," needed or
not, prompt the delivery of medical care services and, hence, curative services are of utmost importance in analyzing any health care delivery system. At present, growing out of historical emphasis, curative medical care
dominates health care delivery.

In spite of past absence, the impact of patterns of individual behavior
and environmental quality on perceptions of health is growing. Health
education, preventive medicine, environmental health, and expanded
primary care services would be more apparent in current health care sys-

tems, if in the past they had been perceived as more important in attaining the "healthy" state of being. The model proposed in this paper includes both the curative aspects of health care and the services required to influence individual behavior, to improve environmental quality, and to redistribute physician efforts in the direction of primary care.

## Health Care Delivery Systems

Following the lines of the preceding discussion leads to a necessary definition:

> Health care delivery systems provide curative services to a segment of the population demanding them and other services which seek to adjust individual behavior and to enhance the physical environment through modification of factors that are believed to promote health.

To be useful in analysis of ongoing systems, methods are required which delimit the population to which the definition is applied and which structure the myriad services implied in the definition.

### Zone of Interest

To delineate the boundaries of populations to be served by one or more health care delivery systems requires that manageable geographic areas be identified. To accomplish this, the analyst needs to be able to create a *zone of interest*, a geographic territory whose borders are set in some systematic way.

Several nations have adopted regional approaches to the development of health service policy, facilities, and service programs [Bjorkman and Schulz, 1981, pp. 205-20]. In the United States, the regionalization fostered by P.L.93-641 follows political boundaries, especially state borders resulting from the constitutional delegation of responsibility for peoples' health to the states. Unfortunately, political boundaries are frequently poor delineators of meaningful health care zones.

The geographic distribution of health care services provides the basis for a holistic definition of delivery systems. Using the proper analytical tools, meaningful geographic arrangements of health care services can be articulated. In a subsequent section of this paper, levels of curative care services will be used to define zones of interest for health care delivery.

### System Operators

Once the analysis of health care systems moves beyond the determination of the zone of interest, sets of activities are confronted which must be considered in terms of the behavioral and input-output approaches. What, for example, are the system or subsystem goals, resources, processes, products, and how are they interrelated?

To answer these questions requires that a point of view be identified. Whose goals? Whose processes? Whose services? *It has to be those pro-*

*vided by the system operators.* Goals or purposes are not inherent in a health care system or subsystem. Outputs and the way they are created and modified through time are not happenstance. System operators determine them.

The point may seem trivial, but is quite to the contrary. The analyst would be adrift without the reference point provided by the system operators, those hypothesized to be controlling key variables such that they are "operating" the system under review. In this analytical model, system operators will be explicitly noted, and where optional operators need be considered, they will be listed. The significance of each system operator to the analysis which follows must also be provided.

### System and Environment

One of the more important decisions in analysis of systems is determination of what is system and what is environment. The drawing of geographic boundaries in setting zones of interest can be done through trial and error until a useful zone is created. Defining care systems and subsystems within the zone of interest poses a problem of greater difficulty. These systems can be defined when the operators and their purposes are known.

System variables will be defined as those whose values are controlled by the system's operators; environmental variables will be viewed as not under operator control, but whose values determine outcomes in conjuction with the system's outputs. Control of variables by operators will be expressed in terms of the probability of setting variables' values in response to operator actions, lack of control being defined as the failure to reach the established, minimum probability criterion. Variables which are neither under operator control nor interact with the system to yield outcomes are extraneous to the analysis.

To obtain a formulation of a health care delivery system amenable to analysis requires, not only the specification of zone of interest, but also of the important care subsystems included within that zone. These subsystems emerge from a process of successive approximation utilizing the operator-centered classification of variables that has been described. To do so is a demanding task involving the consideration of hundreds of variables. Although the full process cannot be described in this paper, various features of the method are provided in sections which follow. Variables which were considered in developing the primary care subsystem are included in condensed outline form in Table 1.

### Health Care Delivery System Models

The matters considered in the preceding sections can be integrated into a model for analyzing health care delivery systems. Development of the model can be clarified through its application to real world situations in this and the next section of the paper. Once again, only partial detail can

**TABLE 1**

**Classification of Variables For a Primary Care Subsystem**

   I. System Operators
     A. Physicians
     B. Other Care Providers
     C. Professional Managers
     D. Governments
  II. Operator Variables
     A. Service Variables
       1. Care production functions
     B. Subsystem Management Variables
       1. Financial and administrative
       2. Communication and data management
       3. Patient routing and scheduling
     C. Provider Role Setting
 III. Environmental Variables
     A. Governmental Programs and Regulations
     B. Reimbursement Policies and Procedures
     C. Professional Licensure Practices
     D. Professional Ethical Standards

be examined as various phases of the model are presented.

*Zone of Interest*

In this model, the geographic zone of interest will be determined by the pattern of distribution of curative services. There are commonly recognized three levels of care: primary, secondary, and tertiary. The definitions of each and the relationship of the levels, one to the other, is shown in Figure II.

Primary care is shown as nearest to the patient and his or her family, while tertiary care, on the other hand, envelops the other care levels. Such is the case when one examines the geographic arrangement of the levels of care. Primary care is provided to small populations in relatively limited geographic areas. Tertiary care is provided to large populations spread over the broadest geographic territory of all the levels. The secondary care zone generally envelops the primary zone, but is a smaller area than that for tertiary care. The care level distinctions blend into one another at their edges, but the conceptual separation is useful to the purposes of this model.

The three care levels can be seen in concept as relating geographically to one another, as portrayed in Figure III. Two tertiary care zones are shown, as are several secondary and primary care zones. The tertiary

Figure II
HEALTH CARE DELIVERY SYSTEM—LEVELS OF CARE

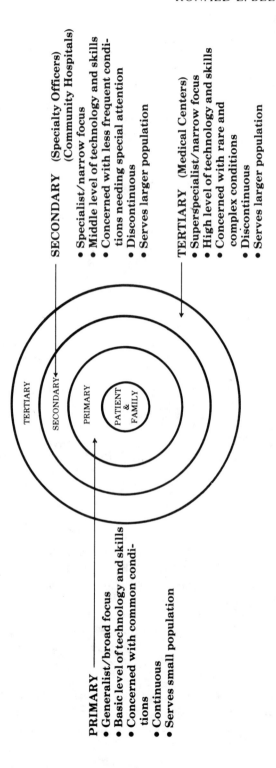

SECONDARY  (Specialty Officers)
              (Community Hospitals)
• Specialist/narrow focus
• Middle level of technology and skills
• Concerned with less frequent condi-
  tions needing special attention
• Discontinuous
• Serves larger population

TERTIARY  (Medical Centers)
• Superspecialist/narrow focus
• High level of technology and skills
• Concerned with rare and
  complex conditions
• Discontinuous
• Serves larger population

PRIMARY
• Generalist/broad focus
• Basic level of technology and skills
• Concerned with common condi-
  tions
• Continuous
• Serves small population

zones are essentially the trade areas of comprehensive medical centers; the secondary zones being the trade areas of community hospitals. The primary zones envelop the several practices of primary care physicians centered on communities located in the territory. For the sake of brevity, not all of primary or secondary care zones are defined in Figure III.

When this type of analysis is extended to the actual geographic area of the United States shown in Figure IV, portions of Tennessee, Virginia and North Carolina, the secondary and tertiary care zones that result are portrayed in Figure V. The primary care zones are assumed to coincide roughly with their respective secondary zones in this diagram.

There is another tertiary care zone centered on Raleigh-Durham, North Carolina, and primary and secondary care zones around all of the communities in the total territory. They are not shown in Figure V, as they do not add materially to this particular analysis. The trade areas for all levels of care zones can be derived from zip code data from patient records. The area's actual shapes will not take the regular form used in the examples.

*Primary Care Subsystems*

Primary care is found closest to the consumer largely because of the type of services delivered and the frequency of need for them. As Rogers indicates [1977, p. 82]:

> "The term 'primary care' is usually used to describe the range of care traditionally rendered by physicians in community practice. It is the point of first contact for an individual with a physician, . . . . But primary care is more than the medical care of individuals; primary care practitioners also have responsibilities for groups of people, usually in a defined geographic area. Finally, its interests are comprehensive: primary care . . . is concerned with the psychological and social as well as the physical aspects of illness . . . . But, however constituted, it is the point of entry into the health system and of continuing contact with it. Its patients are usually ambulatory and able to function at home, although it utilizes . . . some hospital services."

Another definition, paralleling Roger's, is used in primary care planning. Such care [ARCHA, 1980, p. 108]:

> ". . . provides continuous and immediate care not requiring a specialty service, with triage, coordination and referral to secondary and tertiary sources."

Based upon this notion of primary care, the subsystem for its delivery and its connection to the secondary and tertiary care subsystems are shown in input-output format in Figure VI. In addition to the basic input-output flow, feedback loops are indicated between all components of the model which are assumed to possess higher order capability.

The directed arrows in Figure VI are meant to represent patient and data flow; personal services and other resources represented by dollars do not flow between, but directly to the several components of the system. These resource inputs are not shown in order to limit the complexity of an already complicated diagram.

The transformation of inputs to outputs in all levels of care takes place within the components of the subsystems and the yield is either final pro-

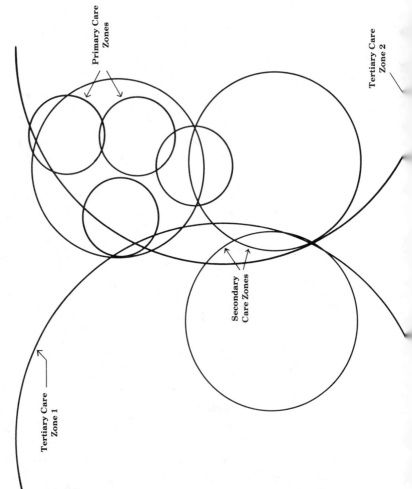

Figure III
Conceptual Zone of Interest Defined by Level of Care Zones

Figure IV
Zone of Interest in United States

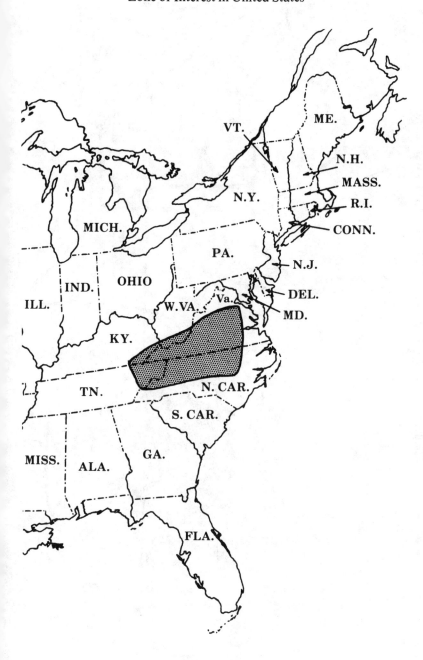

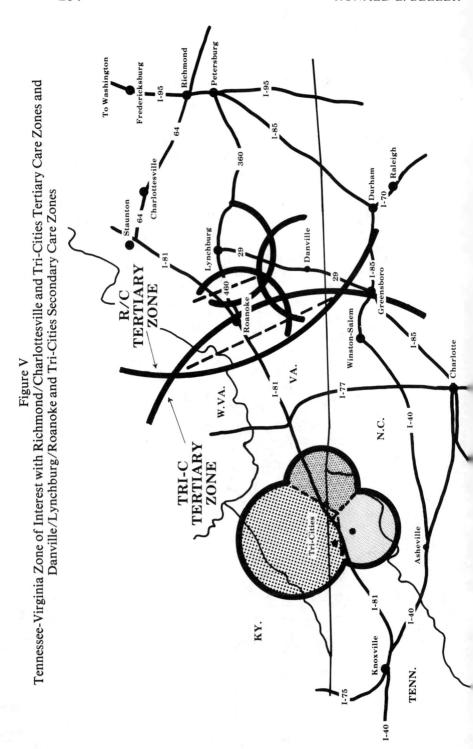

Figure V

Tennessee-Virginia Zone of Interest with Richmond/Charlottesville and Tri-Cities Tertiary Care Zones and
Danville/Lynchburg/Roanoke and Tri-Cities Secondary Care Zones

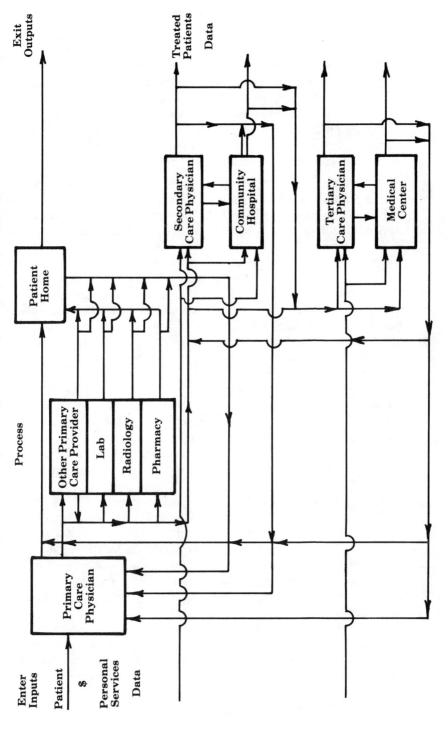

Health Care Delivery Primary, Secondary and Tertiary Care Subsystems

ducts to the environment or intermediate products to other subsystems within the total delivery system. The nature of these transformations is presented in subsequent sections of the paper.

*Secondary and Tertiary Care*

Secondary and tertiary care represent designations along a continuum of science-based, hospital-focused care provided by medical specialists and other health professionals, paraprofessionals, and other staff. These levels of care deal with illness and injury of sufficient degree to require hospitalization up to and including those conditions which require the ultimate diagnostic and therapeutic capabilities of personnel and facilities.

*Subsystem Production Processes*

The general resource transformation processes used in all levels of care can be displayed, as in Figure VII. Although this model was developed specifically for application to secondary care, its general features are descriptive of primary and tertiary care as well [Beller, 1971, pp. 90-137].

This model of the production processes of health care is strongly related to the models proposed by Fetter and his colleagues, which form the basis for reimbursement of care in terms of diagnosis related groups (DRG's) [Fetter, *et al*, 1980, pp. 5-14]. The model in Figure VII shows care as consisting of essential medical services and supplemental care, each divided into stages of the provision of particular services. In addition to these fairly self-evident categories, the patient is shown as an integral participant in his or her own care.

In these approaches, econometric modeling of hospital and non-hospital production functions permits the inclusion of all variables of significance to the particular levels of care. It is possible to structure these models so that optimization of some objective function, such as cost minimization, can be sought subject to constraints that can, through direct and proxy variables, set upper and/or lower quantity and quality standards.

Various behavioral assumptions can be incorporated into the analysis of the inner workings of the levels of care and of the relationships between levels using the models offered by Loomis, Tichy, and Katz and Kahn. When the three levels of care are contrasted using Loomis' elements and processes, a case can be made that the care levels are distinct subsystems along the *gemeinschaft-gesellschaft* continuum, such that their integration into a total delivery system poses major problems of "system-linkage" [Hardy, 1982, p. 38].

Close examination of the provision of primary care in solo-physicians' practices and in HMO's yields evidence of erosion of the strong *gemeinschaft* characteristics of the former mode of delivery. The implications of this, in terms of patient acceptance and system integration, are not clear.

*Non-Curative Health Care*

The model to this point has emphasized curative care, although primary

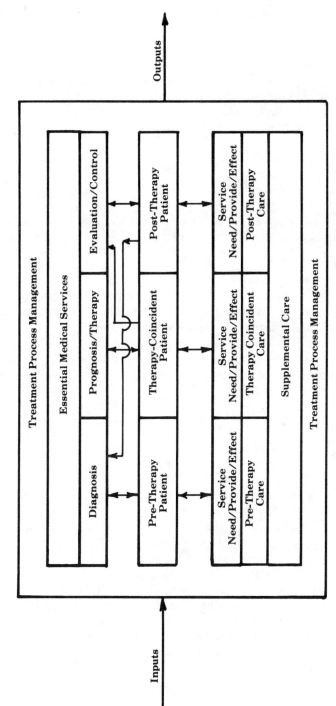

Figure VII
Primary, Secondary and Tertiary Care Production Processes

care includes non-curative services. This results, to a great extent, from the curative emphasis of ongoing health care systems.

Governmental efforts to improve physical environment are underway in several nations. Whether these efforts in environmental health will be of consequence equal to those of the late nineteenth century on the general health of broad populations remains to be seen. If such results occur, they will become apparent in the morbidity and mortality statistics of the populations in zones of interest and, as such, will be environmental variables in health care delivery systems.

Health education aimed at changing individual life-styles and health habits can be incorporated in the model through inclusion of subsystems which deliver these services. To some extent, changes in medical education curricula and the growing emphasis on primary care and family medicine will lead to increasing emphasis on this non-curative service within the primary care subsystem.

### Maternal and Infant Care Delivery

The health care delivery system model that has been developed can be applied to a specific type of health care in a geographic region, in this case, maternal and infant care in northeast Tennessee and southwest Virginia. This area coincides with major portions of Tennessee District 1 and Virginia District III Health Service Agencies' (HSA) geographic areas. Much of the information used to determine the zone of interest and the services provided within it are derived from the Tennessee District 1 health services planning documents [ARCHA, 1980, pp. 142-54; ARCHA, 1981, pp. 11-2].

*Zone of Interest*

The delineation of the zone of interest for maternal and infant care in the subject region depends on the definition of the relevant tertiary care zone. Tertiary care services for the mother can be provided in most modern comprehensive community hospitals. The services that distinguish a center as being truly tertiary in maternal and infant care are those that relate to the infant from fetus to neonate. Thus, in this case, the tertiary care zones are drawn with respect to the so-called Level III services available for infants from prenatal through neonatal stages.

One of these tertiary zones is centered on Tri-Cities; a second on Knoxville, about 110 miles to the west; and a third on Lynchburg/Roanoke, approximately 170 miles to the east. The resultant zone for Tri-Cities is shown in Figure VIII. The secondary care zone for Tri-Cities, shown as the shaded area in Figure IX, reflects the service coverage of the region's several community hospitals. These hospitals provide a full range of secondary maternal and infant care and include three Level II neonatal care units.

Genetics counseling, relative to mother and infant, is offered throughout the Tri-Cities secondary care zone and much of the tertiary zone. The

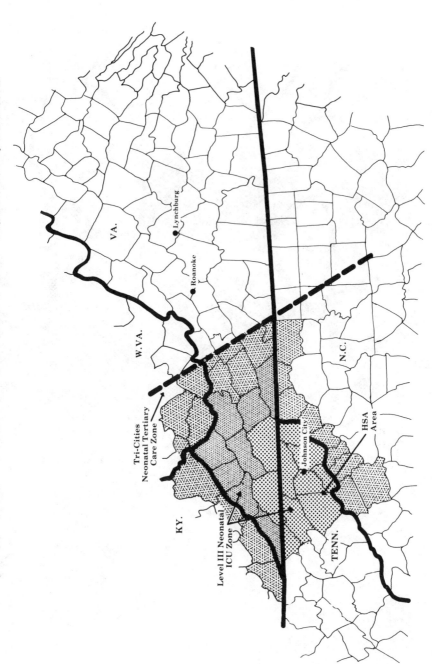

Tri-Cities Maternal and Infant Care Zone of Interest With Secondary and Tertiary Care Zones

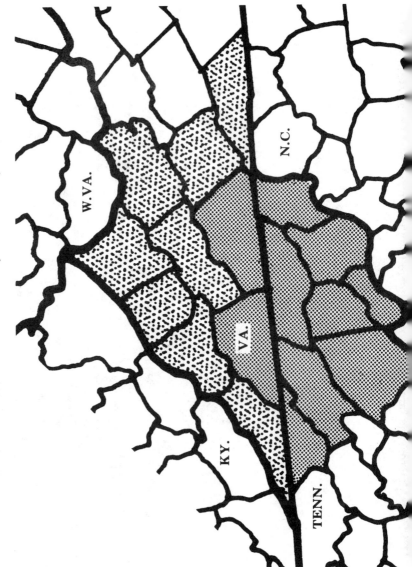

Figure IX
Tri-Cities Maternal and Infant Primary and Secondary Care Zones

nearest alternative centers for genetics counseling are found in Knoxville and Roanoke.

Primary care, in the form of prenatal services, is provided currently within the HSA district by 182 physicians. These practitioners are distributed unevenly, relative to female population of childbearing age, ranging from about 1:500 to 1:1450, with a mean of about 1:600.

These figures do not begin to tell the story of prenatal primary care for indigent women. Public health nurses provide the lion's share of services to these women in all counties in the HSA district. These nurses receive varying degrees of physician oversight and refer all at-risk pregnancies to physicians.

*System and Environment*

Physicians are firmly in control of the maternal and infant care delivery system in the HSA district. During the past 10 years, the nature of this control has been changing in all but a few pockets of resistance because of the establishment and development of a medical college in the Tri-Cities. Now, in addition to community physicians, there are full-time clinical faculty of the college practicing in the community hospitals, alongside medical students and house staff, and in family practice centers with approved residency training programs in each of the three cities.

Though the maternal and infant care system is operated in the main by physicians, public health nurses have a major impact in the system via their services to indigent women. For these women, primary care during pregnancy is provided by the public health nurse. In these cases, up to the point of referral to a physician for portions of prenatal care or delivery, the nurse is "operating" the system, even if with circumscribed authority.

*Operator Variables*

Major operator variables are evident in the provision of maternal and infant care services by physicians, nurses, and other personnel. These variables are either a part of the essential medical services for mother and infant or a part of their supplemental care and, as shown in Figure VII, relate to the expectant mother and fetus during the prenatal period, to the delivery of the infant, and to the mother and newborn infant following delivery. The mother, as patient from beginning to end of the process, clearly assists in all stages of her own and the infant's care.

A full range of models of maternal and infant care, from prenatal through neonatal periods, can be developed from information abstracted from medical records. Fetter and his associates identify six of their 83 mutually exclusive and exhaustive "major diagnostic categories" as relating to various aspects of care of mother and infant [Fetter, *et al,* 1980, pp. 10-1, p. 49, p. 51]. Within their six categories, they construct 16 diagnosis related groups encompassing all of the medically meaningful diagnoses encountered in maternal and infant care. One of the categories, "normal delivery," includes three diagnosis related groups, all of which utilize essentially the same production process in the delivery of care.

Such an approach enables the analyst to model the delivery of curative services. Omitted are the physician services not documented in the medical record, such as patient education, genetics counseling, and public health nursing services. Since these services are important elements of maternal and infant care in the HSA area, they must be incorporated into the overall model in the same fashion as are the curative services variables.

*Environmental Variables*

The population of the region yields a number of important environmental variables crucial to understanding the outcomes of maternal and infant care delivery. In 1980, the proportion of women of childbearing age in the regional population was the same as that in the nation. A higher percentage of women over 35 have babies than is true nationally.

Individual educational attainment for women and the average incomes of their families are below national averages, but both are experiencing relative improvement. Certain remote locations in the HSA area remain resistant to improved education and economic development, having high proportions of families below defined poverty levels. The situation is markedly better in the urbanized areas of the region where national averages for these variables are approached.

In 1976, Tennessee was identified as one of the 13 states contributing to high infant mortality levels in the United States. To deal with a serious regional problem, federal funding was obtained to operate a Towards Improving the Outcome of Pregnancy (TIOP) program. These services were provided primarily to indigent women with at-risk pregnancies, the majority of whom were teenagers. Recently, when federal TIOP funds were no longer available, the program was placed under Medicaid by the State of Tennessee.

**Conclusion**

The facets of the application of the analytical model to maternal and infant care has been presented only in the briefest fashion. Behavioral analyses, using the variety of models proposed in preceding sections, could be made of many of the activities associated with this care, such as the process of acceptance of Level III services by the community physicians and the women of the area.

There are undoubtedly many more features of on-going systems that should be considered in a full-fledged analysis. Different problems would lead to different approaches. The proposed model is believed to possess the power and flexibility necessary for analysis of health care delivery systems of varying size and complexity. Thorough testing in real-world situations will be required to properly assess the model's utility and to remedy weaknesses which are detected.

Much more needs to be done to refine the model. As was stated at the outset, what is proposed is an initial step in what is hoped to be a continuing process of model testing and adjustment.

## REFERENCES

A. Angyal, *Foundations for a Science of Personality,* New York: The Commonwealth Fund, 1941.

Applachian Regional Council for Health Advancement (ARCHA), *Health Systems Plan,* Johnson City, TN, 1980.

Ronald E. Beller, *Toward a Resource Planning Model for Community Hospitals: A Conceptual Model of the Patient Treatment System,* Ph.D. Dissertation, University of Florida, 1971.

_____ and Lowell E. White, Jr., "Long-Range Planning for a Department of Surgery. A Systems Analysis Approach," *Journal of Medical Education,* 47, November 1972.

James Bjorkman and Rockwell Schulz, "On the Implementation of Change in National Health Delivery Systems: A Model and an Application," *Journal of Health and Human Resources Administration,* 4, Fall 1981.

Daniel Callahan, "Health and Society: Some Ethical Imperatives," *Daedalus,* 106, Winter 1977.

C. West Churchman, *The Systems Approach,* New York: Dell Publishing Co., 1968.

Merlin K. Duval, "The Provider, the Government, and the Consumer," *Daedalus,* 106, Winter 1977.

Robert B. Fetter, Young Soo Shin, Jean L. Freeman, Richard F. Averill, and John D. Thompson, "Case Mix Definition by Diagnosis-Related Groups," *Medical Care,* 18, February 1980.

Clyde T. Hardy, Jr., "Healthcare Delivery in the Federal Republic of Germany," *Medical Group Management,* 29, July/August 1982.

Van Court Hare, Jr., *Systems Analysis: A Diagnostic Approach,* 2nd ed. New York: Harcourt, Brace & World, Inc., 1967.

D. Katz and R. L. Kahn, *The Social Psychology of Open Systems,* New York: John Wiley, 1966.

David Kindig, "Different Models of Delivery Care: A Panel Discussion," *The Journal of Ambulatory Care Management,* 2, February 1979.

Herbert E. Klarman, *The Economics of Health,* New York: Columbia University Press, 1965.

John H. Knowles, "The Responsibility of the Individual," *Daedalus,* 106, Winter 1977.

Charles P. Loomis, *Social Systems,* New York: D. Van Nostrand Co., Inc., 1960.

Stanford L. Optner, *Systems Analysis for Business Management,* Englewood Cliffs, N.J.: Prentice Hall, Inc., 1960.

Marc J. Roberts, "Planning and Competition in Healthcare Delivery," *Michigan Hospitals,* 17, March 1981.

David E. Rogers, "The Challenge of Primary Care," *Daedalus,* 106, Winter 1977.

Noel M. Tichy, "Diagnosis for Complex Health Care Delivery Systems: A Model and Case Study," *The Journal of Applied Behavioral Science,* 14, July/August 1978.

Aaron Wildavsky, "Doing Better and Feeling Worse: The Political Pathology of Health Policy," *Daedalus,* 106, Winter 1977.

Irving K. Zola, "Culture and Symptoms An Analysis of Patients' Presenting Complaints," *American Sociological Review,* 31, October 1966.

# Chapter Nineteen

## Case Mix Management System

### R. KENNETH McGEORGE

### Introduction

In 1959, the Canadian government enacted the Hospital Insurance and Diagnostic Services Act as its answer to the perception of the need to stabilize hospital financial operations and to prevent its citizens from financial hardship resulting from hospitalization. The basic principles of the system under the act were: universality of access and comprehensiveness of coverage.

The system was based on the federal government reimbursing provincial governments (based on a formula related to provincial costs) in the neighborhood of 50 percent of the costs incurred by the provinces in operating their provincial plans. To qualify for federal reimbursement, the provincial plans were required to meet the tests of the principles of the federal legislation and their shareable costs were outlined in a document commonly referred to by the provinces as the "red book," a document which specified the services in which the federal government would share the costs. Generally, the shareable services consisted of standard ward care and, generally, all medically-prescribed services required by inpatients. Over time, the contents of the red book expanded to include a variety of outpatient services as well.

Throughout the 1960's, hospitals in Ontario tended to fare rather well. New hospitals were constructed and most older hospitals experienced major expansion and modernization. With the lifting of the financial barrier to hospital care, the demand for services increased in geometric proportions. Throughout this period, there was not only a substantial growth in programs but there was a tremendous growth in union activity, as well. The latter growth has extended into the 1970's, with the result that in Ontario the greatest majority of hospitals now bargain with a multiplicity of unions which represent the majority of their staff.

At the Kingston General Hospital, for instance, there are four unions and nine separate contracts. Out of a total of 2,300 employees (including, for instance, interns, residents, nurses, psychologists, and social workers), only 200 are not represented by a union, these being management and designated confidential positions. The effect of this has been that salary rates for hospital workers have typically exceeded rates paid for similar staff in the United States by a considerable margin. For instance, the 1984 starting rate for a registered nurse (after completion of a 19-month training program) is $26,000 in Ontario, while in Watertown, New York, the rate is $14,000. The unions have also been generally able to negotiate very attractive but costly fringe benefit packages costing hospitals up to 23 percent of payroll.

Throughout the 1960's and 1970's, the method of reimbursing hospitals has undergone a variety of changes.

1. *Line-by-Line Budget Review:* Established in 1959, this mechanism required all hospitals to submit to the provincial government a detailed budget, listing historical and projected costs in great detail, based on the Canadian Hospital Accounting Manual. The detail required was carried to the extent of salary rates for individual staff members. These budget submissions required a large governmental bureaucracy to review the submission, comparing hospital requests with those of other similar hospitals. The government had very strict staffing guidelines which were used for assessment of submissions. The result of this process was that hospitals typically were advised by the government of their approved level of reimbursement on a line-by-line basis. The weakness of the system, as time went on, was that there was no portability between lines so that surpluses in one area could not be used to offset shortfalls in others. A hospital could, over all, end its fiscal year in good financial health, but still incur a shortfall from a reimbursement point of view.

2. *Global Budget:* In 1969, in response to pressures from hospitals and a concern for dramatically rising costs, government introduced the Global Budget System. Under this system, the base year of funding was established, then in each succeeding year government simply announced a percentage increase to the previous year's *approved funding level.* In the main, this system worked well for a few years, and it had the following characteristics: (a) An incentive for hospitals to "work smarter," since surpluses in one area could be used to offset shortfalls in other areas; and (b) Limited requirement for a large governmental staff to review budget submissions.

Moving into the latter part of the 1970's, however, trouble developed with this system. First of all, since hospitals had little, if any, influence over labor settlements, government was called upon repeatedly to make additional funding adjustments to cover labor costs in excess of the approved inflationary adjustment. There have been some serious inconsistencies in approach which have penalized hospitals. Secondly, the explosion of technology in teaching and some nonteaching referral hospitals resulted in cost escalations far in excess of annual inflationary adjustments. This has left this group of hospitals with a serious deterioration of working capital but has resulted in the government creating two new categories of extra-global reimbursement.

(A) Life Support Program Funding: which covers the incremental cost increases incurred by chemotherapy, pacemakers, renal dialysis, neonatal intensive care, and cardiac surgery.

(B) Growth Funding: additional funding is made available to certain hospitals, based on their ability to demonstrate abnormal growth in the volume of high-cost services. These funds are flowed one-year retroactively, and capped at 2 percent of total net expenses.

### Current and Projected State of Affairs

The current and projected problems with reimbursement in Ontario (and probably across Canada) are:

1. There is no organized mechanism for financing equipment replacement and acquisition of new technology.

2. The cost of high technology programs is growing at such a rate that the traditional reimbursement system cannot easily cope with it.

3. There is a perception among some larger referral hospitals that there are serious problems of distribution of funds. That is, the high-cost patients are typically referred to the referral hospitals, with the referring hospitals continuing to operate with the same access to annual budgetary adjustments (i.e., insensitivity of reimbursement to case mix and changes therein).

4. Traditional hospital accounting systems and government reporting forms do not reflect in *any way* the implications of case mix.

5. The working capital of referral hospitals has deteriorated much more rapidly and seriously than non-teaching hospitals.

6. Inter-hospital comparison of operations is impossible with existing data systems, hence, there is no way to determine which hospitals are efficient or inefficient.

7. It is apparent to hospitals that even with the known implications of the costs of new technology and the health needs of the greying population, government simply does not have sufficient resources to make more than modest annual adjustments to reimbursement levels in the future. This has been compounded by the recession, of course.

8. Based on 7, there are two major challenges posed particularly to referral and teaching hospitals:

(A) To be able to demonstrate, clearly and objectively, the *cost implications* of case mix changes.

(B) To be able to involve physicians in a much more intimate and meaningful way in the internal management processes of resource allocation, cost analysis, and cost containment.

### Case Mix Management at Kingston General Hospital

The Kingston General Hospital in Ontario, Canada, is a 508 bed teaching and referral hospital which serves as the largest teaching hospital affiliated with Queen's University Medical School. Unlike some other teaching hospitals, whose roles may tend to be more clearly focused on a few sub-specialties, this hospital serves a variety of roles, providing a comprehensiveness of services unparalleled in Ontario. Indeed, the author has not been able to find another major institution which, in addition to its roles in medical and surgical services, operates a comprehensive Mental Health Program, a Regional Rehabilitation Center, a Regional Perinatal Program, and a comprehensive Ambulatory Care Program.

The hospital, since 1978, has had tremendous problems in articulating its case to government relative to reimbursement. Fundamentally, the problem has been that there are no similar hospitals to use as a basis for comparison for reimbursement, and the hospital's management information system does not reflect its role in terms of output. In managing its affairs, the hospital utilizes the tools which have become standard in hospitals in Ontario; internal cost center budget control system, Canadian Hospital Accounting Manual, Hospital Information System, highly skilled financial and executive staff, and medical staff budget committees, to name a few.

Nonetheless, the hospital leadership claims to be underfinanced relative to its role and some physicians continue to operate with the suspicion that the hospital would be a better place if the administration would work a little smarter!

In the search for better management tools, the hospital began a process of reorganizing and, in this context, recruited financial people to key posts from the industrial sector. The industrial thinking which these executives brought to the hospital included a new sense of cost consciousness and awareness of sound principles of cost analysis. This together with a leading surgeon who had commenced graduate study in Business Administration, and a Board Chairman from the auto industry, started an entirely new environment for cost analysis. People began to ask: What are we producing? (a question seldom posed in a hospital); and, Who causes the costs to rise or fall? The traditional answers, from the hospital sector, to these questions have been: We do not produce anything, but we treat patients. Furthermore, costs are controlled by cost center managers.

In thinking this through and posing many more questions, it became apparent that the traditional approaches were inadequate. With the help of the Center for Hospital Finance and Management at Johns Hopkins University, hospital administrators came to see that there are ways of defining product lines and the new financial executives believed, based on industrial experience, that one could cost the product lines and probably the individual products.

A series of encounters were then put in place to determine if other hospitals had tried to develop a mechanism for product line definition and costing. The results indicated that:

1. U.S. hospitals typically deal with a charge system, not a cost system.
2. U.S. hospitals were now threatened with the advent of a DRG-based

reimbursement system for Medicare and Medicaid patients, and that hospitals without a *cost* system were worried.

3. No Canadian hospital had any experience in this field, except one or two which had developed new rate structures for a limited range of high technology procedures.

This resulted in the Kingston General Hospital deciding to embark upon a research and development program aimed at producing a management information system based upon case mix cost accounting. The project has a coordinating committee consisting of: Chief Executive Officer; Assistant Executive Director (Finance and Administration), serving as Project Manager; and Associate Executive Director, serving as the leader of the product definition component. The project has an advisory committee made up of persons with a demonstrated interest in the project and includes trustees, physicians, administrative staff, finance staff, and nursing representatives. There are two key physician advisors, playing key roles in product definition and quality assurance, together with other physicians representing clinical specialties assisting in the area of product definition.

The research and development has two major components, which in approximately 18 months will come together, namely, product definition and product costing.

1. *Product Definition:* The challenge has been, and continues to be, to find a way of classifying hospital output (discharges, deaths, and eventually, ambulatory care) in a manner which will provide for relatively homogeneous groupings. This has led to a variety of statistical reviews and manipulations. The various approaches researched to date have been:

(A) DRG: Essentially, this does not provide the sensitivity to show variances in the severity of illness between types of cases. By definition, severity of illness relates to consumption of resources, so that the simple use of the DRG is inadequate for analysis of resources used.

(B) CMG: This is the Canadian equivalent of the DRG, and has the same weaknesses in application.

(C) CMG with Severity Adjustment: The Severity of Illness Score, as developed by Dr. Susan Horne at Johns Hopkins, helps to develop a finer classification with a reduction in the variance between types of cases.

(D) CMG with Disease Staging: Again, this methodology shows some promise as one attempts to develop homogenuity among case groupings. Essentially, disease staging allows for a classification of CMG's by reclassifying them to four common stages of disease. It is understood, for instance, that a patient with early diagnosis of Hodgkins disease requires less in terms of resources than a patient with Hodgkins at stage four.

(E) KGH Case Mix Groupings: Kingston General Hospital is now researching the question of developing a unique method of classification which will blend ingredients of each of the foregoing, simply to provide the optimum in homogenuity.

2. *Product Costing:* Running parallel with the attempt to find the optimum classification system has been the costing studies aimed at developing accurate costs for the inputs. Key elements in this activity have been:

(A) Nursing: The hospital has used, for many years, a nursing classification system. This system is not seen to be sufficiently sensitive to provide accurate resource consumption by patient classification grouping. The system will shortly be refined to provide for a finer level of detail as to nursing time per patient. A large number of systems are available commercially and these are being evaluated.

(B) Diagnostic Services: Canadian hospitals have never had accurate costs based on time and motion studies, allocation of overhead, and other variables. Research is showing some interesting things and is already helping departmental managers understand their fixed and variable cost ratios much better.

(C) Overhead Costs: This is an area which is causing some question as the administration searches for a mechanism to reflect accurate and fair allocations of overhead costs. Unfortunately, there are no Canadian precedents on which to base development. It is believed that this will evolve into an allocation of fixed overhead, with further definition of variable overhead.

(D) Hotel Costs: The traditional approach to charging hotel costs has been based on a fixed allocation. However, it is apparent that finer breakdowns are required. It is believed that there is variability by case type relative to hotel costs.

(E) Drugs, Medical and Surgical Supplies: It is imperative to be able to cost supplies out accurately by case mix type, since there is such wide usage variation between case mix groupings. The question under review is at what point to capture the data (i.e., nursing unit or at source; prospectively or retrospectively).

**Management Reports**

This is the point at which, as an executive, the author's heart begins to pound. No longer will the executives and physicians pore over balance sheets and gross revenue and expense summaries. The new routine reporting systems will provide:

1. For the Cost Center Manager: not only cost center revenue and expense statements, but analysis of prime customers. This will be a useful tool for control, planning, and operations analysis.

2. For the Clinical Department Head (who now receives only periodic, overall hospital reports):

(A) A department summary of resource consumption (dollars) by CMG:

(B) A roll-up to total departmental revenue and expense; and

(C) An analysis of resource consumption by CMG, by doctor.

These reports will enable the clinical department head to analyze the economics of his programs in a sensible and business-like way. They will enable him to understand and explain (control?) volume changes, the economic implications thereof, and they will enable him to understand individual practice patterns. The net result should be that the clinical department head will be able to more effectively manage resources, rather than simply respond to issues.

3. Executive Summaries: The Chief Executive Officer now will be able to get a firm grasp on program costs, impact of forecast case mix changes, and physician practice patterns. Finally, he will have information in a form which will enable him to act before the fact and to assure that rational control measures are in place.

**Conclusion**

While in a Canadian context hospitals have tended to be responsive in terms of the marketplace, a Case Mix Management System will enable truly proactive management. The guesswork should be minimized and hospitals will not be able to say "we can't effectively control because we don't have the data." In short, Case Mix Management will bring a new era of corporate management to the hospital sector.

# Chapter Twenty

# Hospital Information Systems

**HELMUTH JUNG**

## Introduction

Every organization undergoes changes and develops in response to its environment. An organization and its managers must be flexible in reacting to changing conditions, otherwise it will no longer be competitive and may even face economic ruin. For management, goal planning is certainly of decisive importance, but the search for effective methods to realize goals—or, in some cases, to speed up development—is equally important.

Organizational changes usually occur at two levels, the level of technical organization and that of social interaction. These two aspects are closely related, and each influences the other. Difficulties for management always arise when changes on these two levels do not take place parallel to each other. In general, resistance to change occurs at the level of social interaction. Sociologists and organizational theorists have already studied this problem in detail. The laments of political leaders in past centuries were perhaps not based on scientific research, but they reflect practical experience, as in Machiavelli's comment [1532]: "There is nothing more difficult to take in hand, more perilous to conduct, or more uncertain in its success, than to take the lead in the introduction of a new order of things."

Organizational development attempts to bridge the gap between achieving management goals and dealing with the reactions of organization members to the proposed changes. Furthermore, organizational development is concerned with the methodology of development: How must organizational changes be planned and carried out in order to arrive at a long-term solution? How can the members of an organization identify with this specific goal and change their behavior and attitudes accordingly?

Organizational development theory proceeds from the assumption that *social change* in an organization can and must be planned, just as technical changes are. Thus, organizational development theory is not limited to the formal structure of an organization, but also includes informal factors (the invisible part of the iceberg) as a significant part of the organizational culture.

Traditionally, top managers have based their efforts to implement

223

innovations on two basic assumptions: (1) that the most certain way to introduce innovations successfully is by imposing them "from the top;" and (2) that the workers in an institution can be manipulated as management desires. With regard to hospitals, this author has shown elsewhere that, under certain conditions, the influence of the lower organizational levels is much more important, representing a greater barrier to innovation than the influence of orders issued from the top [Jung, 1983].

This paper will look at a project currently in progress, where hospital management correctly anticipated this type of behavior and is taking steps to ensure that lasting success can be achieved by working together with the hospital staff.

**The Project**

In a university hospital in Berlin, the installation of a Hospital Information System (HIS) is planned, both to improve communication and information flow and, also, to improve the hospital's financial situation. At this point, it must be made clear that the purpose is not to improve the accounting system but rather to increase the efficiency of patient care. "POINT" is the German abbreviation for "Patient Oriented Information Processing System." This university hospital, with numerous decentralized areas, departments, and laboratories is purchasing a standard version of a Hospital Information System. This product and the organization purchasing it—the university hospital—do not really fit together. However, since modifications in the system are expensive, they are supposed to be kept to a minimum, and the organization itself will have to undergo significant changes.

The project is not only one of major financial importance, which will require a longer period of time to complete, but it will also be an innovation for German hospitals. Computers have been employed for a long time in many areas of administration and laboratory work, but they have not been used in conjunction with patient care. With the exception of IBM personal computers employed in limited areas, not a single hospital in Europe has a Hospital Information System which includes patient care.

This can be illustrated by a brief comparison between the United States and the Federal Republic of Germany. In the United States, implementation of the Hospital Information System began in the early 1970's—at El Camino Hospital in Mountain View, for example [Giall, 1975]. The El Camino project may be considered an outstanding example and studies were done on it very early, as can be seen by the extensive literature available on the subject. At the same time, in the Federal Republic of Germany, hospital accounting systems were just being converted to electronic data processing.

Comparing computer progress in the hospitals of the United States and the Federal Republic of Germany brings one to the decisive problems associated with the organizational change described above.

## Project Problems

What are the general reasons why HIS is not routinely used in the Federal Republic of Germany?

1. The prosperous economy in the Federal Republic of Germany and the methods usually employed to finance its hospitals have encouraged medical and medical-technical progress, but not cost-consciousness or improvements in hospital planning and management methods.

2. Under present conditions, it is not possible to monitor performance or efficiency in the hospitals.

3. Another significant factor is the attitude of doctors and nursing personnel. Reorganization of work routines and computer-assisted communication processes are viewed as endangering professional autonomy.

4. Each member of an organization occupies a specific position and associates it with certain rights, duties, and advantages. Technical or structural changes in an organization represent a latent threat to the positions occupied by its various members. The power, status, and image of individuals can be negatively affected, as well as access to certain sources of information. The general phenomenon of fear is present and, in the specific POINT project, this was also intensified by scepticism about technical progress.

Even though today many areas of the university hospital and jobs are supported by computers, there is no detailed knowledge about the possibilities offered by a uniform hospital information system which encompasses all the areas of a hospital. From the large number of discussions conducted with the future users, it also became very clear that both the doctors and the nursing staff expected no reduction in their work load. Rather, they assumed that there would be still more paperwork and additional tasks to perform.

## Special Reasons for Opposition

In addition to these general reasons, there are also many special reasons for resistance which result from the specific situation of this university hospital. Some of the most important reasons are briefly discussed below.

1. Because the hospital is split into a large number of special disciplines and scientific institutions, each of these units has been able to pursue its own special aims. Thus, each printed form could be created for the specific needs of the individual units (there are presently about 1600 different forms); each department has its own work routines.

2. In addition to a central clinical laboratory which is supposed to serve all the departments, there are also many ward laboratories which perform the same types of analyses. POINT is supposed to encourage laboratory centralization.

3. As in all health care systems, rising costs have led to cutbacks, and in the Federal Republic of Germany these have particularly affected the area

of personnel. At first, university hospitals were less affected by this development but now the situation has changed fundamentally.

This means that the project is now associated with an area of general conflict—the issue of rationalization. Any cutbacks in funds for personnel are seen in connection with the POINT project. This is certainly even more true with regard to those staff members who do not have much information about the project at the moment. Rumors are the best way to foster resistance to organizational changes.

## The Goal Orientation

Even though the initial prerequisites for such a project do not appear to be particularly good, there are some reasons why implementing it is urgently necessary. The danger of an informational infarct, safeguarding the availability of medical care and the financial situation of the hospital, as well as the need to increase efficiency and competitiveness, make implementation unavoidable.

Since the project involves an area where there are definite conflicts of interest—external, internal, and also very individual ones—management has sought effective methods of implementation. Since POINT represents a philosophy or framework which can and must be filled with specific concerns, the basic prerequisite existed for applying the method of organizational development.

It is now the author's task, by using the method of organizational development, to provide support for the social change which occurs at the interactional level and to ensure that no, or at least fewer, discrepancies arise between technical-organizational and structural development.

## Practical Application of Organizational Development

In the first place, any practical applications of organizational development methods are confronted with the basic problems of defining the role of the consultant and his acceptance by the staff. The consultant comes from outside the organization and is hired by management, but by no means should he function strictly in the interest of management, as its extended arm. He is not an expert who develops technical solutions, which management then decides to adopt or not, but rather he enters into cooperative relationship with the client. His place in the organization is peripheral; he is neither a decision maker, nor may he be directly affected by the solutions adopted. However, he plays a number of roles—for example, process consultant, technical specialist, trainer, and proposer of alternatives.

Along with the problem of being accepted by the organization's staff, there is also the question of basic strategy. Where should the consultant begin his work: The choice of strategy often depends on the organizational structures and the way the hierarchy is set up, as well as on continuity at the management level.

It does not make much sense to concentrate on certain levels of management, groups working in specific areas, or individual vocational groups, because these often function independently of each other in separate systems. A top-down or basis-upward strategy is also not very useful. Approaching the lowest and highest levels of management also seems inappropriate, because this puts pressure on mid-level management.

The multiple nucleus strategy has proved to be a useful approach in organizations with many small hierarchies. By this means, all levels are included simultaneously and receive the same amount of attention. However, the consultant must be accepted by everyone in the system if this approach is to be effective.

The first step is to gain the confidence of the staff at the various levels of the hospital hierarchy. Rumors and the political oriéntation of individual groups make this a difficult task. In the current case, the preconception was widespread that organizational development represented a subtle tactic of management and the supplier of the information system to achieve their goals. *Before* the contract was signed, the author tried to change this opinion and gain the trust of the staff. Naturally, in these discussions, it was not possible to achieve a completely open relationship with the staff—this was also not the actual goal. Rather, the point was to create a basis for cooperation.

After the necessary basis for confidence had been established to some extent, it was possible to proceed one step further and collect initial data, analyze, and develop user requirements. The project team employed two strategies in this connection: On the one hand, experts from the electronic data processing (EDP) department of the hospital worked together with the respective departments to define user requirements for admittance of patients and settlement of accounts, as well as for areas with administrative tasks. On the other hand, the doctors and the nursing staff developed their concepts of how the hospital information system could assist them with their work in patient care.

However, the second and much more difficult strategy clearly led to better results. With the reservation that the project is not yet completed and changes could occur at any time, it is nevertheless possible to point to increased staff confidence in the project and to the learning process which has taken place.

During discussions with the future users of the system, no attempt was made to convince them to accept a certain solution. Instead, the problems were presented to the group, and then there was a mutual search for solutions. During these group discussions, any conflicts were discussed for the purpose of resolving them and not pushed aside for the time being, as is so often the case. The role of the consultant was to transmit information between the users on the one hand and the EDP department and management on the other hand.

These group discussions have not only resulted in the formulation of highly detailed user requirements; in addition, the users have taken further, very significant steps toward implementation of the system. First, their own attitudes about why it makes sense to implement a hospital information system have changed. These staff members, in turn, pass on information to others. Second, as a preliminary step toward implementing the HIS, a uniform method of keeping patient records has been introduced at the hospital—a goal which the nursing management had been trying to realize for some time with very little success. Third, the discussion groups have said that they would like to document the organizational changes and that they want to analyze the degree of goal achievement for themselves. This means that the foundation has been laid for self-examination, i.e., for critical observation of what takes place and for making necessary corrections. This represents the beginning of activity research.

## Goals and Planning

This brief survey shows that one is still at the beginning of a long project, and at this point it is only possible to provide a general outline of the methods to be employed. Because of the hierarchical structure to be found in a university hospital, the contingency approach of Lawrence and Lorsch [1969] seems most appropriate. In this approach, the hospital is viewed as a complex organization and its efficiency is seen as dependent upon having organizational structure and management practices directed at specific organizational situations. In this case, organizational development means a change in behavior throughout the entire system [Sievers, 1979]. The contingency approach is also compatible with the philosophy of the project.

During further development of the project, there will be three main areas of emphasis, namely promoting: (1) acquisition of knowledge about the system; (2) the ability to cooperate; and (3) group solutions to problems. In this context, knowledge about the system does not mean passing on information about systems software or hardware, but in understanding the system and learning how to work with a hospital information system on a day-to-day basis. In addition, being informed about organization structures and work routines is also involved. This area of concern, which in a narrower sense is directed at implementation of the POINT system, requires intensive staff training in computer operation and, also, must take existing structures and work routines into account.

The other two areas of emphasis may at first seem less directly related to the POINT project, but these actually represent the prerequisite for the success of this project. Weisbrod [1974] has described the communication and cooperation relations in university medical institutions convincingly and in great detail, and anyone who has ever worked in a university hospital can confirm what Weisbrod has to say. Realization of the Point project will require practice in cooperation and a search for group solutions to concrete problems (while avoiding the zero solution approach). The time framework and subject matter will be determined on the one hand by the implementation concept and on the other hand by the conduct of the hospital staff involved. In the past, the staff was simply confronted with a new system; now it is not only supposed to help modify and adapt a new system, but it is also expected to have a lasting effect on organizational structures and management attitudes.

## Conclusions

The project is setting out on a long and difficult journey and the participants will probably often wonder whether they have chosen the most effective method of carrying it out. They are proceeding from the basic assumption that nothing can be put into practice if the members of an organization are opposed to it—instead, the staff must identify with the new system. However, the organization members will only accept solutions if they have played a decisive role in developing them. The decisive changes in the project will not take place so much at the management and technical levels, but rather on the interactional level. However, this means that the perceptions, attitudes, and behavior of all (or at least most) of those involved will have to change.

The idea of organizational change cannot remain limited to individual subsystems; instead, it must encompass the entire system. Only the most important aspects of the strategies employed to effect social change can be outlined here, and these strategies will depend on the attitudes and behavior of the organization's members. Here the openness of this method can be seen: Organizational development is always responsive to what is happening, i.e., it must involve research on activities.

At the beginning, the author spoke of the dichotomy inherent in organizational change: On the one hand it is unavoidable, while on the other hand there are many barriers to change. In the author's opinion, both these problems can only be solved successfully if the methods of organizational development are applied, for doctors and nurses are specialists in search of their own organizational structure and management practices. They are being supported by experts, while seeking to define *their* solutions to the problems confronting them. Let us return to the question at the beginning: Is organizational development the way to salvation? In the author's opinion, it may not be salvation but it is still a very efficient method for solving organizational problems!

## REFERENCES

John E. Giall, *et al, Demonstration and Evaluation of a Total Hospital Information System,* Final Project Report, December 1975.

Helmuth Jung, *Koordinationsaspekte in der stationaren Krankenversorgung,* Berlin, 1983.

Paul R. Lawrence and Jay W. Lorsch, *Organization and Environment: Management Differentiation and Integration,* Homewood, IL., 1969.

Niccolo Machiavelli, *Il Principe,* Florenz, 1532.

Burghard Sievers, "Organisationsentwicklung," in *RKW-Handbuch, Fuhrungstechnik und Organisation,* Berlin, 1979.

Marvin R. Weisbrod, "A Mixed Model for Medical Centres: Changing Structure and Behavior," *Theory and Method in Organization Development: An Evolutionary Process,* John D. Adams, ed., Arlington, 1974.

# Chapter Twenty-One

## Behavior Modification For Health Care Delivery Systems

### MARTHA S. ALBERT

Puzzling, intriguing, frustrating, and promising are all meaningful ways of describing the potential relationship of behavior modification to health care systems. Behavior modification theory developed historically within psychology as part of the research tradition involving animals and people. Its relevance to health care systems rests on the possible changes individuals choose to make as they seek or avoid obtaining health care. The puzzling problem is that of developing incentives relevant to people with widely divergent personal characteristics and motivational patterns. While psychology and behavior modification deal with individual behavior, health care systems deal with mass behavior. Experience with HMO's shows that individual choice patterns are difficult to describe or predict in advance, and that there are many problems related to the grouping of "people in general" for purposes of estimating "incentives" to selectively utilize health services.

What is most challenging is the search for common variables associated with more intelligent use of available health services. Potential factors may include: age, education, socioeconomic status, urban-rural location, area of the country, religion, ethnicity, sex, occupational status, physical health, third party reimbursement schedule, perception of receptivity by health care personnel, and the health belief model subscribed to by the individual. With so many variables potentially interacting, the researcher is tempted to succumb to paralysis rather than search for factors which determine whether and when individuals choose to consult health care practitioners. It is possible to speculate about the generation of a few crucial variables capable of reinforcing new behaviors. Most commonly, the current dialogue centers around higher deductible and the use of HMO's for health resource conservation to affect individuals with widely varying characteristics.

Frustration on the part of social scientists has arisen from observations of health practitioners who encourage client dependence and ignorance, leading to overutilization, and because of client unwillingness or inability to question the system or to modify their demands. For many groups, including the poor, no incentives for health care maintenance and disease prevention have been discovered yet. Experimentation is highly desirable,

231

but funding for this purpose has not been forthcoming. Society tends to deal globally with the public "in general," while health behavior is idiosyncratic, highly individualistic, and often reflective of life-style.

What is promising is the current mood of experimentation among the public at large, a thrust which may escalate to the point where new structures are created to find and develop health maintenance and disease prevention alternatives for broad populations. Certainly the system is under such siege that the motivation for devising new structures to meet new behaviors is higher than ever. It may be that, in the search for more workable incentives for health maintenance, one will discover that new structural types arise to satisfy newly defined needs. In brief, structures and incentives may fit like hand in glove. Older structures may be the products of regulatory constraints, non-profit status with open-ended reimbursement, and the notion that there are economies of scale in the health care industry.

In an economic environment where cost containment prevails, where multihospital corporations operate for profit, where reimbursement is curtailed, and where competition seeks to contain overutilization, small, atomistic, decentralized, cohesive units with high staff and client loyalty may become the norm. Where, then, will behavior modification be employed? Clearly, current momentum is to modify third party payment mechanisms to encourage fuller use of HMO's, with higher deductibles as promotional devices. There is considerably less certainty concerning health promotion incentives, because it is more difficult to deal with individual life-styles. Further, society's mass marketing and bureaucratic and structural orientation facilitates changing behavior in large, measurable, and quantifiable groupings. Changing life-styles for health may be akin to using solar systems for heat—the lack of organized constituencies or corporate beneficiaries does not fit with the basic directions in which economic and political changes occur in Western nations. A compromise between the rugged individualist's focus upon life-styles and third party payor's emphasis on HMO's are the many corporate health improvement programs reported in industrial nations.

This paper will examine the major strategies in behavior modification today: (1) HMO's, (2) self-improvement, and (3) corporate health improvement plans. These strategies will be assessed in terms of constituencies, relative success, and future potential. Other strategies will be considered and obstacles to successful health behavior modification will be offered for discussion. It should be noted that all of these strategies encounter resistance because they ask individuals to accept relatively more responsibility for their own health than has been the case in many years in industrial nations. In addition, for mainstream members of Western nations, less healthy life-styles are frequently built into work and home life, including alcohol and rich food at business lunches and parties, smoking as part of camaraderie, and a frenetic pace with ample business travel disrupting exercise habits and plans. The perception of future benefits must be high to delay current gratification.

Smoking is a good example. A recent book, *The Economic Approach to Human Behavior,* describes the cost-benefit ratio; Professor Gary S. Becker writes that [Goodman, 1983], "There are two costs of smoking— the current price and the anticipated cost. People will smoke or not smoke depending on the relative importance to them of these two prices." Rationality governs, according to this theory, but high taxes on cigarettes or alcohol would reduce consumption by changing the cost-benefit ratio.

Less murky in its invasion into the human psyche is the notion of HMO's. The theory is simple: If an organization receives a set price to deliver health care to individuals, its practitioners will have ample reason to be judicious in performing tests, doing surgeries, and recommending additional medical appointments and treatments. Certainly, there is some evidence that regionalization of services within a multihospital HMO can result in more outpatient-oriented services and fewer technologically based services, with the latter concentrated in larger hospitals. Prepaid group practices are less costly, though the reasons are still obscure and can include style of medicine practiced, geography, and lesser demands of enrollees (for example, if the elderly and the poor are not represented in great numbers) [Luft and Crane, 1980, pp. 231-47].

Certainly the experience of private sector HMO's has not been consistent with that of public sector HMO's; failure to increase enrollment and to reach self-sufficiency has been reported, in large part because disincentives existed, especially entitlement to free care from other sources, as well as the inability to choose a physician freely or to receive care at the closest geographic source. Comprehensive and continuous institutional provision of care was not viewed as a real incentive [Meier, 1981, pp. 328-38].

HMO's developed exclusively for Medicaid patients have differed widely from the characteristics of middle class HMO's as evidenced by unethical marketing practices, inadequate services, and excessive administrative costs. Access to mainstream medicine has not really occurred. Bruce Spitz, of the Urban Institute, believes that the explanation rests with the political process which generated Medicaid recipients' HMO's, exaggerated claims for prepaid group practices, and policy distortions and peculiarities of the Medicaid program itself. Insufficient services are linked to patient docility and provider cost cutting, and high administrative costs are linked to the expense of frequent disenrollment and a lack of governmental oversight. As part of a welfare bureaucracy, Medicaid is hemmed in by cumbersome regulations [Spitz, 1979, pp. 497-518].

HMO enrollments have varied greatly among the states, with higher hospital costs and mobile populations encouraging HMO development. Unionization and availability of prepaid group practices are also significant contributors to HMO growth [Goldberg and Greenberg, 1981, pp. 421-38]. The potential for a voucher system for Medicaid patients may greatly affect the disposition toward HMO's, depending upon the level at which the voucher is set, with age, physical condition, and region of the country as variables to be considered [Iglehart, 1982, pp. 451-54].

Studies of HMO's do not seem to address the issues which enrollees and "resistors" discuss and which remain unresolved in some organizations. For example, what happens when an enrollee has an accident or illness far distant from the HMO headquarters and requires immediate treatment? What if a patient is really ill and the HMO's physicians refuse to make tests to determine the nature and extent of illness? What if treatments do exist (and are reimbursed by other third party payors), but they aren't "done" by the HMO's physicians? Who is the patient's advocate within the HMO system and how strong is this ombudsman, if he or she exists at all? What are waiting times like at HMO's, and is service delivery deliberately limited by a "queuing system" requiring tenacity, persistence, and endless waits to obtain health care? The free choice system at least kept practitioners aware that patients could always go elsewhere and that some did.

These questions are important because a certain naivete permeates HMO discussion. The assumption is that people will use the least costly system to save money. In the short run, many people may do just this. Unless HMO's facilitate obtaining rapid, sufficient, and timely care, they may be unable to keep patients who have the choice of going elsewhere. People are motivated to seek quality care and want the sense of attachment to individual practitioners when they are ill. HMO's will have to accommodate these needs. Institutional behavior may require more modification than individual behavior for HMO's to become a more prevalent and significant method of health care delivery. Medicaid and poor patients will undoubtedly fare better in integrated HMO's, with patients drawn from a variety of socioeconomic groups.

Individual life-style improvement has been occurring in some industrial nations as more educated people belong to exercise clubs and spas and practice sports activities regularly. In the United States, this trend has enormous economic significance, with physical fitness as a major budget item for many members of the upper middle class. The virtue of such activity is well accepted by most Americans, despite the flourishing of sports medicine, a growth specialty addressing the varied ailments of Sunday athletes. There is a great deal of sorting out still to be done concerning appropriate type, level, and frequency of exercise, if improved health is the objective.

There are always risks—for example, that cardiovascular fitness pursued so actively may lead to knee surgery! Nevertheless, Americans in record numbers are reducing hard liquor consumption, salt and sugar intake, meat in the diet, and caffeine consumption, with dramatic effects on the food and beverage industry. Demand for high fiber foods and for corporate exercise plans have increased, with the potential for disease prevention enhanced. To date, no incentives have been discovered for health promotion among the poor. Vouchers may be necessary for health clubs or cooking classes (dietary experimentation), methods wich have not been widely debated by policymakers.

Corporate health improvement activities are probably the most clearcut experiment in successful behavior modification. Peer relationships, regularity, and medical supervision are advantages as new habits are formed. A major complication is the limited knowledge available concerning the health belief models followed by members of the general public and, of course, the frequent divergence of belief and behavior. People vary in the extent to which they regard their health status as self-determined; many think that luck, environment, or heredity are very important, despite ample evidence that diet, exercise, and life-style lengthens the healthy life span for most people.

The concept of health protective behavior may be particularly helpful in defining individuals as producers and not simply consumers of health care. Unfortunately, most of the research to date has dealt with patient compliance with recommendations of health care providers or the extent of direct contact with health care professionals for routine health maintenance activities, such as immunizations, prenatal care, and the like. The notion of health protective behavior is broad enough to encompass the self-defined behaviors engaged in by people which they believe promote health. Health protective behavior is defined by Harris and Guten [1979, p. 18] as: ". . .any behavior performed by a person, regardless of his or her perceived or actual health status, in order to protect, promote or maintain his or her health, whether or not such behavior is objectively effective toward that end."

The current model views health-related behaviors in terms of motivation to perform them, perceived value in reducing the threat of disease, belief that one's own health action potentially reduces the threat, and modification of the above by demographic, structural, and enabling (institutional) factors [Harris and Guten, p. 19]. A recent research effort concluded that most people are performing some behaviors which they think protect their health, with nutrition, sleep and relaxation, and exercise as most frequent. Most health protective behaviors do not involve contact with the formal social system and are part of a personal habit system. Interestingly, Harris and Guten interpret their statistics to mean that [p. 24] "those in 'poor' condition less often consider proper food and nutritional habits and physical exercise to be important health protective behaviors, but that they more often mention health care system use, taking medication, and performing or refraining from performing some types of physical activities."

Sick role behavior contrasts sharply with the health protective behaviors of the healthy. Health protective behaviors were most often performed by those perceiving themselves as most or least likely to become ill. Both groups apparently believe that health requires hard work! The Health Belief Model was only moderately predictive of health protective behavior (HPB) scales. Dimensions of HPB include: (1) personal health practices; (2) safety practices; (3) preventive health care; (4) environmental hazard avoidance; and (5) harmful substance avoidance. Compliance with the medical-scientific health behavior model was not necessarily related to HPB's, suggesting that HPB's should be examined to understand health in a life-style context [Harris and Guten, pp. 17-29].

The experience of corporate health programs is an excellent application of health protective behavior in the work place; it usually involves harmful substance avoidance, personal health practices, and preventive health care. The most frequent target has been smoking cessation, where a variety of behavior modification techniques have been employed, from electric shock to excessive cigarette smoke and covert sensitization. High success, in one instance, was partly attributed to the presentation of a variety of cessation methods for individual choice [Powell and McCann, 1981,. pp. 94-104]. One theory holds that smoking cessation occurs more easily for individuals with "psychosocial assets" or personal security (the individual's belief that he can control what happens to him) [Ockene, et al, 1981, pp. 623-38]. Clearly, the work context can foster a sense of control supported by peers, facilitating cessation and its maintenance.

Several other work site behavior modification programs have been effective. Individuals screened at the work site for hypertension control did get medical follow-up and their knowledge was significantly greater if they received educational materials which indicated their blood pressure or extent of risk. Failure to follow through by patients has, however, been a significant obstacle to treatment after screening at other locations [Bloom and Jordan, 1979, pp. 500-06]. Whether the work place experience itself was most instrumental or whether this particular work place package was carefully designed to alert health care avoiders is unclear; it is known, however, that the least compliant are usually patients who are white, young, male, and employed.

Community-wide and school programs have also been reported in the literature with some long-range retention. One example is the Weight-A-Thon, a six week fund raising event sponsored by the American Cancer Society of Allegheny County, Pennsylvania. Thirty-two hundred people lost an average of 8.3 pounds, and seven months after they still had an overall weight loss of 4.5 pounds. Another program of this sort for obesity is the Stanford Heart Disease Prevention Program, a mass media campaign focused on cholesterol and saturated fat consumption, affecting communities with a total of about 42,000 people. The German Federal Republic, with the Max Planck Institute of Psychiatry, produced a seven-part series on weight control for prime time television which reached an estimated 7.8 million people, 2.8 million of whom were overweight, producing an average weight loss of 5.5 pounds.

Behavior modification for obesity has been the thrust of community interventions directed toward supermarket shopping behavior, cafeteria food choices, vending machine selection, and exercise habits. After reviewing the related studies and their own data on Weight-A-Thon, Wing and Epstein concluded that continued social support and skills for weight reduction maintenance are both necessary for weight loss retention [Wing and Epstein, 1982, pp. 245-50].

Several programs in child health education have reported success. Screening for chronic disease risk factors in children from 15 countries showed that factors leading to success included acceptability of the screening, children's enjoyment in participation, and the prevalence of risk factors. Major concerns were dietary habits and substance abuse prevention [Wynder, et al, 1981, pp. 121-32]. One program includes health screening, the Health Passport, a behavior-oriented health curriculum, and special intervention for high-risk students—the Know Your Body (KYB) program. This approach holds promise because the stages from screening through information distribution and behavior modification are encompassed [Williams, et al, 1980, pp. 371-83]. Another unusual program was life skills training for early adolescents in New York to increase students ability to cope with direct pressures to smoke, indirect social influences to smoke, and to improve their ability to cope with anxiety. Allied health professionals used group discussion, modeling, and behavior rehearsal [Botwin, et al, 1980, pp. 135-43].

As one explores the relationship of behavior modification to health, it is clear that social support and knowledge dissemination are crucial to the modification of behavior. Such modification can occur due to programs at the work site, in schools, and in communities. It seems likely that programs are more effective if the entire cycle from screening, to knowledge, to behavior change occurs within a single effort. Further, it will not be promising to identify individual, idiosyncratic variables statistically related to predicting outcomes, since it isn't feasible to screen people in and out of programs based on their psychological makeup; rather, it makes sense to engage in health behavior modification in groups where members value their associations and peer group support can develop.

The linkage of behavior modification to health care systems presents a more difficult dilemma. Employers can't be quoted exact figures for cost savings if employees change their life-styles. Until employers pay differential health insurance premiums, based on the risks presented by individual employees, there will not be sufficient social pressure for many individuals to modify their own behavior. Dr. John H. Knowles, the late president of the Rockefeller Foundation, said in 1977 that [Kristein, 1982, pp. 729-32] "...the costs of individual irresponsibility in health care now becomes prohibitive. The choice is individual responsibility or social failure." Both social unacceptability and assistance in quitting will be needed for massive change to reduce American health care costs.

Where the health care system can be involved is in the generation of a variety of related screenings and physical fitness programs with quality leadership, carefully devised motivational schema, convenience of participation, and social support of enrollees [Pate and Blair, 1983, pp. 632-43]. In the final analysis, the popularity of behavior modification programs rests upon organized public and private support for "owning" one's own health. Individuals paying differentially for self-imposed risk legitimates this notion. Spreading the risk among individuals, regardless of their behavior, tacitly supports irresponsibility of health care habits. Further, "bonuses" for sick role behavior would have to be eliminated. Sick leave should be viewed as paid vacation for basically healthy people. Sick leave could be computed as part of annual (vacation) leave.

For the poor and the disadvantaged, significant peer groups and health maintenance incentives must be devised so that they are brought into the new system. This may include health speakers at community churches, ethnic groups promoting sceening of their members, and vouchers for poor people for athletic clubs and spas. Behavior modification is based on the notion that individuals "own" their own behavior within limits and should be expected to "carry themselves" rather than expect society to assume the burden of self-imposed illness. Social policy must reflect this philosophy; at this time, sick leave encourages the belief that illness among basically healthy people is a result of bad luck rather than self-care.

In the long run, more information will emerge concerning the cost effectiveness of health promotion, facilitating third party support. One problem is that of comparability of data, because definitions vary with respect to such terms as health education, disease detection, and health protection. Multiple health promotion strategies employed together will probably yield much greater cost benefits than singular strategies [Rogers, et al, 1981, pp. 324-39]. Overall cost effectiveness will probably vary by age, sex, geography, socioeconomic status, health status, setting and peer group for health promotion exposure, previous health practices, and attitudes. Carefully controlled and replicated research with international generalizability remains difficult to fund, design, conduct, and coordinate.

At this point, employee fitness programs show the greatest promise for applications of behavior modification theory. Such programs are directed toward the least health-conscious segment of the population who are "captured" by a highly valued institution, the work group. People at work can be subjected to peer pressure with predictable frequency, intensity, and regularity. A recent study indicated that the cost of exercise and program development for an employee program is $100 to $350 per participant a year. With a 20 percent participation rate, the benefit would be a savings of over $700 per year for each labor force member. Thus, a $40,000 cost for 200 people in a company with 1,000 employees would yield $650,000-700,000 in benefits per year [Shephard, 1983, pp. 644-53].

The task for health care policymakers is to sell such programs to third party payment sources, including government, insurors, and employers. The largest obstacles thus far are the absence of nationally recognized marketing strategies, the absence of belief by third party payors that fitness saves on health costs, and the lack of legal vehicles to pay initial costs of health and fitness programs.

One means of generating needed capital for health and fitness programs is by assessing individual risk and setting differential premiums or higher deductibles for high risk individuals (smokers and other substance abusers and individuals who have not engaged in activities which are known to reduce risk from identified health problems). Employers and third party payors could provide economic pressure, forcing individuals to assume responsibility for self-imposed risk. For this to occur, sophisticated risk identification, estimation, and reduction methods consistent with sound financial managemet should be developed. Risk profiles may be very appealing to Americans as part of life-style counseling [Bernstein, 1983, pp. 882-87]. Counseling, which brings together health knowledge and perception of life expectancy, can have an impact on individuals' health behavior choices [Hamermesh and Hamermesh, 1983, pp. 911-14].

Innovative methods for health behavior modification should be attempted. For example, incentives could be developed for television and other media to consistently show characters in dramas and soap operas practicing good health habits. Prime time programs frequently show people engaged in eating, drinking, and activities which negatively affect health status. According to Gerbner, *et al* [1981, p. 904]:

> "television . . .may well be the single most common and pervasive source of
> health information. We know that television tends to monopolize the free time
> of less educated, lower-income individuals . . . these groups have the poorest
> opportunities for health and nutrition and are the most in need of valid infor-
> mation about health. [A General Mills] study also found that next to doctors,
> television was the most frequently cited source of information about health."

Gerbner's research showed excessive television watchers are more complacent about eating, drinking, and exercise as well as expressing higher confidence in physicians. The authors concluded that "The cultivation of complacency, coupled with an unrealistic belief in the 'magic of medicine,' is likely to perpetuate unhealthy life-styles and to leave both patients and health professionals vulnerable to disappointment, frustration and litigation."

For available behavior modification techniques to be used to change Americans' health habits, individuals, families, employers, and municipalities must assume responsibilities for wellness [Plyman and Perkins, 1983, pp. 6-9]. Mass marketing for structural innovation (such as HMO's) must be accompanied by methods of arousing individuals to act in their own behalf. Life-style change is a question of values, and values reflect goals and resources. Goal setting, for satisfaction with one's own health, must be accompanied by management of key scarce resources, time, and psychological energy [Schowengerdt, 1983, pp. 17-20].

Health behavior for individuals is a function of priorities within life's momentum. For countries, health behavior is a consequence of economic, social, and political forces, as well as beliefs about self and societal responsibility. In the final analysis, health behavior is the burden of individuals and of countries.

## REFERENCES

James E. Bernstein, "Handling Health Costs by Reducing Health Risks," *Personnel Journal,* November 1983, pp. 882-87.

Joan R. Bloom and Stacey C. Jordan, "From Screening to Seeking Care: Removing Obstacles to Hypertension Control," *Preventive Medicine,* 8, 1979, pp. 500-06.

Gilbert J. Botwin, Anne Eng, and Christine L. Williams, "Preventing the Onset of Cigarette Smoking through Life Skills Training," *Preventive Medicine,* 9, 1980, pp. 135-43.

George Gerbner, Larry Gross, Michael Morgan, and Nancy Signorielli, "Health and Medicine on Television," *The New England Journal of Medicine,* October 8, 1981, p. 904.

Lawrence G. Goldberg and Warren Greenberg, "The Determinants of HMO Enrollment and Growth," *Health Services Research,* 16, No. 4, Winter 1981, pp. 421-38.

Walter Goodman, "In Theory: Cost Benefit Analysis Putting a Price on Life's Miscellanea," *The New York Times,* Sunday, December 18, 1983.

Daniel S. Hamermesh and Frances W. Hamermesh, "Does Perception of Life Expectancy Reflect Health Knowledge?" *American Journal of Public Health,* 73, No. 8, August 1983, pp. 911-14.

Daniel M. Harris and Sharon Guten, "Health-Protective Behavior: An Exploratory Study," *Journal of Health and Social Behavior,* 20, March 1979, p. 17-29.

John K. Iglehart, "The Future of HMO's," *Health Policy Report,* 307, No. 4, August 1982, pp. 451-54.

Marvin M. Kristein, "Health Care Costs and Preventive Medicine," *Preventive Medicine,* 11, 1982, pp. 729-32.

Harold S. Luft and Steven Crane, "Regionalization of Services within a Multihospital Health Maintenance Organization," *Health Services Research,* 13, No. 3, Fall 1980, pp. 231-47.

Gitta Meier, "Prospects for the Contra Costa Health Plan, A Public Sector Health Maintenance Organization," *Journal of Health Politics, Policy and Law,* 6, No. 2, Summer 1981, pp. 328-38.

Judith K. Ockene, Ronald Nutall, Robert C. Benefari, Irving Hurwitz, and Ira S. Ockene, "A Psychosocial Model of Smoking Cessation and Maintenance of Cessation," *Preventive Medicine,* 10, 1981, pp. 623-38.

Russell R. Pate and Steven N. Blair, "Physical Fitness Programming for Health Promotion at the Worksite," *Preventive Medicine,* 12, 1983, pp. 632 - 43.

Jeffrey S. Plyman and Lyndon D. Perkins, "Fitness Monitoring," *Public Management,* August 1983, pp. 6-9.

Don R. Powell and Barbara S. McCann, "The Effects of a Multiple Treatment Program and Maintenance Procedures on Smoking Cessation," *Preventive Medicine,* 10, 1981, pp. 94-104.

Peggy Jean Rogers, Elizabeth K. Eaton, and John G. Briehn, "Is Health Promotion Cost Effective?" *Preventive Medicine,* 10, 1981, pp. 324-39.

George C. Schowengerdt, "The Why, What, and How of Life Planning," *Public Management,* August 1983, pp. 17-20.

Roy J. Shephard, "Employee Health and Fitness: The State of the Art," *Preventive Medicine,* 12, 1983, pp. 644-53.

Bruce Spitz, "When a Solution is not a Solution: Medicaid and Health Maintenance Organizations," *Journal of Health Politics, Policy and Law,* 3, No. 4, Winter 1979, pp. 497-518.

Christine L. Williams, Betty Jean Carter, and Anna Eng, "The 'Know Your Body' Program: A Developmental Approach to Health Education and Disease Prevention," *Preventive Medicine,* 9, 1980, pp. 371-83.

Rena R. Wing and Leonard H. Epstein, "A Community Approach to Weight Control: The American Cancer Society Weight-A-Thon," *Preventive Medicine,* 11, 1982, pp. 245-50.

Ernst L. Wynder, Christine L. Williams, Kristina Laakso, and Marcia Levenstein, "Screening for Risk Factors for Chronic Disease in Children from Fifteen Countries," *Preventive Medicine,* 10, 1981, pp. 121-32.

# Chapter Twenty-Two

## Cost Containment: Successes, Failures, New Initiatives

### EDWARD P. ROBINSON

## Introduction

The initial purpose of this paper is to identify and define the two sides of the health care financing coin as it exists today. The first side of the coin regards the ability of the U.S. government and the third party payors to adequately finance the present health care delivery systems, while at the same time maintaining their own fiscal integrity. The other side of the coin involves the ability of the health care providers to maintain their own fiscal integrity, through adequate reimbursement for their services, so that they can continue to maintain the quality, availability, and appropriate level of care sought by the American public.

This paper will provide a short description of the present programs, with a brief review of Public Law 98-21 and the Social Security Amendments of 1983. The proposals of many non-governmental, third party payors, involving concepts such as health maintenance organizations, preferred providers, and prospective payment systems will also be considered. There may be possible side effects and fallout from these programs that can have an effect on the quality of care.

Finally, in conclusion, the author shall seek to place these various strategies in proper perspective by suggesting additional and alternate courses of action.

## The Problem

In April 1983, a new Medicare prospective payment system was included in the Social Security Amendments of 1983 and the rules of implementation for Public Law 98-21 were published in the September 1, 1983, *Federal Register*. This constituted a sweeping and quite dramatic change in the method of government reimbursement to hospitals. By the end of 1984, practically all acute-care hospitals that come under the Medicare program will be operating under the prospective payment system, utilizing Diagnostic Related Groups (DRG's).

Beginning with a three-year phase in, started October 1, 1983, payment to hospitals for Medicare services will be based upon pre-established rates, as determined by the 467 DRG's approved, rather than upon the retroactive payment system that had been in existence since the inception of

Medicare. The prospective payment system is programmed to work in the following manner [Davis, 1983]. Payment to hospitals for Medicare services now will be based on a unit of payment—a pre-set rate for kind of illness treated. Each of the 467 DRG's is constructed from: Statistical and clinical analysis of all cases treated; Patient age and sex; Treatment procedure; and Specific diagnosis.

The DRG's were developed under contract with the Health Care Financing Administration and the Yale University Center for Health Studies over a 10-year period. Under the new system, rates for DRG's will be set annually and will be based on rural and urban differentials. If hospitals provide treatment at a lower cost than the DRG rate, they make a profit. If the hospitals provide treatment at a higher cost than the DRG rate, they suffer a loss. Medicare will pay, in behalf of its beneficiaries, only the DRG rate. Beneficiaries cannot be billed beyond that level, except for normal deductible and co-payment amounts. Additional payments are provided to hospitals if cases involve unusually high treatment cost or long lengths of stay. Medicare's share of a hospital's capital and medical education expenses will continue to be paid on a hospital-specific basis. The rate of payment for over-all medical education costs will be increased.

It has been evident for some time that the increasing expenditures in health care are rapidly draining the ability of the Social Security system to generate sufficient funds to meet the demand. In 1982, $322 billion, 10.5 percent of the gross national product, was spent on health care. Forty-two percent or $135 billion went to hospital care. Health care is the nation's second largest employer, after education, and is the third largest industry in consumer spending, after food and housing. This subject has been well-covered and well-documented in many papers and discussions throughout the country during the past year. Therefore, the author will not dwell on the details of this subject at great length.

It is generally accepted that new and innovative programs must be implemented during the 1980's if the health care system in the United States is to remain healthy, maintain financial integrity, and be able to continue to offer the present quality of care that the American public desires.

Granted, there is agreement by all concerned that a major crisis exists in health care financing. Granted, new programs must be instituted to substantially alleviate the situation. Therefore, the first premise of this paper (i.e., to identify and define the problem) has been satisfied. The next section looks at some of the implications the new system will have on health care delivery in this country.

**Reactions and Repercussions**

The next premise to be addressed will be a brief description of the present programs and their objectives, with consideration given to reactions and repercussions that these programs may create throughout the health care delivery system. They may produce unwanted fallout. It still remains a valid theorem that for every action there is an opposite (and sometimes equal and sometimes unequal) reaction.

The objective of the prospective payment mechanism and the changes in the present reimbursement are all designed to decrease the cost of hospital care to the consumer. This is a noteworthy goal. The creation of Health Maintenance Organizations and the Preferred Provider concept are other mechanisms to reduce the amount and cost of hospitalization. It may even be true that healthy competition among hospitals will weed out the inefficient and the unneeded. Many of these programs are intended to foster and heighten the competitive concept.

However, the author believes that one must be careful not to throw out the baby with the bath water. If hospitals are not compensated fairly and properly, a reaction will be triggered. The hospital that cannot recover its legitimate expenses and costs is in dire trouble. The cost of care provided to the truly medically indigent patient must be considered and included in all reimbursements to the health care delivery system.

If a hospital cannot recover its legitimate costs, it has few alternatives but to reduce the quality of care, not to admit the truly medically indigent, or, as a last resort, to declare bankruptcy. Many hospitals will declare bankruptcy in the coming years and the number of hospital beds and, consequently, hospital services, will be reduced.

One must be concerned, however, that the question will not run from "How many unnecessary beds do we have in the United States?" to "Do we have *enough* necessary beds to provide the quality of care we desire?" Therefore, one must approach a real two-headed dilemma. How does one reduce hospital costs, maintain the fiscal integrity of both the consumer and the provider, reduce the number of unnecessary beds and services, and still maintain the medical standards desired? Some alternatives and future directions are discussed in the following section.

**Alternatives**

Concerned citizens and groups need to take heed of possible reactions to the present system and to look to additional alternatives. The following programs are some suggested alternatives for consideration.

1. The concept that hospitals must increase their emphasis on cost containment is a valid approach. It would be recommended to acute-care facilities that patient-care programs receive the primary dollar to the detriment of the non-patient support services, if necessary, in order to put the health-care dollar where it has the most impact.

In addition, private industry must realize that it also has a dual relationship and responsibility with the provider. Industry, through the third party payor, has a valid interest in hospital cost containment. Increasing costs of energy, medical supplies, food, and the like, all contribute directly to the increasing cost that the hospital provider must bear and then charge back to the third party payor. Ironically, the very firms that supply and service the hospital, also are responsible for a considerable share of the hospital's costs.

2. Increased use of outpatient services must be stressed. All areas of admission to inpatient care must be thoroughly scrutinized to assure that, whenever possible, the same procedure can be accomplished on an outpatient basis, rather than an inpatient basis. This will enable the patient and the third party payor to benefit tremendously by lowering costs through outpatient services. At the same time, the third party payor, industry, and the government all have an obligation to add a financial incentive that would increase outpatient utilization.

3. Home-care services must play an ever increasing, important part in discharge planning. If the provider is expected to promptly discharge the patient who no longer needs acute hospital care, then there must be some place that is financially feasible for the patient to go. In many instances this discharge may be delayed, not because of medical reasons, but simply because either the patient has nowhere to go that he or she can afford, or the family does not have the financial or physical resources available to take care of the patient at home.

The reimbursement for the home-care services has been spotty and minimal, at best. Homemaking services are not included in reimbursement mechanisms. The overwhelming majority of patients do wish to leave the acute-care facility at discharge time. It is the cost factor *after discharge,* to them or to their family, that is the deterrent. The author believes it would behoove third party payors to analyze home-care services carefully, with a view toward reimbursement.

For the sake of argument, if it is assumed that a particular hospital per diem is $700 per day and a patient stays five days over the actual discharge and this excess can somehow be justified, the additional cost to third party payors is $3,500. If payment arrangements could be made for home-care services which would include private duty nursing, a live-in companion, physical therapists, and so forth, this would enable the patient to return to his or her own home or to a family member's home.

For example, approximately $1,500 for a 30-day period could be allotted for home-care services. In this hypothetical instance, the third party payor would save $3,500 in hospital costs and $2,000 overall.

At the same time, the patient would be able to return home and have 30 additional days of care at less cost to everyone. At the present time, all reimbursement plans call for payment while the patient is *in* the hospital. Why not institute a reimbursement program to cover home-care services and make payments to keep the patient *out* of the hospital?

4. Simplify the 467 DRG prospective payment system by having hospitals establish an all inclusive, per diem rate. Each service of the hospital, such as medical service, surgical service, obstetrical service, ICU/CCU

service, pediatric service, nursery, neonatal service, and so forth would have its own all inclusive daily per diem. Thus, there would be approximately 8 to 10 services and, therefore, only 8 to 10 reimbursement groupings, instead of 467.

This would eliminate a great deal of bookkeeping and billing procedures. It would also enable the third party payors to compare all inclusive daily per diem rates, by hospitals, in a similar region. The third party payor could then establish a usual and customary fee to be paid to all hospitals per day in that region. The length of stay would be determined by the utilization review committee. Lengths of stay in excess of the utilization review committee guidelines would not be paid. This is where the home-care reimbursement mechanism would start to give the patient an incentive to leave the hospital. Hospitals who were being paid below their per diem rate would have additional incentive for increased cost containment.

5. The present program of prospective payment includes the acute-care facility but not the physician. While it is true that it is essential to have physician and hospital cooperation, it is felt that if the physician shares the same reimbursement concept with the hospital where, as a team effort, both would be rewarded or penalized *together,* this cooperation would be greatly strengthened and decreased costs to the patient would be a result.

6. The impact of the investor-owned hospital will cause reimbursement to the not-for-profit hospital to suffer. There are, indeed, two sides of the health reimbursement coin to be considered once again. The investor-owned group has the luxury to choose between the financially responsible patient and the medically indigent patient. The not-for-profit hospital group does not have this same luxury but must become involved with all financial classes of patients, regardless of the ability to pay.

It becomes evident that as one group continues to absorb more of the financially responsible patients, the other group must then absorb more than its share of those unable to pay, with the subsequent financial consequences. The not-for-profit hospital finds itself in a financial competition that it cannot win because of a position of significant disadvantage under the present rules. This problem must be addressed.

7. No new or present program can function, nor succeed, without *all* third party payors and hospital groups assuming equal responsibility with the not-for-profit hospitals for the unpaid balances of the truly medically indigent patient. Not-for-profit, acute-care facilities must care for the truly medically indigent. The private payor sector is justifiably concerned that cost and price shifting will put the entire burden on it. Many industrial groups are considering DRG prospective payment systems similar to that of the Medicare program.

If all third party payors pay cost or below and none of the third party payors include the expenses of the truly medically indigent in their reimbursement programs, the author is hard pressed to understand how the not-for-profit voluntary hospital system can continue to exist.

The author recommends that all third party payors agree to include expenses of the truly medically indigent patient in their cost reimbursement formulas. It is also recommended that each county be expected to provide, through a tax-supported base if necessary, funding for these patients, either in a private acute-care hospital or through the establishment of a county hospital.

It would be said by some that the cost to the third party payor is excessive and prohibitive, but who is to say that this cost is not excessive and prohibitive to the voluntary hospital which must carry the entire burden alone? The other, more drastic alternative, is that the voluntary acute-care hospital will collapse under this weight and not only will the quality of care suffer and be lowered, but the availability of care may be drastically curtailed or, indeed, even disappear. Who, then, will provide the necessary care?

### Conclusion

The author has attempted to identify and define the very real reimbursement problems facing both the third party payors and the acute-care facilities. An analysis has been made of the present programs coming into effect. Unwanted fallout that may be concurrent with these programs and concepts have also been discussed. The concluding portion concerned itself with a review of several particular programs and considerations that the author feels can be productive or need addressing. There is no doubt that this is an issue that cannot be solved quickly nor simply, but people of goodwill in government, in the private sector, and in the hospitals must remain concerned.

REFERENCES

Carolyne K. Davis, *Medicare Prospective Payment,* Washington, D.C.: Health Care Financing Administration, August 31, 1983.

# Part Seven

**Fraud and Third Party Reimbursement**

# Chapter Twenty-Three

## Third Party Reimbursement for New Medical Technologies

### LEWIS FREIBERG

### Introduction

It is well-known that market pricing of goods and services generally includes a component for risk or uncertainty. Indeed, the business of the insurance industry is the pricing of products according to the risk of payment. Likewise, a portion of the price associated with the development, production, or sale of a good or service is generally acknowledged to include a component for the uncertain profitability of the activity—the more uncertain the activity, the higher this component.

When exchange prices are determined by the market interaction of buyers and sellers, the resultant market price accounts for this risk or uncertainty. When initial prices are set too high—above that required to cover resource costs and uncertainty, given demand—competition will result in a bidding down of prices until these are appropriately evaluated.

Such may not be the case when third parties, to market transactions, attempt to establish market prices through negotiations with sellers. A case in point is the pricing of new medical technologies. The pricing of these services is heavily influenced by approval processes of governments and negotiations with third party payors, such as Blue Cross plans.

Importantly, there is no market mechanism which will automatically tend to correct "excessive" prices. Once established, these prices tend to be inflexible downward because of the political difficulty of negotiating price decreases and because of the prior acceptance of the methodology used for calculating prices. For this reason, setting initial reimbursement rates becomes especially crucial for third party payors and all consumers in general.

This paper examines a general price-setting mechanism—negotiation between providers and third parties—when uncertainty is particularly high due to a lack of information. Such conditions are cogent when the process involves price setting for new medical technology.

### Negotiation

In the medical sector, it is common for third parties to negotiate the price of a service or good with providers. Indeed, because of the dominance of third party payors in this sector, the negotiated price often becomes the price to all consumers of the service, e.g., direct pay patients, whether or not they were a party to the negotiation. For example, state agencies may negotiate with third parties not only over the right of a provider to offer a service, but also over the price which may be charged. Often, these two decisions are interrelated. That is, whether or not a service is approved depends upon the price estimate of the provider. Blue Cross plans negotiate with providers on whether or not and how much they will pay for a service.

There are two bases of this negotiation process. One is the objective discovery of information so that the economically efficient price can be determined. The other is the political give and take among participants so that the fair, equitable, or just price can be determined. The more uncertain the relevance of the information, the more vigorous and important is the political basis of the negotiation. Since the fair price is a subjective concept, third party and provider perceptions of fair may be widely divergent. Negotiations then center around compromise—reaching a decision acceptable to all parties.

This process is complex, depending upon local or regional institutional relationships, personalities, and philosophies of important individual participants and institutional incentive structures faced by the participants. Since these factors are generally unrelated to an objectively-determined, economically efficient price, there is no presumption that the outcome of the negotiation process is an efficient price.

This paper abstracts from the political basis of negotiation and examines a model of negotiated pricing where the relevance of the available information is highly uncertain. The goal of this process is presumed to be the selection of a fair price. However, it is assumed that fair to the third party payor means economically efficient, while fair to the provider means something else.

## Information and Uncertainty

The negotiation process results in the presentation and consideration of information which is used as a basis for price setting. This information contains data relating to the cost of production and the level of expected utilization. Generally, there are three sources of such information. First are the individual provider generated data. Such data may contain information on purchase prices, renovation costs, staffing costs, interest costs, expected utilization, and prices to be charged. Second are similar data on the operations of other providers or third parties. These data may be compiled by third party negotiators and provider negotiators. Third are data gathered from research and experimental sources. These data are usually introduced into the process by third party negotiators, although provider negotiators may find it advantageous to introduce such information.

The uncertainty of the information is a function of the degree to which that data are based upon *ex ante* expectations or *ex post* results. When a procedure or service has been widely used for a significant period of time, the information introduced tends to be a more certain representation of expected outcomes for an individual provider. Not only do the data come from actual practice, but they also cover a large number of providers. Thus, the provider-negotiator's estimate of his own costs is likely to contain less error (be more certain) and, therefore, is likely to more closely coincide with the third party's notion of the efficient price. In such cases, the outcome of the negotiation process is less likely to revolve around price and more likely to revolve around need.

When much of the data introduced into the negotiating process is based upon *ex ante* expectations, however, the degree of uncertainty is significantly higher. Such is the case when providers propose to offer a new service. Since the service is new, third parties have little *ex post* information and the range of such information which they do have (research and experimental data) is limited to a few providers who are not likely to be representative of the type of providers who serve the general public. From the perspective of providers, their cost and utilization estimates for the new service are based upon *ex ante* expectations and are, likewise, subject to a higher degree of uncertainty.

As this level of uncertainty increases, the information introduced into the negotiation process will include a compensatory component designed to protect the negotiator. For example, provider estimates of cost, utilization, and prices will be designed to protect the provider from the higher expectation of losses caused by the uncertainty. Likewise, third party negotiators build such components into their data in order to protect themselves from the expectation of excessive payments caused by the uncertainty. The end result is a relatively large divergence between the third party's efficient price and the providers' fair price. Generally, each party will argue that their data are more reasonable and accurate for the problem at hand. If the situation is successfully negotiated, so that the service is provided, the resulting price will depend upon the relative bargaining and political strengths of the negotiators.

### Shifting Risk of Production

The above process can be interpreted as an attempt by the participants to shift the risk of production to the other party. This section develops such a model. To clarify terminology, one may think of a "risk" as a quantifiable uncertainty. The measurement of actual risk requires knowing a probability function of actual outcomes. When one is dealing with a new service, this cannot be known. However, by adding some assumptions to the model, the maximum risk facing the participants can be defined and estimated.

*Assume:* (1) The subject under consideration is a new service which has not previously been widely used; (2) This service is capital intensive, with a high fixed-cost component; (3) Both parties base their pricing position on information which is adjusted to fully compensate them for the uncertainty of producing or paying for the new service; (4) Once the price is set in the negotiating process, it becomes inflexible downward; and (5) The agreed upon decision rule is price equals average cost.

Assumption (1) implies that the information brought into the negotiation process is of an uncertain nature. Assumption (2) results in a decreasing average cost function. This tends to reflect the economics of much new medical technology. It certainly reflects the case of CAT scanners. Assumption (3) implies that both parties recognize the high degree of uncertainty, and it presumes that the third party goal is to minimize payments for a given level of utilization, while providers seek to minimize losses from the provision of service. Assumption (4) recognizes a tendency in the regulation of medical services—once prices are set, they tend to be inflexible downward. Assumption (5) suggests that providers and third parties agree on the overall goal of the negotiation process. That is, to set a price where the provider is fully compensated, but just so, for the cost of providing the service. Both agree that the provider should not suffer losses, but neither should he reap a monopoly profit. The average cost of production may include a return on investment in the case of for-profit providers.

The certain case can be represented, as in Figure I. The decreasing cost curve depicts the relationship between utilization and unit costs (and according to the decision rule, price).

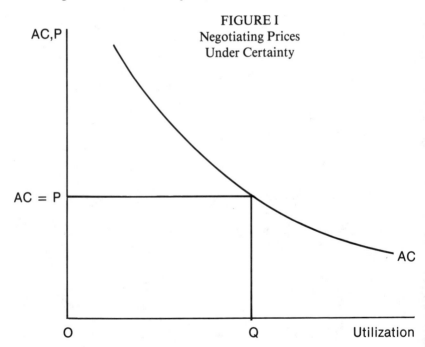

FIGURE I
Negotiating Prices
Under Certainty

If this cost curve were known with certainty and if the level of utilization were known with certainty, then the negotiating parties could easily agree on a price. Both would agree to a price of $0P$. The total annual payments would be equal to $0P,0Q$, which is equal to total cost to the provider, $0AC,0Q$. In this case, the provider's fair price would be equal to the third party's efficient price.

Introducing uncertainty into the model changes this simple result. Two basic sources of risk are the market risk and the technology risk. The market risk is related to the degree of uncertainty associated with predicting the future level of utilization. With a new service, this uncertainty will be high because of the lack of information. This risk can be analyzed by considering different points along the average cost curve.

The technology risk is associated with the uncertain useful life of the production technique. The capital will be depleted over time and possibly new technology will replace the existing technology, thereby rendering the service or its quality obsolete. Accurate price determination requires that this technology risk be appropriately incorporated into the average cost curve. Again, because of the paucity of reliable information, the risk is expected to be high and difficult to measure. This risk can be analyzed by considering the positioning of the average cost curve in the $AC/P,Q$ space.

Figure II represents the negotiating problem under uncertainty. Consider first the market risk. Since the level of utilization, *ex post*, is unknown both parties must estimate an *ex ante* level of utilization. Third parties have an incentive to generate high utilization estimates, while providers have an incentive to generate low utilization estimates. This behavior is merely an attempt to shift risk. Assume, for the moment, that AC is accepted as the "correct" average cost curve and assume that the third party negotiators select $q_0$ as their *ex ante* value, while providers select $q_1$. Further, assume that the values selected are such that the market risk to each party is zero (or nearly so), if that value is granted in negotiation.

The maximum risk to the third party of accepting the provider's estimate can be easily determined. If the *ex post* level of utilization is $q_0$, then the decision rule is satisfied at a price of $P_0$—the amount paid for services is $P_0$, $q_0$ (area $A + B$) which is equal to the total cost of providing services, $AC_0 \cdot q_0$. If, however, $q_1$ and hence $P_1$, is accepted and *ex post* utilization is $q_0$, then total payments are $P_1 \cdot q_0$ (area $A + B + C + D$) and far exceed actual costs of $P_0 \cdot q_0$. Accepting the provider's estimate, then, results in a potential maximum risk of excessive payments of $(P_1 - P_0)q_0$, areas $C + D$.

The situation is reversed from the provider's perspective. If the provider accepts the third party's *ex ante* utilization of $q_0$, and hence $P_0$, and *ex post* utilization is $q_1$, then the revenue he receives is $P_0 \cdot q_1$, area $A$, and his cost of providing the service is $AC_1 \cdot q_1$, area $A + C$. Hence, he suffers losses of $(AC_1 - P_0)q_1$, area $C$.

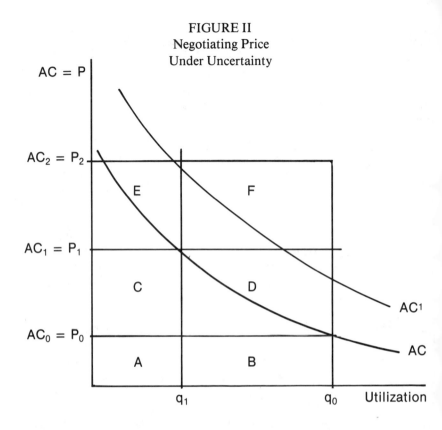

FIGURE II
Negotiating Price
Under Uncertainty

The negotiation process, then, becomes one of risk shifting behavior. Providers seek higher prices by understating utilization, while third parties seek lower prices by overestimating utilization. As the negotiated level of $q$ increases or $p$ decreases, the risk of third party overpayment decreases, while the risk to providers increases, and vice versa.

Finally, it should be noted that the risk is not symmetrical. The third party risk of overpayment is higher than the provider risk of losses. If the third party accepts the provider's *ex ante* $q$ of $q_1$ and *ex post* $q_0$ occurs, then third party overpayment is the area $C + D$. If, however, providers accept the third party's *ex ante* $q$ of $q_0$ and *ex post* $q_1$ occurs, then provider losses are the area $C$.

The technology risk arises from a potential divergence between the expected useful life of the production technique and its actual useful life. This is a dynamic problem which is handled on an annual basis by establishing a rate of depreciation for the capital investment. Under conditions of certainty, the annual depreciation would be such that the cost of capital would be recovered at the end of that capital's useful life. This implies (assuming variable costs are recovered) that, over the useful life of the capital, total revenue from the provision of the service will equal the total cost of providing the service, and the decision rule of negotiation would be achieved.

Under conditions of uncertainty, however, the useful life of the technology can only be estimated. Thus, the actual rate of depreciation may diverge from the rate which would just allow for the recovery of capital costs. This potential divergence is the technology risk. If the useful life of the capital is underestimated, then depreciation will be overestimated and third party payors will suffer. If the useful life is overestimated, then depreciation will be underestimated and the providers will suffer a loss from providing service. In the negotiating process, then, both parties will attempt to shift the technology risk by obtaining a favorable depreciation rate.

The technology risk can be isolated in Figure II by assuming that the *ex post* level of utilization is known—assume it to be $q_1$. The depreciation becomes a fixed cost in the average cost function and thereby positions the curve in the $AC/P, q$ space. Lower rates of depreciation shift the cost curve down.

Now assume that the zero-risk depreciation rate for the third party results in the cost curve $AC$, while the zero-risk depreciation rate for the provider results in the $AC^I$ curve. The maximum annual technology risk for the third party, if he accepts the provider's preferred depreciation rate, is $(P_2 - P_1)q_1$, area $E$. That is, the third party will overpay by an amount represented by $E$. The maximum overpayment over the useful life of the capital is

$$\sum_{i=1}^{n} (P_2 - P_1) \cdot q_1 \cdot (1 + r)^i$$

where, $n$ is the useful life of the capital and $r$ is the opportunity cost of funds. The maximum annual technology risk for the provider, if he accepts the third party's rate of depreciation, is also equal to $(P_2 - P_1)q_1$, *area E*, and the risk over time is identical to the third party's maximum risk. In other words, if the provider accepts the third party's preferred depreciation rate, and his own *ex ante* estimate of useful life is accurate, then he faces annual losses of $E$ over the useful life of the capital.

Unlike the market risk, the technology risk is symmetrical for both parties. That is, the provider's potential maximum loss is equivalent to the third party's potential maximum loss.

It is now possible to consider the total maximum risk stemming from both the market and technology risks. Assume that the third party's *ex ante* estimates of utilization and useful life ($q_0$, $AC$) prove to be accurate *ex post* values, and assume that the third party accepts the provider's *ex ante* estimates ($q_1 \cdot AC^I$). The third party will pay $P_2 \cdot q_0$, area $A + B + C + D + E + F$, while the cost of service production to the provider will be $P_0 \cdot q_0$, area $A + B$. The third party will overpay for the service by an amount equal to $(P_2 - P_0)q_0$, area $C + D + E + F$.

If the provider's estimates prove to be accurate, *ex post,* and he accepts the third party's *ex ante* estimates, then he will receive $P_0 \cdot q_1$, area $A$, in payments, but it will cost him $AC_2 \cdot P_1$, area $A + C$ m $E$, to produce the service. Thus, he suffers losses of $(P_2 - P_0)q_1$, area $C + E$.

The maximum risk to the negotiating parties is not symmetrical because the market risk is not symmetrical. In fact, the third party faces significantly higher risk than the provider. His maximum risk is $(P_2 - P_0)q_0$, while the provider's maximum risk is $(P_2 - P_0)q_1$. Thus, the third party's risk exceeds the provider's risk by $(P_2 - P_0)(q_0 - q_1)$, area $D + F$.

The negotiations will be bounded by the zero-risk, *ex ante* estimates of the parties, $(q_1, P_2)$ for the providers and $(q_0, P_0)$ for the third party. The agreed upon values (if an agreement is reached) will depend upon the relative bargaining strengths of the parties, and this, in turn, depends upon the political arena within which the negotiations take place. The more uncertain is the available information, the higher are the risks, and the more the participants seek to protect themselves from that risk. This risk-avoidance behavior, then, increases the divergence between the *ex ante* values as the uncertainty increases.

The risk to all parties can be minimized if expected outcomes $(q, AC)$ are known. In general, this requires knowing the frequency distributions of $q$ and $AC$ across a large number of providers. However, this is exactly the information which is not known *ex ante.* If it were known, third parties could set prices at their expected value, and while they would pay some providers more than cost, (the efficient ones), they would pay others less than cost (the inefficient ones). From the provider's perspective, this would be equivalent to paying each individual provider a price equal to his average cost. Providers would face a known price, be able to evaluate costs, *ex ante,* and make the decision of whether or not to provide the service depending upon their estimation of risk. The allocative benefit of this "ideal" process is that inefficient providers would face higher risk and would be less likely to offer the service. In any case, if the service were offered, the incentive would be to offer that service efficiently. Unfortunately, by the time such expected outcomes are known, prices have already been negotiated.

## Empirical Analysis: CAT Scanners

This section uses the above model to estimate the market and technology risks associated with the introduction and dispersion of CAT scanners. The data are those that were available in 1977—shortly after scanners were becoming widely used.[1] It represents one of the largest sets of cross-sectional data available to decision makers during the time important pricing decisions were being made. The sources of the data are

---

[1] These data were gathered while the author was a research economist at the National Association of Blue Shield Plans.

four: (1) individual provider estimates developed for certificate-of-need negotiation; (2) actual experience of general providers; (3) experience of providers who had been performing scans on an experimental basis; and (4) research activities on scanners and their costs. The total number of sources is 17. Cost and utilization estimates are presented in Table 1.

One factor that this table masks is the degree of heterogeneity in the source data. In fact, the data from the individual sources are quite diverse and difficult to standardize. Cost breakdowns varied significantly, with respect to both detail and terminology. The cost categories presented are a standardized set into which individual cost estimates were placed.

Aside from this, other sources of heterogeneity are apparent. While hospitals are the major source of information, other sources include a university, physicians, and a clinic. The type of scanner also varied, not only by type (body and head), but also by size and capability. The basis of the cost and quantity estimates also varies, with 10 sources being based upon experience, while six (6) are based upon estimates. Finally, many sources contain omitted variables. Noteworthy is the fact that eight sources provided no data on utilization, even though such information is extremely important for negotiating prices.

All of these factors introduce significant uncertainty regarding the accuracy and relevance of the available data in the negotiating process. Attempts to more fully standardize the data would merely remove observations from the already limited number available and it is not clear that doing so would improve the information available to negotiators or reduce its uncertainty.

Faced with this highly uncertain data, the model suggests that a provider's *ex ante* estimates will diverge significantly from the third party's estimates. This is indeed the case, as is pointed out below.

These data include technical costs only: they exclude the professional fee paid the radiologist for reading the scan results. Interestingly, in 1977 the Conference of Blue Shield Plans recommended that payment for the professional fees and the technical costs be determined independently. In terms of the above model, this can be viewed as a method of reducing the overpayment risk faced by these third parties. Essentially, this decision recommended partitioning the payment mechanism into two components whose information varies significantly with regard to reliability. The highly uncertain nature of technical cost is easily seen in Table 1.

While information on professional fees for CAT scans, *per se,* was likewise in short supply, there existed a method of estimating appropriate fees which embodied much less risk to the third party. This was simply a relative value approach. Interpreting the results of a CAT scan is merely interpreting the results of a sophisticated X-ray. One can determine a "fair" price by comparing the relative human capital required for the scan interpretation. Since there was accurate information on prices for reading ordinary X-rays, this could be used to set price limits on the interpretation

TABLE 1

Cost of CAT Scanner Facilities Per Year By Major Cost Category — Geographical Area

| Area | Location[1] | Type[2] | Source of Numbers[3] | (1) Equipment, Rennov.,etc. | (2) Personnel | (3) Supplies | (4) Maintenance | (5) Overhead[5] | (6) Total Tech.Cost | Number of Procedures |
|---|---|---|---|---|---|---|---|---|---|---|
| New England | hb | bs | E | $614,000 | $57,155 | $42,240 | $37,613 | $NA | $289,280 | 3200 |
| East 1 | hb | bs | E | 670,000 | 36,000 | 8,000 | 27,000 | NA | 237,160 | NA |
| East 2 | pb | bs | A | 560,000 | 30,000 | 12,000 | 40,000 | NA | 220,880 | NA |
| Atlantic 1 | hb | hs | A | 403,000 | 54,300 | 21,600[4] | NA | 45,090 | 220,934 | NA |
| Atlantic 2 | hb | bs | A | 555,875 | 48,587 | 37,674 | 44,054 | 22,291 | 290,463 | 1350 |
| Atlantic 3 | univ. | hs | A | Leased | 43,000 | 50,000 | 60,000 | 71,600 | 398,600 | 1500 |
| Atlantic 4 | hb | hs | A | 427,000 | 129,400 | 33,800 | 45,000 | 72,000 | 386,096 | 2000 |
| Atlantic 5 | hb | hs | A | 469,523 | 64,567 | 35,799 | 41,697 | 29,092 | 287,597 | 2530 |
| Southern Border States | hb | hs | LX | 425,426 | 37,500 | 40,671 | 21,271 | 45,000 | 249,948 | NA |
| Southeast | hb | bs | E | 574,400 | 36,000 | 51,000 | 30,000 | NA | 259,451 | 1300 |
| Midwest 1 | hb | hs | E | 450,000 | 45,000 | 18,750 | 21,000 | 50,000 | 244,910 | 1500 |
| Midwest 2 | pb | hs | A | 500,000 | 27,500 | 27,000 | 27,000 | 43,800 | 249,300 | NA |
| Southwest 1 | hb | bs | E | 553,500 | 19,728 | 30,660 | 40,000 | 16,358 | 243,146 | 2148 |
| Southwest 2 | hb | bs | E | 501,500 | 15,434 | 9,307 | 20,000 | 17,986 | 187,099 | 3667 |
| Northwest 1 | hb | hs | A | Leased | 24,000 | 9,000 | 24,690 | 14,000 | 182,190 | NA |
| Northwest 2 | cb | hs | A | 380,000 | 35,000 | 50,000 | 30,400 | 95,000 | 304,640 | NA |
| Northwest 3 | hb | hs | A | 372,962 | 40,000 | 27,000 | 27,055 | 66,000 | 252,550 | NA |
| Average | | | | 497,146 | 43,716 | 29,676 | 33,549 | 32,627[6] | 264,955 | 2244[7] |

[1] hb – hospital based, pb – physician based, cb – clinic based
[2] bs – body scanner, hs – head scanner
[3] E – estimated, A – actual, LX – limited experience
[4] Supplies and professional fee were combined at $121,600. It was assumed that $21,600 was the supplies cost.
[5] Where overhead was not given, no estimate was made.
[6] Because of unavailable data, the average overhead figure contained error. For this reason, average overhead was "forced" to equal average total technical cost

of CAT scans. The resulting price had a high degree of certainty and, hence, a low degree of risk. In addition, control of these fees over time could be more effectively exercised because they were not hidden in the technology costs. The analysis then excludes the determination of professional fees.

The market and technology risks are estimated using the average cost data (across providers), shown in the last row of Table 1. Average cost, $AC$, of scans is estimated as

$$AC = \frac{FC}{q} + AVC,$$

where, $FC$ is fixed cost, $AVC$ is average variable cost, and $q$ is the level of utilization—number of scans. Fixed cost is that cost which does not vary as the level of utilization varies. Variable cost does change with the level of utilization.

The fixed cost is estimated by aggregating annualized equipment and renovation, overhead, maintenance, and personnel. At the limits of operation, very low or very high personnel costs may be somewhat variable. But, in general, staffing needs tend to be constant over the relevant range of operation. In any case, because of the uncertainty involved, there were no rules for adjusting this assumption. Maintenance and overhead costs tended to be estimated on a fixed basis, such as cost of annual maintenance contracts, percentage of purchase price, space occupied, and the like. While this might to some extent vary, in the main they are fixed.

The equipment and renovation costs were used to account for the technology risk. Totals must be allocated (depreciated) on an annual basis in order to determine annual average cost. As pointed out above, selecting depreciation rates is the way that the parties attempt to compensate for the technology risk. In 1977, providers argued that rapid technological change would reduce the useful life of scanners that were then available. Thus, they sought a rapid rate of depreciation. While some variation may have occurred, providers argued that a five year write-off period was fair. This assumption is used to estimate the average cost curve which results in zero technology risk to the provider. Third parties, on the other hand, were skeptical of such rapid depreciation. One third party who generated the most information (from scanner manufactures, experimental operations, and research) argued that eight years was the reasonable write-off period. Since this was the most informed third party at the time, the eight-year period is used to calculate the average cost curve which results in zero technology risk to the third party. Eight percent was assumed to represent financing costs, since this percentage was used in many cost estimates.

The variable cost of providing scans is the supplies cost, shown in Table 1. This cost includes items such as contrast medium, syringes, magnetic tape, film, and the like. Offhand, one would think that this would be the

easiest cost to estimate and that it would be closely associated with the
utilization estimates. However, an examination of the data indicates that
this is not the case. The average supplies cost estimate is $18.78 and
ranges from $2.54 to $39.23. Such variation indicates a high degree of
uncertainty regarding *ex post* costs. Third party cost estimates, based on
consultation with radiologists and manufacturers, ranged from $2 to $5,
while a survey by researchers yielded an average cost of $14.60 [Evans and
Jost, 1977; AHA, 1977; *Health News Report,* 1977]. This analysis assumes
an average cost of $15. In any case, the significance of potential error is
small since variable cost makes up such a small percentage of average
cost. The zero-technology-risk average cost curves for providers and third
parties are estimated using the above assumptions.

$$AC_1 = \frac{\$233,184}{q} + \$15$$

and

$$AC_0 = \frac{\$194,406}{q} + \$15.$$

The zero-market-risk levels of utilization were similarly estimated for
providers and third parties. The average utilization from Table 1, for
those sources providing the information, is 2,244. Many providers, however, argued that 1,500 was the reasonable utilization. If the one high-
estimate outlier is removed, the average utilization is 2,066. When the
basis of the utilization figures are considered, the 1,500 seems to represent
*ex post* results. The average number of scans for these sources reporting
actual experience is 1,345, while that based upon *ex ante* estimates is
2,563. This may well indicate a negotiating strategy on the part of providers seeking third party approval. Providers might have viewed 1,500 as the
zero-risk level of utilization but, because of expected third party opposition in the negotiation process, might have opted to bear the market risk
of the higher estimate. For purposes of this analysis, 1,500 is assumed to
be the zero-market-risk for providers, and 2,244 will be used to estimate
the amount of market risk which providers choose to bear at the beginning of negotiations.

The zero-market-risk level of utilization for providers is assumed to be
the capacity limit of the scanner operation, assuming one shift of personnel. Estimates of capacity limits are highly uncertain because of differing
types and sizes of scanners, differing queuing mechanisms, and differing
types of practice. In addition, since CAT scanners were relatively new,
even the *ex post* information did not adequately account for the expected

increases in efficiency, due to gaining experience. The well-informed provider, mentioned above, estimated that 5,000 scans per year were reasonable to expect. However, it based this estimate upon examination of extremely efficient facilities and in consultation with manufacturers anxious to have their products approved. For these reasons, this analysis will scale down that estimate to 4,000.

All of the above assumptions were used to estimate the maximum market and technology risks of providers and third parties. This was done by evaluating the cost curves at the zero-risk levels of utilization. The results are shown in Table 2.

## TABLE 2
### Maximum, Annual Third Party and Provider Risk: Market, Technology, and Total

| Participant | Maximum Market Risk | Maximum Technology Risk | Maximum Total Risk |
|---|---|---|---|
| | $(P_1-P_o)q_0$ | $(P_2-P_1)q_0$ | $(P_2-P_o)q_0$ |
| Third Party | $324,000 | $36,000 | $424,000 |
| | $(P_1-P_o)q_1$ | $(P_2-P_1)q_1$ | $(P_2-P_o)q_1$ |
| Provider | $121,500 | $37,500 | $159,000 |

For the third party, the maximum market risk is $324,000 per year and the maximum annual technology risk is $36,000. The maximum total risk is $424,000. For the provider, maximum risks are considerably smaller. The market risk is $121,500, the technology risk is $37,500, and the total risk is $159,000.

Four points about these results should be considered. First, the market and total risks are lower for the provider because the potential errors result from overestimation of utilization, while the potential third party errors result from underestimation of utilization. If the third party overpays because the utilization is underestimated, then this overpayment is made on each scan provided. If, however, the provider is underpaid because utilization is overestimated, the cost of this underpayment is less because the actual utilization is less.

Second, the maximum total risk for the third party is more than the sum of the individual market and technology risks. This occurs because the potential overpayment of the technology risk is paid on each additional unit of utilization arising from the market risk. The total risk for the provider, however, is merely the sum of the market and technology risks.

Third, the technology risk is slightly higher for the provider than it is for the third party. This is due to the asymptotic nature of the decreasing average cost curves. At low levels of utilization, the cost difference between the curves is greater than it is at higher levels.

Fourth, it should be reiterated that these dollar risk estimates do not represent actual outcomes. Rather, they represent worst-case scenarios for each party. That is, if one party concedes to the zero-risk assumptions of the other party, then the one party's worst potential loss is the estimated values, shown in Table 2. The actual risk will be determined when prices are set in the negotiating process and will depend upon the relative bargaining strength of the two parties. The stronger party will obtain more favorable prices and, thereby, shift some potential risk to the other party.

## Implications

The analysis presented above is an attempt to describe the price-setting under a high degree of uncertainty—in this case, new medical technology which is characterized by decreasing average cost curves. In addition, it provides estimates of magnitudes of risk faced by parties in the price setting negotiations. Several inferences may be drawn from the results.

First, the commonly-heard charge that society is overpaying for new medical technology may well have a basis in logic, and, indeed, in fact. Certainly, the potential for significant overpayment exists. However, if such overpayments are significant, it is because of the failure of a political process, not a market process.

Second, errors made by third party bureaucrats (approving excessive prices) are potentially more costly than those made by providers (approving inadequate prices). The charge of significant overpayment suggests that bureaucrats are not tough enough in price negotiations with providers. This, however, is a function of the political system and is subject to incentive structures within the system. Merely changing the basis of what is negotiated, without changing bureaucratic incentives, will not likely improve the price-setting mechanism.

Third, from a negotiating strategy viewpoint, some factors deserve mention. One, because of the lower technology risk, third party negotiators may be well-advised to buy a reduction in market risk with an increased willingness to accept a higher technology risk. This would entail bargaining for a reduction in price by granting an increase in the depreciation rate. It will be recalled that zero market risk for providers occurred around 1,500 scans per year, while providers on average estimated utilization at 2,244. This indicates that providers are willing to assume about $76,500 in market risk before negotiations even begin. This shifting of risk (voluntarily) alone reduces the market risk to third parties by $184,000. Two, third parties might stage negotiations over time, obtaining agreement to set initial prices low with the promise to cover losses or adjust prices upwards as more certain information is developed. True, such retrospective reimbursement reduces the incentives for efficiency. However, in lieu of the significant potential overpayment, it may well be a small price to pay. Essentially, this is a means of reducing the third party risks to the level of the provider risk. Since risks are asymmetrical, a net reduction in total payments would occur. Three, third parties might profit from reliance on data from research and experimental facilities, rather than provider estimates. The latter are biased by the degree of uncertainty and reflect an attempt by providers to shift risk.

## REFERENCES

R. G. Evans and R. G. Jost, "Economic Analysis of Computed Tomography Units," *American Journal of Roetgenology*, July 1976.

*CT Scanners: A Technical Report*, American Hospital Association, Chicago, 1977.

*Health News Report*, Systems Corporation, Chicago, July 1977.

National Association of Blue Shield Plans, *Report*, PA-77-41, August 29, 1977.

# Chapter Twenty-Four

## Correction of Fraud, Abuse, and Waste in Health Insurance Programs in Puerto Rico

### FRANK W. FOURNIER

In order to control fraud, abuse, and waste in health insurance programs, all parties involved must begin to study the data that have been accumulated during the last decades. This paper will attempt to provide some suggestions on how to deal effectively with the problem of fraud, abuse, and waste in health insurance programs. It is based on the experience and wisdom that Seguros de Servicio de Salud de Puerto Rico (SSS), the largest health insurance carrier in Puerto Rico, has gained since it was founded in 1959.

Freiberg, in a previous chapter, pointed out two areas of abuse in health insurance programs. First, the charge that society is overpaying for new medical technology may be well-founded. Certainly, the potential for significant overpayment exists. However, if such overpayments are significant, it is because of the failure of the political process, not a market process. Second, errors made by third-party bureaucrats (approving excessive prices) are potentially more costly than those made by providers (approving inadequate prices). This charge suggests that bureaucrats are not tough enough in price negotiations with providers. However, as a function of the political system, it is subject to incentive structures within the system. Merely changing the basis of what is negotiated without changing bureaucratic incentives is not likely to improve the price-setting mechanism.

Freiberg shows the application of economic theory to an actual case of pricing for a new medical technology that could cause abuse and waste. In this case, in particular, the possibilities of abuse and waste appear in the initial stage of price negotiations between insurers and providers. The shadows of abuse and waste hinge not on wrong economic criteria but on weak negotiating skills of the third-party bureaucrats.

Freiberg is prescribing a new incentive structure that, on the one hand, could improve the negotiating skills of people in the third party and, on the other hand, would prompt reliance upon data from research and experimental facilities rather than provider estimates. This case involves an interactive relationship among four major components of the health care system: (1) the employer or purchaser; (2) the insurer; (3) the provider; and (4) the consumer.

At the conceptual level, all four components of the health care system will wholeheartedly agree that cost escalation, due to inflation, fraud, abuse, and waste is a common problem that must be tackled by all groups within the system. However, the mere recognition of a common problem or issue, although necessary, is not sufficient to deal effectively with the problem. It is also necessary to agree on the *type of intervention* needed and the *instruments* and *mechanisms* that could be utilized in intervening within the health care system.

The following section provides recommendations about the type of intervention and some of the mechanisms that could be utilized to reduce fraud and abuse.

Any intervention must be based on the principle that abuse, fraud, and waste are common problems and that, just as all components of the system must share the costs of these negative factors, so also should they enjoy the benefits when a reduction or correction occurs. Thus, a set of instruments or mechanisms of intervention should be designed and implemented that will assure fair and just distribution of costs and benefits among the four major components of the system. Those instruments generally fall into two broad categories: (1) regulations and punitive actions (negative); and (2) incentives (positive). Substantial progress has taken place in the first category. There is abundant discussion and written material on regulations against offenders. This does not imply, however, that new refinements and up–to–date approaches are not needed. On the contrary, that is a priority task. However, more time and consideration should be devoted to the development of a set of incentives geared to assure the appropriate distribution of benefits among the system's major components. Existing laws and regulations assure the allocation of costs but neglect the benefits side of the equation. If a system could be designed and implemented whereby incentives could be translated into direct monetary benefits for all parties involved, then the issue of fraud, abuse, and waste would be seen as a problem common to all components and, thus, incorporated as a common concern and priority.

SSS is trying to devise and implement a set of incentives geared to the eventual distribution of monetary benefits to its insured. The development of incentives is based on the following objectives:

1. A wise utilization of health services and facilities through preventive medicine and modification of human behavior and nutritional habits to reduce the probability of sickness, while stressing the advantages of wellness.

2. A conscientious utilization of services and facilities through ascertaining that the provider is billing for services really offered at the moment of delivery of the services.

3. An informed decision making process regarding hospitalization through open and frank discussion between physicians and patients regarding the pro's and con's of hospitalization versus ambulatory care.

The insured would receive benefits as a class, as well as individually. As a class, the insured would get more services for the same premium, less premium for the same services, or more services for less premium. The real benefits for the group will materialize in the long run. Of course, this will ultimately depend on success in communicating this strategy. In any event, this strategy is so realistic and easy to grasp, that SSS is very hopeful its insured will welcome this new approach. However, specific groups of insured could benefit in the short run, depending on their commitment to this strategy.

Electronic data processing capabilities will allow SSS to obtain accurate and timely data to assess experience by group or individual plans. This permits two modes of benefits distribution: (1) reimbursement of a portion of the premium paid at the anniversary of the contract; and (2) reduction in the premiums to be paid. The insured will become part of the solution rather than part of the problem.

Such an approach, combined with regulations and due prosecution in cases of violation, could assure the fair and just apportionment of the cost and benefits referred to before.

The incentives cannot be devised exclusively for the insured; the provider must also be given incentives. The most direct of these for the provider is a revision of the prevailing rates structure. However, any revision of the prevailing rate structure should embody some sort of deterrent for excessive use of services. The practice of ordering an excessive battery of tests and X-rays as a possible defense in a malpractice suit is pervasive. A doctor may be forgiven a more than average use of X-rays in cases where he is demonstratively protecting himself against a potential charge of malpractice. But, the consistent practice of overt abuse and waste must be detected and corrected immediately.

The adoption and implementation of a coherent set of incentives requires conciliation between the expectations of the insured and the provider. The incentives to be offered to the provider must harmonize with those offered to the insured. For instance, SSS recognizes that a greater utilization of ambulatory care, whenever adequate and appropriate, would result in cost reduction. Therefore, SSS is considering compensating doctors for the reduction in cost that a greater use of ambulatory care would produce. A preliminary estimate of the savings to be passed on to doctors is between 20 and 30 percent of the cost reduction attributable to greater use of ambulatory care.

The same approach will be utilized in other cases. For example, there are dozens of surgical procedures that can be safely performed in outpatient facilities. A portion of the reduction of costs resulting in the performance of this type of procedure outside the hospital will also be passed on to physicians. Another example is excessive prescription of medications. This practice also increases the cost of health care. There is no need to prescribe medications in excess of those required to help the patient.

Above are some techniques and approaches that may be implemented as mechanisms of intervention from the perspective of incentives. In the following section, the regulation and monitoring of activities are considered as a way of deterring fraud, abuse, and waste in health insurance.

SSS is a firm believer in incentives as a way to contain costs. Nevertheless, it recognizes that there is a need to regulate and monitor in order to avoid fraud, abuse, and waste. A great deal has been accomplished, but more must be done to crack down on abusive practices. SSS has taken several measures along these lines. Specifically, it has:

1. Established a medical service department to audit diagnostics, treatments, and procedures;

2. Identified some physicians with a persistent history of overutilization and taken measures to decertify them;

3. Reconsidered the practice of admitting all physicians that request participation in the insurance plan;

4. Considered establishing a hot line through which persons could provide information in cases of fraud, abuse, or waste. This would be in coordination with the office of the Inspector General;

5. Established a coordination mechanism with the office of the Inspector General to combat fraud and abuse in the Medicare system;

6. Considered developing computer analysis facilities to the maximum permissible by current available technology to detect cases of abuse, fraud, or waste.

In addition to these steps, SSS is aware that some legislation is necessary to eradicate the fraudulent use of insurance cards. There is an indication that unscrupulous persons are using cards belonging to other persons to obtain medical services and medications.

There is one final issue that is quite important for cost containment. Medical and hospital equipment are subject to excise and sales taxes of up to 25 percent. This alone increases tremendously the cost of operating medical facilities and contributes to increases in costs of medical services. Serious consideration should be given to exempting medical equipment from these taxes. The fiscal impact would be relatively minor, yet it would represent a big relief for consumers and providers.

Prevention is the key to correcting fraud and abuse in health insurance programs in Puerto Rico. The local medical community must be made fully aware of the proper course it should follow in the health insurance market through sustained publicity in all media. Such communication should voice an appeal to professional ethics and also publicize the effective checks utilized in post-pay systems to identify provider abuse.

The systems established to transfer money from premiums and taxes to payments for health services carry with them a responsibility to build processes to assure that money is spent only for covered services on behalf of eligible individuals for health care medically required. There is a need for stiff penalties for those who defraud or abuse the privilege of drawing on health care funds.

# Part Eight

Marketing Health Services

# Chapter Twenty-Five

## Psychographic and Life-Style Analysis in Marketing

**WILLIAM J. WINSTON**

### Introduction

Most marketing activities in health and human service organizations are implemented randomly and haphazardly. It has only been during recent years that health marketers have started to target their potential clients with any form of marketing sophistication in marketing planning activities. This sophistication has included refinement of the segmentation and targeting process in planning. This paper discusses the basic principles of using psychographic and life–style analysis for two of the most important steps in developing a marketing plan—that of segmenting and targeting. The subdividing of a human service market into distinct sections is known as "segmenting." The action of evaluating and concentrating on those segments of the marketplace which appear to be the most cost–beneficial is called "targeting." From these refined segments and targets, individualized marketing strategies can be created and implemented. In this way, the health organization can attempt to maximize its marketing efforts.

### Historical Methods of Segmentation

Segmenting a marketplace is similar to cutting a pie into many different pieces. Each piece becomes a segment which can be addressed by the health care organization. Whether one is dealing, for example, with psychiatric facilities, outpatient services, counseling agencies, hospitals, clinics, or alternative forms of health delivery systems, it has become vitally important to direct marketing endeavors to the most cost–beneficial individuals or groups.

Traditionally, segmenting a market was directed towards mass appeal. Health care attempted to be all things to all people. Unfortunately, resource constraints prevented one from being able to serve all the health needs of society. This led administrators to be more selective in allocating their precious resources. As the health industry grew, competition expanded. This stimulated health organizations to differentiate their services within the community. Human services began to identify their uniqueness in comparison to other forms of human services in the same geographic area. This differentiation was accomplished by physical features of the facilities, quality of care, types of care and service provided, types of providers involved, and even the image or positioning of the organization within their marketplaces.

Segmenting a marketplace has typically limited itself to the variables of:

*Geographic Location.* Regionalization, city size, and density;
*Demographic Factors.* Age, sex, family size, and educational level;
*Economic Factors.* Occupation, income, and wealth; and
*Social Factors.* Religion, nationality, and social class.

All segmentation variables are important in dividing up a consumer and provider marketplace. Once these segmentation processes are completed, the targeting or segment prioritizing begins. Targeting attempts to pick out primary and secondary individuals or groups within the marketplace which the health organization needs to communicate with through marketing.

Targeting has usually been divided into three main approaches:

1. *Undifferentiated Targeting:* Attempts to market services to a mass audience and to as many potential clients as possible;

2. *Differentiated Targeting:* Narrows the approach to several market segments with a common denominator of characteristics; and

3. *Concentrated Targeting:* Emphasizes marketing to a select segment(s).

Typically, segments selected are divided into primary groups which have the greatest cost–benefit ratio and potential return. Secondary segments are also grouped for long-term marketing attention.

**Classifications of Psychographics**

Marketers have long used demographic characteristics for estimating the client's propensity to consume or utilize a health service. Most of these analyses are based on "who" and "what" characteristics rather than "why" clients use services. Psychographics and life–style variables attempt to complement demographic, economic, and social variables in selecting the promising target groups.

*Psychographics* may be viewed as the practical application of the behavioral and social sciences to marketing characteristics of clients and patients based upon their life–style, attitudes toward health services, interests and opinions, and personality traits and perceptions of the services and products' attributes. These characteristics definitely cross the socio-economic boundaries to develop a *client profile* of consumer belief and attitude towards select services. This analysis is especially useful in the initial stage of marketing planning.

*Psychographic and life–style* analysis can be divided into four specific categories:

1. *Psychological Attributes:* These answer basic questions related to: (a) What kind of individual a client is?; (b) How does a client perceive him-

self?; and (c) Why do clients do the things they do? Most of the attributes include *personality* traits. These traits are related to populations being: aggressive, gregarious, ambitious, creative, risk–taking, passive, depressed, abused, disciplined, competitive, resistant to change, and others. For example, stereotypic comments, such as, "Clinics are to be used only by those of lower social classes" and "Only seriously ill individuals use hospitals" are derived from people's psychographic attributes.

Some examples of targeting these characteristics include:

(A) Targeting employee assistance programs to human relations oriented corporations;

(B) Targeting mental health programs to those sectors which do not possess barriers or mental stigmas in terms of being receptive to mental health;

(C) Preventive dentistry programs to career–minded groups;

(D) Cosmetic surgery to groups who possess a need for ego-gratification;

(E) Family physicians to people in the community who are security–minded and want a long–term relationship with a family doctor;

(F) Risk reduction programs to anxiety–minded groups; and

(G) Home–care diagnostic equipment to inventive or self–disciplined groups.

2. *Life–Style Variables:* Life–style attributes of a client population involves an examination of people's allocation of time and resources for themselves and their families. The various activities that an individual participates or not participates in becomes the framework for developing a *life–style profile.* Some life–style variables that become important are: relaxation activities, dress, athletic activities, political involvement, work habits, daily routine, eating and drinking characteristics, travel, community involvement, hobbies, and cultural endeavors. These attributes formulate a *life–style sketch* or *portrait* of individuals or groups in their interests, opinions, and attitudes.

Some examples of targeting these characteristics are:

(A) Sportcare programs to the athletic sector of the community;

(B) Weight control programs to those exhibiting poor eating habits or those interested in appearance;

(C) Stress programs to workaholics in the workplace;

(D) Occupational safety programs to high–risk occupations in the community;

(E) Portable exercise equipment to frequent business travelers; and

(F) Biofeedback and wellness programs to those interested in relaxation as part of their life–styles.

3. *Behavioristic* or *Purchasing Variables:* These variables evaluate a person's purchasing habits. A person can obtain a health service based on

their: regularity of purchase, user status, loyalty strength, level of need for service, benefits of service perceived, and motivation for utilization. Clients develop characteristic utilization patterns for different reasons. These purchasing variables can mean the difference, for example, of a client returning or making a referral.

Examples of targeting include:

(A) Target to heavy users based on their commonality of demographics, personality traits, and so forth;

(B) Target media ads to heavy users for continuation of referrals. There is an 80/20 rule usually in health services which depicts that 20 percent of a patient base makes 80 percent of the referrals. This group is usually neglected;

(C) Target select benefits of the service to cost–conscious and benefit–seeking groups. Bundling of services for one price can be effective in marketing to these cost–benefit minded groups;

(D) Target more educational strategies to those groups who are not aware of the service or motivated yet to use it; and

(E) Target strategies to constantly remind groups who are sporadic users about the existence and usefulness of the service. It usually takes four to five repetitions of communicating with the same groups before they try your service.

4. *Service Attributes and Perceptions:* Lastly are the perceptions people develop towards select physical or psychological characteristics of a service. For example, price and value aspects are the foundation for the question of "Are these trips to the doctor worth it?" Taste factors are depicted in the comment that, "This cough medicine tastes like cherry." Quality is the basis for the comment, "Only the best physicians are associated with this health center." Benefits derived from the service are important in the statement, "I feel so much better after my physical." Trust is the underlying factor in the statement, "I need to rest daily as my doctor prescribed."

Examples of targeting include:

(A) Market the quality of the medical staff to quality–conscious groups;

(B) Market the ease of parking and public transportations to those groups interested in access;

(C) Market the availability of monthly payment plans or credit to cost–conscious groups;

(D) Market the professional image of the service to those groups interested in the trust factor;

(E) Market the pleasant surroundings to groups interested in atmospherics;

(F) Market the modern technology available to groups identified as interested in quality of care and receiving the most modern techniques and service; and

(G) Market the lack of waiting time to get services to groups interested in speed of service or smooth triage systems.

## Benefits

By psychographic and life-style marketing, the health administrator can construct an operating model of the attitudes and activity processes that the organization's marketing and technical capabilities can serve. This approach can provide an orientation to the health service's market that no statistical description of its demographics can provide. This gives the health administrator a chance to not just *know* the markets, but to virtually *become* part of the market by understanding its humanistic characteristics.

The results of using this type of targeting are to:

1. Restimulate existing services which are being utilized below their capabilities;

2. Identify and develop new client needs and, thus, new services; and

3. Strengthen the financial viability of the health organization and serve the clients and patients cost-effectively.

Psychographic and life-style marketing are rooted in market needs. Since these characteristics are built up over a period of years, they can be researched, modeled, planned, and marketed to over a period of time. Understanding emerging life-styles and forecasting their impact on developing market segments is becoming a major concern of health marketers.

One manifestation of a psychographic and life-style change is the emergence of smaller segments within the health marketplace. Health marketers are gradually learning that they need to measure the performance of new services whose only differences may be positioning. Gradually, there will be fewer really new breakthroughs in health services. New services are likely to be in existing categories, with only minor benefits differentiating them in the eyes of the consumer. Positioning, target identification, and media effectiveness will dictate service success. As health service positioning becomes more precise, target identification will become very important. The main question will be "Who is the real user of the services and have we communicated to them and motivated them positively?" The answer to this key question will require the use of understanding and relating to the consumer through psychographic and life-style analysis.

The process that was described is the first step in a new service development phase that attempts to meet the needs of the clientele. By identifying the population target by socio-demographic characteristics first, life-styling the group based on the four categories of psychographic profiling, and discerning what service opportunities can be generated to fill health gaps, new service development is initiated. These new services can supplement, complement, or replace existing services.

When psychographic and life–styling has been identified, it is divided into distinct life–style roles. These outcomes are the net result of life–style marketing. Thus, these roles become the select target groups which the health organization must address. Each target group is then prioritized and ranked according to its apparent potential and organizational constraints. By targeting in this fashion, the health organization is able to reposition itself in the marketplace. Repositioning allows the organization to be perceived in a fresh, new light by its clients and patients. Repositioning could, for example, make the organization the leader in a specific new service.

**Conclusion**

Life–styles are changing very quickly during this current decade. These pressures for change create major impacts on people's attitudes, perceptions, and life–styles. The alterations in people's psychographics leads to a need for sensitivity when marketing health services.

Psychographic and life–style information can complement each other. The demographic information can describe the physical attributes, while psychographic and life–style data can analyze the psychological and emotional aspects of the health consumer. Each marketing strategy can be organized to meet the needs indicated in the psychographic and life–style profile. In other words, the marketing mix components of price, product, place, and promotion can be specifically designed to meet the psychographic and life–style needs of the consumer.

Psychographic and life–style targeting is an essential ingredient for a successful marketing program. This is especially true in today's environment of scarce financial resources for health care. As health marketers become more adept in analytically selecting marketing targets, the use of psychographic targeting will increase. Based on these advanced statistical tools, it will be constantly possible to determine market information about the relationship between the consumer's life–style and health service utilization.

# Chapter Twenty-Six

## Entrepreneurial Aspects of Health Care

**PAUL F. DETRICK**

Is there a crisis in health care today? One frequently hears this thought projected. Frankly, this author does not believe that there is a crisis. One only has a crisis when situations develop that people are not able to deal with; but the author believes that health care professionals are capable of handling problems they are faced with today. For the most part, society feels that it is probably uncontrolled, increasing costs and poor management in health care institutions. In some cases, this might be the situation. As costs increase, many third parties are endeavoring to control them by merely tightening the purse strings of reimbursement. One needs to look at the entire picture when talking about the cost of health care.

As one looks at the crunch being placed on hospitals and health care delivery in general, several things must be recognized. The inflationary factor of increasing costs and the technical advances have been fantastic in the last 15-20 years. In fact, health care as it is delivered today, is nowhere comparable to the type of care that was delivered just 20 years ago. The industrial community that has negotiated health care for the employees of their various firms must be looked at. When health care was first included in union contracts, it was an inexpensive item that could be added to company benefits without greatly affecting overall cost. Also, in many cases, health institutions were financed, in large part, through charitable contributions. However, as it became necessary for hospitals to stand on their own financial legs, as technical advances came about, and as salary increases became effective, costs became an important factor to every business in the world, especially in the United States. Tremendous pressure was being placed on more efficient operations to cut fat out of the delivery system; if purse strings could just be tightened, hospitals would operate more efficiently. If this were the case, to the extent that it was believed, government agencies endeavoring to cut health care costs would not have encountered the extreme difficulties that they have. Only now are government officials beginning to recognize that hospitals are not expensive because of inefficiencies, but because of the quality and the unique type of service rendered.

The intent here is not to complain about the pressing problems of realities: the tightening of purse strings, or the fact that people do not understand the situation. It is absolutely necessary, as it was in 1965 with the advent of Medicare and Medicaid in the United States, that a hard look be taken at health organizations. What are the problems? What are the strengths and weaknesses? What is being done and what can be done?

In the past, the hospital fairly well maintained its activities within the four walls of the physical plant. This cannot be the case in the future. It is necessary for survival that expansion and movement into the community and other activities occur.

Health care institutions of the present are changing shape. The business magazine, *D and B Reports,* states [Swartz, 1983, p. 14]: "The days of America's nonprofit hospitals as just hospitals are over." Figure I shows the typical hospital as an independent entity and a centralized organization with a single purpose: care of patients admitted into the hospital [MacEachern, 1962, p. 84]. This purpose must be maintained as the primary objective of hospitals, even today. In order to survive, reevaluation and readjustment of organizational structures and ways of thinking must take place.

Many individual health care institutions typify the dramatic changes occurring in the industry. One example is Baylor Health Care Systems in Dallas. It is a holding corporation that controls, not only the Baylor University Medical Center, but also three professional buildings, a construction company, a 75-room hotel, a high volume gasoline station, two restaurants, a post office, a laboratory, a visual testing center, a physical fitness center, and an off-shore insurance company [Swartz, 1983, p. 14]. Another example is Fairview Community Hospital in Minneapolis. It is the parent corporation for eight wholly-owned hospitals with more than 40 other participating hospitals under contracts in nine midwestern and western states, in Western Europe, and the Middle East [Fairview, 1982]. Other diversified enterprises include contracts for management information systems and materials management. Fairview Community Hospital has also invested in retirement housing projects.

In the for-profit sector, which was, at one time, a bad name in health care delivery is one of the fastest growing corporations in America today, Hospital Corporation of America (HCA). The corporation successfully challenged the myth that the bigger the company, the more apt it is to be inefficient and complacent. HCA was founded in 1968, as an attempt to infuse more capital for expansion into Park View Hospital in Nashville, with the thought of entering the hospital management business to spread cost. Within 10 years, HCA grew to over 100 hospitals. Today, it is a giant of the industry, owning or managing more than 370 hospitals with over 53,000 beds around the world [HCA, 1982].

In the early 1950's, the Kaiser Health Program of California was thought by many to be a radical program which certainly was not something with which to be affiliated. Today, this type of program serves, in many cases, as the ultimate example. What has really prompted this kind

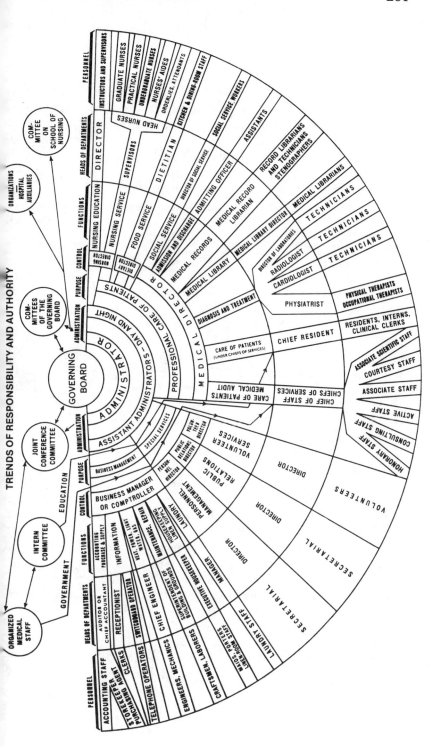

of growth and diversification in the health care field? A great deal can be traced back to the fact that hospital finances must be stabilized. A hospital must carry its own weight and stand on its own feet. Leaders, of these and other successful health care institutions, have long been aware that the hospital average of .8 percent return on gross revenue leaves no room for expansion [Swartz, 1983, p.14]. Even the more select subset of hospitals, which has been profitable for the most part, has shown only an aggregate 5 percent return on gross revenues over the past few years. The outlook for the solitary acute institution standing alone is not bright. A report by the American Hospital Association (AHA) predicts the following results through prospective payment controls [AHA, 1983]:

> "By capping the amount of money paid to hospitals and establishing linkages between the product purchased (DRG) and the price paid, the Health Care Financing Administration expects the new payment system to reduce expenditures by $1.5 billion in fiscal year 1984."

This new method of payment is the Prospective Reimbursement or DRG (Diagnosis Related Groups), wherein a fixed price would be established by a government agency to reimburse hospitals (and physicians in the future) based on diagnosis, rather than length of stay or individual service rendered. This will draw the financial solvencies of individual hospitals into even more critical review. These fiscal realities of life have prompted health care institutions to branch out into other enterprises, which are usually related, but not necessarily, to health care or its delivery. These ventures are usually separate from the acute care institution, but are legally affiliated, either by partnerships, overlapping boards of directors, restructured holding companies and subsidiary organizations.

This is what was done at Christian Health Services Development Corporation in St. Louis! These ventures appeal to many health care managers because of the promise of a higher return on investments. The profits from these enterprises provide capital which may be channeled back into the acute care system, not only for the delivery of care, but for the development of additional opportunities. This diversification gives strength in many ways. It makes it possible to deal with third party reimbursement groups from a stronger position. It strengthens purchasing program, because it generates larger contracts for such items as linen, food, and drugs. It gives the corporation political strength in dealing with legislation. It also gives the corporation financial strength in dealing with the money market and capital financing.

Certain changes came to Christian Hospital of St. Louis, which improved its corporate restructuring. Founded in 1903 as a 12-bed hospital, it grew over the years, and later merged into Christian Hospital Northeast-Northwest, which is now a two-division hospital consisting of

---

¹ The author would like to express appreciation to Bruce Gosser, Assistant Administrator, Christian Hospital Northeast-Northwest, who assisted in the research for the chapter.

725 acute care beds. About 10-12 years ago, maintenance contract costs became quite high, and it was decided to undertake maintaining the equipment in house. More skilled technicians were hired to maintain the equipment, and some of these services were marketed in order to spread the cost. From this idea, a very active shared service program was developed.

In 1980, it became important for Christian Hospital Northeast-Northwest to diversify because of possible changes in public policy; financial viability would not be maintained through operations of acute care hospitals alone. Objectives were defined, along with the manner of achieving those objectives. After studying what was to be accomplished, a holding company was organized. Figure II shows the parent corporation and its six subsidiaries. These include a two-division, acute care hospital (Christian Hospital Northeast-Northwest); a life care center, with a skilled nursing home facility (Village North, Inc.); a network of ambulatory care centers (CH Allièd Services, Inc.); a contract management company, which manages other small hospitals in the surrounding region (Christian Health Care Systems, Inc.); a preferred provider organization (Metro-North Health Care Corporation); and a real estate company in which ownership of much of the property rests (Christian Health Services Properties Foundation). The parent corporation, Christian Health Services Development Corporation, has overall responsibility. General, overall direction of activities, overall corporate financing, and long-range planning and development is the responsibility of the parent company.

Many organizations are successful in adjusting to the changing economic environment. To ignore these changes can only lead to disaster. Diversification is a must. Diversification or reorganization, however, is not a remedy for all the ills of every institution, nor is it the thing that every institution ought to do. The life of a free-standing hospital is limited in the United States, and, in the years to come, it will become necessary through various types of affiliations and associations for hospitals to bind together. Financial advisor, Fred Hyde, is among those who has cautioned against hasty or ill-timed reorganization in the health care field. He raised six critical questions [Hyde, 1983]:

1. Does the move to diversify help the hospital system, or other institutions, fulfill its basic mission?
2. Will this effort divert management talent from the basics of running a good hospital?
3. How will success be measured in the new or newly organized fields?
4. Is the organization ready to spend a dollar to earn a dollar?
5. Is the business organized properly?
6. Are the right people involved?

These are primary items that need to be investigated, prior to moving into reorganization.

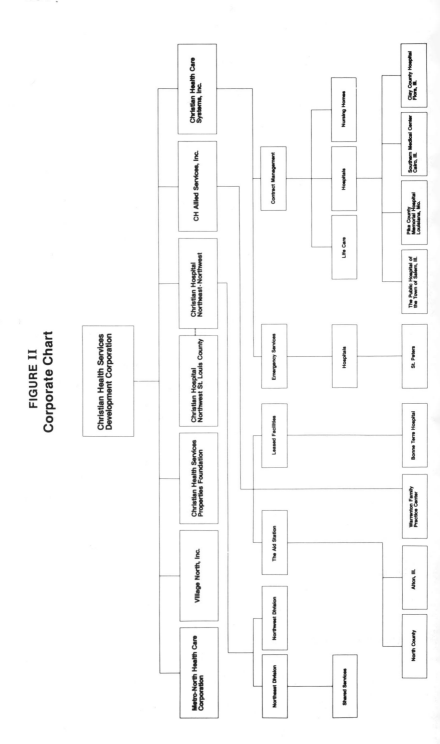

FIGURE II
Corporate Chart

There are many advantages for hospitals moving toward diversification and reorganization:

1. Political strength.
2. The ability to spread costs over a broader base, thus reducing per diem or per patient cost.
3. The opportunity to bring services to smaller institutions that might not have been able to afford them.
4. The ability to preserve financial stability.
5. The opportunity to limit liabilities.
6. The ability to develop management personnel.
7. The ability to employ and develop highly specialized and skilled personnel.
8. The ability to present life-time employment to personnel through advancement, thus reducing cost of turnover.

To the contracted hospitals, it is felt that it is now possible for them to have services they might not otherwise be able to afford. These hospitals have political strength through association. The hospitals can obtain expertise in a particular field, whether it be medical, technical, administrative, or financial, that they would not have been able to afford. Much needed services have been brought to small communities which would have had a difficult time acquiring them otherwise. Life care programs have been brought to a group that is many times forgotten.

Health executives should not ring their hands in despair and feel that the world is caving in. There are problems that need to be met. The author has the greatest confidence in health executives, not only of the United States, but throughout the world, in their ability to meet and solve these problems. It is absolutely imperative to grow and develop within changing external and internal environments. Health executives must look outside the four walls of their institutions to what the community needs, what its strengths and needs are, and determine whether the hospital can develop, modify, or change some of its activities to fill a need in the area. It is absolutely necessary that each new service be evaluated and viewed as any other business would evaluate a new service or a new product: is it needed; can it be delivered practically; and is this a financially viable undertaking?

The lesson to be learned is that health executives have to get out of their offices, out of the traditional image, and into the business world. Health care is one of the largest industries in the world today. There are many ways in which health executives are needed and many challenges to be met. They must constantly scan the horizon and not be afraid to do the unusual or the different. Evaluate it well and be ready to adjust to changing times.

## REFERENCES

American Hospital Association Report, "The Impact of the Medicare Prospective Payment Systems and DRGs on Hospital Leaderships," *The Hospital Research and Educational Trust,* 1983.

Fairview Community Hospitals, *Annual Report,* 1982.

Hospital Corporation of America, *Annual Report,* 1982.

Fred B. Hyde, "The Financial Exchange," *Trustee,* November 1983.

Malcolm T. MacEachern, *Hospital Organization and Management,* Berwyn, Illinois: Physicians' Record Company, 1962.

Herbert Swartz, "Hospitals Diversify to Beat the Budget Crunch," *D and B Reports,* September/October 1983.

# Part Nine

Case Studies and Analyses

# Chapter Twenty-Seven

## Technique for Cost Effective Patient Scheduling

KYTJA K. S. VOELLER,
WILLIAM CLEGG,
ETHEL M. WILCOX,
ROBERT STRAUB,
CHRIS ELEVICH

## Introduction

The time available for outpatient appointments represents an expensive commodity: there are fixed costs (heat, light, space, telephone, and manpower costs), as well as variable costs (generating letters and processing laboratory specimens). Because most of the costs are fixed, losses are likely to be substantial if the clinic does not run close to capacity. On the other hand, consistent overbooking carries with it other costs: patients may walk out and seek care elsewhere; the staff may become overwhelmed, tired, and inefficient. The problem is analogous to that of an airline which faces heavy fixed costs if a jet liner takes off half–full but must pay penalties for overbooking. There have been various methods suggested to devise an optimal booking level for a given clinic—but these generally do not attempt to develop a formula to predict a no–show rate for a given clinic day, but rather assume, if anything, a fixed no–show rate. This often results in erroneous predictions because the no–show rate can be so variable.

The present study describes a method of developing an overbooking formula, using a statistical analysis of multiple variables. Although tailored to a specific clinic population, the technique is applicable to any clinic setting, permitting the calculation of an appropriate level of overbooking, thus minimizing the costs of under– and overutilization.

## Methods

Two thousand consecutive patient appointments to a busy university hospital subspecialty ambulatory care unit which took place over a 10 ½ month period were reviewed. Patients who resided in institutions or came under a court order were excluded from consideration. The study ultimately focused on the appointment-keeping behavior of 351 patients. The following variables were recorded for each patient: location of residence from clinic in miles; phone/no phone at home; type of medical insurance; father's and mother's occupation using a modified Hollingshead scale; father's and mother's educational level in years; and new or return clinic appointments.

An estimation of the severity of the patient's medical problem was pro-

289

vided by the "physician severity rating" in which the physician's assessment of the need for medical care was assigned a numerical rating. The dependent variable was the ratio of missed to kept appointments (mean $0.229 \pm 0.200$, Skewness 0.933). The data were then subjected to a multiple regression computer analysis utilizing the SPSS program. A formula was then developed which made it possible to determine the number of patients to overbook by determining the probability of no–shows for any given clinic day, by summing the individual no–show probabilities, and using that to calculate the appropriate number of patients to overbook. The formula was then tested by applying it retrospectively.

### Results

*Place of Residence.* The patient's residence had been categorized as ranging from 0–to–1; 1–to–2; 2–to–3; 3–to–5; 5–to–7; and 7–to–10 miles from the hospital. Thereafter, increments of 5 miles up to 30; 30–to–50; 50–to–75; and 75 and over, were used. From Figure I, it can be seen that there was a bimodal distribution with 18 percent of the patients living in the 3–to–5 mile zone and 19.7 percent living within a 30–to–50 mile zone. A somewhat smaller number (10 percent) lived within the 25–to–30 mile zone.

*Type of Third Party Insurance.* Type of insurance was broken down into none (only 2 percent of the patients had no insurance); insurance in which there was likely to be a self–pay component (22.8 percent); medicaid–welfare–ADC (25.6 percent); the state Crippled Children's Insurance (10.5 percent); and other forms of commercial insurance, which often picked up an outpatient charge (38.7 percent). Thus, only a small number of patients had no insurance and approximately equal numbers had some form of state or federally funded payment for medical care or commercial insurance, which generally covered outpatient costs.

*Father's Educational Level.* Of those studied, 42.7 percent of the fathers had 12 years of education and approximately 30 percent had an educational background above that level.

*Mother's Educational Level.* The average educational attainment of the mothers was also at a high school level and, again, 30 percent had some college or technical school thereafter.

*Age of Patients.* The patients ranged in age from infants to those over 21 years of age. Those under 5 years were 22 percent; 50 percent were in the 5–12 year old bracket; and 27.7 percent were in the 12 years and above bracket (this category of patients was included because of the possibility that it might be easier or harder for an adolescent to attend the clinic).

*Significant Variables.* Two variables were identified as significant: the physician's severity rating (the greater the severity of the illness as viewed by the physician, the less likely the parent was to miss the appointment); and the mother's education in years (the higher the educational level, the less likely the mother was to miss the appointment).

FIGURE I

RELATIONSHIP OF OVERBOOKING TO COST

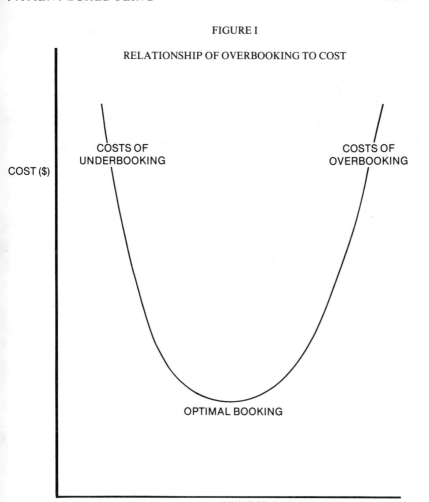

These variables were then placed into the following equation: Y = a - b - c, where Y = ratio of appointments missed; a = constant; b = severity as perceived by physician (the greater the severity, the *less* likely to miss); and c = mother's education in years (the higher the educational level, the *less* likely to be a no-show). The results were:

$$Y = 0.44543 - 0.0156 - 0.01265.$$

The formula was then applied retrospectively to a number of clinic sessions and the question was asked: had the clinic overbooked according to the formula, would it have run the sessions closer to an optimal level? The method was as follows: (1) The no-show probability for each individual was determined by reading off a table constructed for this purpose (the physician's severity rating was on the X-axis and the mother's education in years was on the Y-axis); (2) The individual no-show probabilities were summed and divided by the total number of patients scheduled for the clinic, the total number of patients scheduled was then divided by, 1.00 - average probability of absence (from Step 2).

The probability of missing an appointment ranged from a high of .329 (mother's educational level 8 years; physician's severity rating 1) to a low of .068 (mother's education level 20 years; physician's severity rating 8). However, these extremes were rarely encountered.

Table 1 shows the information obtained from the overbooking formula, retrospectively. The use of the formula would be to increase the number of patients scheduled. Thus, had the clinic staff utilized the overbooking formula, we would have scheduled 20 patients for Clinic Session #1, 16 patients for clinic session #2, and 21 patients for Session #3.

### TABLE 1
#### Overbooking Formula with Retrospective Data

| Clinic Session | Av. No. Show Probability | No. of Patients Scheduled | Calc. No. of Patients | No. of Patients Predicted | Actual No. of Patients |
|---|---|---|---|---|---|
| #1 | 0.239 | 15 | 19.7 | 11.4 | 13 |
| #2 | 0.237 | 12 | 15.7 | 9.2 | 10 |
| #3 | 0.245 | 16 | 21.2 | 12.1 | 11 |

### Analysis

There is a large literature on effective methods of patient scheduling. Patient scheduling relates to two general factors: (1) the total number of patients relative to the no-show rate; and (2) the sequencing or timing of patient visits. The studies on factors governing no-show rates generally relate to specific causes for failure to keep scheduled appointments and methods (such as mailed or telephone reminders) to improve appointment keeping. There are few studies which attempt to establish a probability of no-show within a given clinic setting and overbook on the basis of that probability. The studies which deal with appropriate booking of patient visits generally ignore the issue of the no-show rate or assume that it is constant.

Based on a population in which the no-show rate is generally better than average, it is not rational to attempt to assume that it is constant from day-to-day. To make this assumption will result in costly under- or overutilization of the ambulatory care resources. To underbook means that one may not even reach a break-even point because of the high-fixed costs inherent in an ambulatory care setting. However, at a certain point, overbooking (unless one is dealing with a virtual monopoly) results in a loss of patients. With the current market situation in medicine becoming more competitive, it is appropriate to scrutinize some of the variables which result in optimal numbers of patients to be booked within a clinical setting. Unless there is an appropriate number of patients to schedule within a given time slot, there is little sense in developing an elaborate method of sequencing patient appointments.

It was of particular interest that some of the variables which would seem to be of great significance had, in reality, little effect on the no-show rate. Such factors were the distance the patient lived from the clinic or the financial (insurance, self-pay, federal-state funding) status. Even very great distances did not appear to have any effect on the patients' reliability in keeping clinic appointments; or were such factors as self-pay, third party, or federal-state health care funding. The age of the child appeared to have little bearing on appointment-keeping. The father's educational level, although identical or close to that of the mother, also did not appear to have a bearing. The mother's educational level, however, was an important factor. This further supports the observation that women in the United States are selectors of health care settings. It would appear that women are also the prime movers when it comes to bringing a child to a clinic. The physician's severity rating was also an important factor.

The factors that the authors identified and the overbooking formula that has evolved from them involves some complex sociological and socio-psychological variables. It is probably not surprising that only one of the factors (the physician's severity rating) has anything to do with the patient's medical status. This further substantiates the impression that there are many other factors besides medical care involved in the practice of medicine.

There has been an extensive study of the determinants of failed appointments. The most thorough recent review that the authors were able to locate was that of Deyo and Inui, which summarizes the current information available on the subject. They were able to identify a list of factors which are determinants of broken appointments. These involve general categories of demographic, socio-behavioral features related to the provider; features of the disease and of the therapeutic regimen; patient-therapist interaction; access factors; facilities and administrative process; and environment. Deyo and Inui report that low socio-economic status correlates in a fairly consistent fashion with broken appointments. Race, *per se,* is probably unimportant when one accounts for other variables such as age, education, and socio-economic status. There appear to be inconsistent results with regard to the source of payment, but there is a trend that the amount of out-of-pocket payment at the time care is sought is of some importance, while the source is not.

The patient's understanding of his therapy appears to correlate with appointment keeping, so that educational efforts seem to improve broken

appointment rates. Very little information is available for provider characteristics (such as continuity of care, sex and age of clinician, racial differences in patient–therapist care, physicians versus nurse practitioners, or
physician assistants). Features of the patient's illness appear pertinent.
Patients with psychiatric diagnosis have a higher rate of failed appointments. Duration of illness is generally unimportant, but patients with
chronic disease have been found by other investigators to have fewer
broken appointments than patients with acute illnesses. Deyo and Inui
also pointed out that distance from the clinic did not affect appointment
keeping, which is consistent wth this study's findings.

The other issue relates to the presence of symptoms or a specific concern (called by Sackett a complainent patient—symptomatic—or a lan-
thanic—asymptomatic—patient). With clinical improvement, there is a
trend to higher dropout rates. There is a good correlation between the
provider's view of the importance of the appointment and failed appointment rates and this study certainly supports that observation. If the provider felt this was an urgent situation, the rate of appointment keeping
was generally higher. When medication is prescribed there are generally
higher rates of appointment keeping, but these are depressed with cost
duration and side effects. It is worth noting that compliance with a medication regimen does not appear to be related to the frequency of keeping
appointment visits. Administrative factors, such as clinic waiting time,
also appear to be an important determinant.

It is obvious that when one is dealing with such a multitudinous array
of factors, which also appear to vary in their impact on appointment
keeping from situation to situation, that probably not all the factors operate within a specific clinic. For this study's clinic population, the authors
approached this empirically by attempting to see which of a number of
factors were critical determinants in a patient's appointment–keeping
behavior. A whole array of considerations was reviewed and subjected to
a statistical analysis of multiple variables, which automatically discarded
factors of relatively little importance in this particular setting. It is obvious
that a clinic which deals with children, many of whom are on chronic
medication, would probably have a different array of factors determining
appointment keeping than either an adult psychiatric or medical clinic.

**Conclusions**

The power of the present method is that it enables the manager to
identify the factors that are operating for a specific patient population and
work them into a formula which permits one to determine, for a given
clinic setting, the likelihood of no–shows and overbook accordingly. This
particular formula would not work for any other setting, but the overall
approach can be applied in general. It provides a rational way of predicting patient visits, on any given day, and estimating the number of additional patient visits that need to be scheduled.

Although laborious by hand, this can be easily programmed into a computer and, once the data are in place, the information can be obtained within just a few minutes.

Several comments are in order. First, it appeared that there was little variability in the probability of no-shows in the clinic studied; this fell in the range of 0.237 to 0.245 for the particular clinic sessions examined. Future studies will evaluate a number of clinic sessions, both retrospectively and prospectively, to see if there is a major change in the probability of no-shows from one clinic session to another. An estimate will be made of the probabilities of no-showing for those patients would be in the range of 0.03, according to an intuitive estimation, and this would be built into future clinic schedules.

Second, one could not have identified the probability of not keeping appointments by retrospectively calculating no-show rates from previous clinics, as the no-show rate in the clinic studied varied from 0 to 20 percent. If one were to attempt to use an average value, it is likely that there would be frequent miscalculations for a given clinic day.

There are obviously several problems with information that is used to calculate the probabilities for individual patients. First, in certain circumstances, it is not the mother that brings the child, and this will result in perturbations in the calculations. It may be possible to calculate what factors would determine a relative's willingness to bring the child if there were a significant number of children in this category. Another factor is that the mother's educational level is not one that is regularly part of the data base in every pediatric specialty clinic setting. The authors have this information in their files because of a data base that parents are requested to fill out as they enter the system.

A third factor is that the physician's severity ratings can shift rather abruptly, in some instances. A patient who was initially quite ill can be reclassified in a less acute category and one who is not seriously ill may suddenly become so. Fortunately, these factors, which would weaken the validity of the overbooking formula, do not occur frequently enough to have a significant effect on the calculations.

The usefulness of the present overbooking formula is that it permits a relatively easy and reliable method to calculate the number of patients that should be overbooked for any given clinic session. In a clinic in which there is a relatively small number of patients scheduled for a given session, the application of the formula probably has little impact on the total fiscal scene. However, in larger clinics where a large number of patients are seen daily, the application of the overbooking formula (which can be facilitated by using a computer) would provide an inexpensive and cost-effective method of utilizing the resources of the clinic. When combined with the more sophisticated methods of scheduling patients for given appointment slots (utilizing a linear programming technique or a variable time slot system), there is the potential for substantial cost savings and effective utilization of the available resources. Certainly, as health care delivery becomes more competitive, it is likely that these factors will become of increasing significance.

At the present time, the investigators are developing a three–variable model and are seeking to apply it prospectively to the booking problem.

## REFERENCES

Richard A. Deyo and Thomas S. Inui, "Dropout and Broken Appointments: A Literature Review and Agenda for Future Research," *Medical Care*, 18, 1980, pp. 1146-57.

D.L. Sackett, "Magnitude of Compliance and Non-Compliance," *Compliance with Therapeutic Regimen*, D.L. Sackett and R.B. Haines, ed., Baltimore: Johns Hopkins University Press, 1976.

# Chapter Twenty-Eight

## Labor Productivity In a Rural Hospital

### P. DONALD MUHLENTHALER

### Introduction

This study took place in a 144 bed, general–acute, county–owned hospital on the western edge of a major midwestern metropolitan area. The hospital is 24 years old and is governed by a Board of Trustees appointed County Commissioner. The institution started with 50 beds and has grown steadily in order to meet the needs of the county's population of 35,000 with a service area reaching to the west totaling 50,000.

The extended service area is extremely rural. There is heavy industry and a developing suburban base close to the hospital. The institution is the only hospital in the county, with the nearest hospitals to the west, over 50 miles away. The nearest hospitals to the east are located 20 miles away, in the metropolitan area and are major medical centers.

The hospital has prided itself in keeping a low–cost profile and in keeping rate increases below that of inflation. In 1978, the institution's volume dropped significantly, the hospital was not prepared to deal with it, and thus lost money. At the same time, the hospital was also in the middle of a $6 million building project which was underfunded by $200,000. It was hoped that this funding would be created from depreciation, however, with the loss in volume, the depreciation was used to cover payroll.

In 1979, the first mortgage payment of over $300,000 was due and there were no funds available. The writer became Executive Director of the hospital in December 1978. A large price increase in March 1979, a much higher volume than anticipated, a cost reduction program, and a hiring freeze during 1979, caused the hospital's financial position to be much improved.

### Problem

In mid–1979, the hospital was extremely busy and volume was much higher than anticipated. The hiring freeze was being maintained in order to stabilize the financial base. The 1980 budget was in preparation and many of the department heads were demanding more personnel to handle the higher volume. However, justification for these additional employees was weak.

The Executive Director knew that he must control the hospital's labor cost because the rising volume may not hold and may, in fact, return to 1978 levels. He wished to put in place a management system to control the payroll with the fluctuating volumes of the institution.

The Executive Director had worked previously in New Jersey with that Hospital Association's Productivity Audit and Review (PAR) System. He felt that this system gave good labor cost control to the administration and wished to implement a similar system at the hospital. However, he was aware that in this area it would be most difficult to get people to accept a system that was developed in New Jersey and implemented by individuals from that area. He knew that the system needed to grow from this region in order that department heads and the Board of Trustees could take pride in the ownership of it. Another anticipated difficulty was the overall attitude in the institution, based on a "we have always done it that way" philosophy.

He was also aware that the system was needed much faster than could be totally grown in-house. Alternatives, therefore, were sought for the system's development and it was found that in the metropolitan area one of the large medical centers had significant experience in the management engineering approach to the overall operation of a hospital. This medical center agreed to provide management engineering consultation to the hospital. It was to be on an as needed basis in the beginning and decreasing to approximately one day a week upon implementation.

### Decision

The Executive Director then had to obtain approval from the Board of Trustees of the hospital, consisting of four small businessmen, to hire consultants for the purpose of implementing a labor productivity monitoring system. The board was leery of this kind of system but followed the Executive Director's advice and approved employing the consultants necessary to implement the system.

In implementing this decision, a meeting was first held with the consultants and the hospital's department heads to explain the general approach to the system. The system was to measure a department's productivity by calculating hours needed to do the work and measuring it against hours actually taken to do the work. It was explained that since the system was volume related it would assist the manager in doing his job. It would tell him or her when he or she should think of adding people due to rising volume and, on the other side, notify him or her when it would be necessary to cut back hours due to decreasing volume. This would become a tool for communication, justification, and measurement for the management staff.

Following this meeting, the engineer in charge of the project met with each of the management staff members individually to further describe the system and how it would relate to their particular departments.

Next, each department head was asked to keep certain statistics and further meetings were held to work out time frames that various tasks would take to complete. When feasible, standard times that were already developed by the engineering firm were used. In other instances, times had to be verified at the hospital with slight modifications made. In a few cases, individual time studies were necessary to properly measure and record the various tasks done throughout the hospital.

The Nursing Department had to deal with a patient classification system with associated times for each of the categories. In this case, the system was taken directly from the engineering firm as it was used in the Medical Center. There were slight modifications made to adjust the system to this hospital but, by and large, it was taken as presented by the engineer and verified.

In order to show the administration's interest in the system and intent to use it as a management tool, one of the administrative secretaries was chosen and trained as the system's data recorder. This meant that all input for recordings on a monthly basis had to be given to administration and all reports came from administration. This, in and of itself, helped keep the system's development on track.

The system was developed during 1980 with the larger departments being examined. The system was then used in 1981 budget planning but only for those departments where standards were complete and a track record established. The budget was adjusted downward, through use of the system, by approximately $100,000. This adjustment was not only reported to the board but also to the state's Rate Review Committee.

During this time, all personnel requests, both new and replacement, were reviewed in light of the system and of the productivity changes that it would make. The hospital was beginning to operate using the system and it appeared that the managers were beginning to understand it.

### Results

By the beginning of 1981, all of the major departments had developed standards. These departments covered about 90 percent of the hospital's work force. Monthly monitoring was taking place but all the actions in use of the system were coming from the top down. It had become a good administrative control system but the individual department heads were not really using it as a management tool for their departments. An example of this was in mid-1981 when census took a dramatic down turn. The Executive Director felt that action was necessary to maintain the institution's financial position. Work hour reduction programs were instituted. The productivity program was used to determine how much each department had to contribute to this overall reduction. Many department heads had problems with this approach and felt reductions should be equal among all departments. Employee unrest resulted and meetings had to be held to explain why the reductions were taking place and how the system was being used. As a result of this experience, the administration set out to develop a partnership concept with its employees and a greater sense of responsibility for the program on the part of the management staff.

The system had worked to assist the Executive Director manage the hospital's payroll during these times of fluctuation, but it took well over a year for the department heads to grasp its usefulness and even longer to accept it and use it as a tool for their own management.

In 1981, the state legislature passed an amendment to the County Hospital Law, permitting county facilities to pay productivity incentive compensation as long as every employee was eligible. This bill was introduced and guided through the legislative process by the area's state senator, who was also a member of the hospital's Board of Trustees.

Because of the law, the senator's interest in productivity, and the Executive Director's interest in developing a partnership feeling among the employees in the hospital, the management engineering consultants were asked to develop an incentive concept around the current productivity system. This system, through much study and consultation, and guidance from the Executive Director and the hospital's Chief Financial Officer, developed in the following manner:

1. The average productivity of each department for the previous 12 months was calculated.

2. The average productivity of the highest three months of productivity in the last 12 months was calculated.

3. If the average of the high three months was within 6 to 8 percent above the average of the 12 months and at least 4 percent above the budgeted productivity level, it became the incentive target. Those departments with three month averages that were below 6 percent above the 12 month average had their targets adjusted upward to 6 percent. Those departments with three month averages above 8 percent above the 12 month average targets were adjusted downward to 8 percent. All targets were at least 4 percent above budget.

4. Any department having a productivity at or above the target level for a calendar quarter was paid an incentive check. This check amounted to 4 percent of the individual's hourly wage, times the number of hours worked in that calendar quarter.

The payment of an incentive system was then presented to the hospital's Board of Trustees in December 1981, with the idea of implementation as of January 1, 1982. The Board accepted this concept. It saw the long-term benefit for higher productivity and of the partnership that would be developed between the institution and its employees. The board treated the incentive as an unbudgeted expense because it would be paid from savings when payroll was under budget.

As the system was developed and implemented, educational meetings were held during January, first with the hospital department heads to again explain in detail the productivity system and how it worked for them. Interest at this time was much higher than before because there was a direct financial impact on every employee of the hospital. Once the hospital department head understood his own productivity and how the system worked, he then held individual departmental employee meetings to explain the system. There were many questions but employees took a wait and see attitude.

In the summer of 1982 a low volume period was seen, but in this case no action from the Executive Director had to be taken because individual department heads were making day–to–day volume adjustments in their work force.

By the end of the year, all but two departments had received a productivity incentive check for at least one quarter. The final results were: $58,000 in productivity incentive money paid out from a calculated payroll savings of $278,000.

The productivity system has worked. It has been continued in 1983 and 1984. Individual standards have been adjusted on an ongoing basis as departmental operations have adjusted with new modalities of treatment and methods of operation. The board is pleased with the system and its savings, and the employees now feel a partnership with the hospital's operational success. The system has contributed to the continued health and growth of the institution and the development of its management staff.

# Chapter Twenty-Nine

## Impact of the State of Ohio Funding For Geriatrics

### JOHN P. KEMPH

### Introduction

Six years ago the State of Ohio passed a law to establish geriatrics programs at each of its seven medical schools, with modest funding for the support of this new development. Before describing the impact of that action, it seems appropriate to review briefly the benefits provided to the elderly by the federal and state governments, with particular emphasis on health care. During the great economic depression of the 1930's, the ability of several sectors of society to feed and clothe themselves was greatly impaired, particularly for the elderly. As a result of this great need, local governments, as well as state and federal governmental agencies, began to emerge to provide programs for the needy elderly. By 1934, approximately half of the states in the United States had developed public charity programs for the aged.

The Social Security Act of 1935 established joint programs between the federal and state governments, named the Old Age Assistance Program (OAA). The states determined the benefit levels and the federal government matched funds. By 1940, all of the states in the United States had OAA programs in place, with more than 20 percent of persons age 65 and over receiving payments. OAA payments varied widely from state to state, from $79 to $434 annually. Furthermore, the aged population varied considerably from one state to another. For example, in New Mexico, only 8 percent of the people were aged 65 and over, while in New Hampshire, 15 percent were over 65. Then came Social Security Disability Insurance in 1954, Aid to the Blind, and Aid to Dependent Children.

In 1956, amendments to the Social Security Act clarified the federal Old Age Insurance Program, that the purpose of the federal Old Age Assistance Program was to enable each state to assist aged individuals to attain self-care through appropriate welfare services and financial aid when needed. Congress makes a single appropriation for all of the grants in Aid for Old Age Assistance, Medical Assistance for the Aged, Aid to Dependent Children, Aid to the Blind, and Aid to the Disabled. The Administration On Aging serves as a clearing house for all information from other federal agencies and state commissions on aging, and the universities and local voluntary agencies to inform the general public, includ-

303

ing the elderly, of services available to them.

Total elderly benefits continued to burgeon until 1960, when the total expenditure was $12.8 billion. Expenditure for each aged individual was $768, and the percent of the gross national product was 2.52 percent, with the percent of the total federal budget being 13 percent. By 1978, the total expenditures had climbed to $112 billion total for the elderly, with $4,678 expended per each aged individual. The percent of the gross national product was 5.3 and the percent of the federal budget was 24. At the same time there was a nine fold increase in total dollars spent for the elderly between 1960 and 1978, the actual number of people over 65 increased only by 43.6 percent, from 16.7 million in 1960 to 23.9 million in 1978 [Clark and Meneff, 1981]. It is estimated that in the year 2025 the expenditure will be $635 billion in 1978 dollars. Furthermore, it is estimated that the ratio of males aged 65 and older to males ages 21 to 64 is expected to increase by 66 percent by the year 2025 and 100 percent by the year 2050.

The increase in the federal support of the elderly has improved their living standards but at considerable cost to society as a whole. It should be further noted, however, that if the allocations just described are to be provided, they would require a 60 percent increase in the proportion of the gross national product allocated to the programs for the elderly by the year 2025.

The motivation for the increased public assistance to the aged may be due to the altruism of the taxpayers. There is some evidence to support this hypothesis in the form of a large survey of more than 2,000 persons in the State of Alabama [Klemmack and Roff, 1981]. Approximately 6 percent of the respondents indicated that they believed that the government spends too much money on older people, however, a majority (over 61 percent) reported that categorical programs for the elderly are necessary for the elderly to share equitably in our resources. Also, a majority, over 54 percent, believed that the government is obliged to help the elderly obtain food and medical care. The respondents ranked benefits to older people second to national defense among a list of 10 possible choices of spending federal tax dollars.

Another motive for increased supports to the aged is their increased voting power. A comparison of these two motives has been made by Parsons [1982]. If voting power is significant, states with large percentages of elderly in their populations should be developing stronger programs for the elderly.

**Health Care for the Aged**

Providing health care for the aged antedates all of the other forms of support previously mentioned. Aid to voluntary hospitals has been well established since colonial days. An early example is the Pennsylvania Hospital, receiving 2,000 pounds from the provincial assembly with its charter in 1751 [Stevens, 1982]. This was a matching grant for an equal amount being privately subscribed. Although not specified for the elderly, they nevertheless received major benefit from the care provided at nominal cost or no charge at all. During the great depression of the 1930's, when Social Security was spawned and aid to the aged was begun, it became obvious that there was a great need for public assistance for the health care of the aged. The large city hospitals were burgeoning with elderly patients with no resources to pay for their hospitalization and medical care. However, direct support of the health needs of the aged was not directly provided by the federal government until 1960 when the Medical Assistance for the Aged Act (MAA) authorized grants to the states for medical assistance to the aged. Then, in 1965, Medicare and Medicaid were enacted, replacing the MAA.

Medicaid is a grant-in-aid program, with the federal and state governments paying the costs of medical care for people with low income. In the federal government, the Medical Services Administration in the Social and Rehabilitations Service of the Department of Health and Human Services administers this program. The ultimate goal of the program is to provide medical care to those individuals in the United States who are unable to pay for it. The states are entrusted to provide the quality control of the medical care for the poor. In most states, the administration of this function is within the Welfare Department. The elderly are eligible for this program in all states which provide it.

Medicare is a broad program of health insurance for Americans 65 and older and severely disabled people under 65. There are two parts to this insurance, one part reimburses for hospital care and the other for doctors' services (Parts B and A, respectively).

Long term care for the elderly is provided through Medicaid if the individual requiring the care has insufficient funds to pay for the the nursing home costs from his own private funds. It has become increasingly easier for long-term care of the aged to occur in nursing homes, rather than at the homes of relatives of the elderly, for a variety of reasons. In 16 states, the elderly living at home are not eligible to receive Medicaid no matter how high the cost of their care may be unless they are already receiving public assistance. In the 34 other states, persons receiving cash assistance can receive Medicaid only if their medical expenses are large enough to reduce their remaining income below Medicaid eligibility standards. Since these standards are quite low, persons are encouraged to utilize nursing homes. These and many other rules established by Medicaid encourage nursing home care for the elderly.

The costs of the health benefits provided by Medicaid and Medicare were known to be high in the 1960's when the programs were initiated. However, at that time, it was felt that this was a natural evolution of the federal programs already initiated with the Social Security Act in 1935. Federal programs to develop scientific research and health care facilities were already underway. Much of the federal legislation in the late 1960's dealt with specific programs, such as the mental health programs, neighborhood health centers, and regional medical programs for heart, cancer, and stroke. This might be interpreted as a period when federal legislation was designed to provide access to health care [Lewis, 1983].

Health care programs have burgeoned, in the meantime, with great scientific progress and new technology, all of which have become extremely costly. This cost had become so great that by 1980 it became clear to responsible legislators that greater access in medical care was really not possible until it could be paid for. This has led to much speculation with regard to the access to health care as the federal government aims at reducing its funding of health care programs and to the concern that health care systems would not provide the same quality care to patients. An interesting study performed in the California system, however, showed that imposing limits on physicians' charges to all patients could limit spending without a concomitant reduction in the willingness of the doctors to take the program beneficiaries [Lee and Hadley, 1981].

Therefore, it became essential that an attempt be made to reduce the costs of medical care in the Medicare program. Accordingly, the Tax Equity and Fiscal Responsibility Act (TEFRA) was enacted by Congress in the summer of 1982 and the legislation was passed in March 1983 concerning Medicare prospective payments. These radical changes in the payment of health care services by Medicare establishes a total amount which will be paid based on the previous years' expenditures. Furthermore, the payments to the hospitals will be based on the number of discharges of patients with specific illnesses. There will be a narrow margin for individual differences in patients with the same diagnosis. Dollar amounts have been ascribed to each patient with a specific diagnosis. This series of diagnoses, 367 in all as recognized by Medicare, are referred to as Diagnostic Related Groups (DRG's). It should be noted however, that the elderly will receive particular attention. The hospital will be paid a larger amount for an elderly person with the same diagnosis as a younger person [Medicare Program, 1983].

The major intent of all of the new changes in Medicare is to reduce the cost to the government. The Health Care Financing Administration (HCFA) was established to develop the regulations for prospective payment. Many of the changes being recommended by HCFA will definitely reduce costs rapidly. However, they are causing great fear among hospitals and physicians by making broad sweeping changes which may be deleterious to health educational and service programs which have been developed over the last two decades.

### Health Care for the Aged in Ohio

Ohio is supportive of health programs for the elderly. Its Medicaid program has been one of the largest in the United States. The Ohio legislature has always been cognizant of the need for special programs for the elderly. One program which has been well-funded is the Ohio Soldiers Home, a long-term care facility provided for Ohio citizens who are also veterans of the armed services. Prior to 1977, the Ohio legislature was searching for ways in which it could benefit its elderly citizens.

On August 15, 1977, Ohio House Bill (Ohio HB) 252 was passed by the legislature. This law stipulated that a division of geriatrics must be established in each of Ohio's seven medical schools. The legislation also provided $500,000 to be allocated to the seven medical schools for the purpose of initiating the geriatrics divisions. It was assumed by the legislature that establishing these divisions would provide educational, research, and service programs to improve the status of the elderly in the State of Ohio. Furthermore, placing these funds in medical schools would provide opportunities for students and residents in training to obtain information which could inculcate a desire to treat elderly citizens of the state. In budget year 1984, six years thereafter, this fund supplied by the legislature to the seven medical schools has increased to $1.13 million annually. This remains a modest amount of funding for the support of seven medical schools' geriatrics activities. However, considerable productivity has been achieved.

The funds were allocated to each of the seven medical schools by means of an incentive system utilizing 11 evaluative parameters which were reported by each of the schools in the general areas of service, research, and education. The mechanism of disbursement was established by a committee composed of a representative from each of the seven medical schools. Recently, the deans of the schools reviewed this evaluation process and felt that it was still appropriate for future allocations.

The initial distribution was made under the supervision of Dr. Richard D. Ruppert, at that time the vice-chancellor for health affairs of the Board of Regents for Higher Education of the State of Ohio. Initially, a geriatrics resource center was established at the Medical College of Ohio (MCO), with increased library holdings and a continuing education program established immediately. This was followed by recruiting efforts to hire a geriatrician and other personnel to staff a geriatrics clinic. A survey of faculty interest was completed, followed by an injection of new geriatrics information in the curriculum of the medical school. In the first year, 18 hours were set aside in the curriculum for clinical geriatrics.

Since then, a geriatrics clinic has been established with a full-time geriatrician serving as director, a full-time social worker, and several part-time faculty providing coverage for the clinic to be open 40 hours per week, five days a week, with back-up services on a 24 hour a day basis in the emergency room and in the in-patient unit of the hospital. Eight pilot research projects have been funded and a geriatrics dentistry program has been initiated. A dental program has outreach to a long-term care facility, where one of the faculty of the Department of Dentistry of the Medical

College of Ohio has a dental office on the premises of the facility providing care to the residents of the nursing home. The stroke program has been initiated which has outreach through a public spirited group of volunteers in the community. Volunteer workers are trained to visit the homes of stroke patients to assist them in their rehabilitation by improving their skills for independent self-care in their own homes.

Also, nursing faculty are providing assistance to nursing homes by having nurse clinicians visit these homes and assist with planning and implementation of quality patient care, providing additional stimulation for increased patient activities.

A program has been initiated to stimulate those patients with Alzheimer's type of senile brain disease. A combination of sociopsychological stimulation and pharmacological agents help to prevent patients from slipping into senile dementia through stimulation of memory functions.

The MCO Department of Surgery has a special interest in early mobilization of the geriatrics surgical patient to reduce morbidity and length of stay in the hospital. In the same department, the Section of Ophthalmology operates a low vision clinic which treats primarily elderly patients.

The Department of Family Medicine provides supportive medical care to the patients of two nursing homes. The Department of Neurology also provides coverage for neurological disorders and a local long-term care facility. The Department of Psychiatry provides a consultation service with one of its faculty members specializing in geropsychiatry. The Department of Rehabilitative Medicine has a specialized program for geriatric amputees.

The geriatrics clinic provides ambulatory care training and inpatient training for both residents and medical students as part of their didactic and clinical curriculum.

In the teaching programs, trainees are taught about all forms of conditions which may replicate the signs and symptoms of senile dementia but which can be caused by diseases other than pure senility. Many of these conditions can be meliorated, either through drugs or other forms of treatment. For example, depression in the elderly produces confusion and memory loss and mimics the Alzheimer's type of dementia. Appropriate medication can relieve all of these symptoms. Another example is the moderate overdosage of a variety of medications which are metabolized slowly in elderly patients. By obtaining blood levels of medications periodically during the course of the treatment of the elderly, this problem can be prevented.

In the area of research, six papers have been published by members of the MCO geriatric faculty and four research grants have been obtained from extramural sources. There have also been 51 presentations made either at scientific meetings or at continuing education programs by the staff of the geriatrics program in the last year [Medical College of Ohio, 1983].

A review of the annual reports of the Offices of Geriatric Medicine at the six other medical schools in the State of Ohio show similar accomplishments by their offices to those previously described by the Medical College of Ohio [*Annual Reports*, 1983].

How could so much have been accomplished with a small subsidy of funds from the state legislature? Primarily because the medical schools realized the need for increased activities in the patient care services, educational programs, and in both basic and clinical science research programs. The modest financial supports from the State of Ohio provided the stimulus to develop those programs. The funding was timely and only a small amount was needed to serve as a catalyst to trigger the activity in all the schools.

The main reason for the low cost for this high level of productivity is the absence of payment for hospital costs or physicians' fees. The only patient care support was directed at outpatient clinics where only faculty salaries were paid, not the fees for medical services. Long-term effects of this program are not known because it has been in effect for a relatively short period of time. However, it might be anticipated that the students and residents in training will have achieved a greater familiarity with the elderly patient than their counterparts who graduated earlier. Certainly, the patient care aspects of this program have provided many elderly citizens in the State of Ohio with outpatient care at the seven medical schools for the last six years.

## Summary

The public benefits provided to the elderly by government programs have been reviewed, with particular emphasis on health care benefits. The State of Ohio has passed a law which required that an office of geriatrics be established in all of the seven medical schools in the State of Ohio. Initially, seed money was established for planning, followed by gradually increasing amounts provided to each of the medical schools, based on the activities in geriatrics in each of the schools. As a result of this law with its financial allocation, the development of geriatrics throughout the State of Ohio was well-established and greatly expanded. The amount of funds which each school received in each succeeding year was based on the 11 evaluation parameters in clinical services, teaching, and research.

This program stimulated a massive increase in the activities of all seven medical schools in the State of Ohio in the areas of patient care, educaton, and research. In this report, the development of geriatric programs in one of those seven medical schools, the Medical College of Ohio at Toledo, has been reviewed in detail. During the course of the last six years, the basic science and clinical teaching programs were sponsored and a geriatrics medicine section has been developed.

The patient care aspects of this expansion were most impressive. A full-fledged outpatient clinic was formed, utilizing the services of a full-time medical director, several part-time medical positions, a full-time social worker, and other supporting nursing and clerical staff. The outpatient clinic established a full-time program, being open 40 hours per week, Monday through Friday, with 24 hour per day services available through the Medical College of Ohio Hospital. The geriatrician headed a team of professionals, including students from each of the health care disciplines. One of the specialties of this clinic was to treat patients with the Alzheimer's type of senility, which frequently progresses rapidly to dementia. Particular emphasis has also been given to rehabilitating the patient with neurological and psychiatric diseases caused by problems originating with diseases affecting the central nervous system and the cardiovascular system. Funding for the programs has been obtained from resources other than the state since the inception of the program.

A substantially increasing interest on the part of the health care professionals in the Medical College of Ohio has been stimulated as a direct result of resources made available by the passage of Ohio HB 252. Surprisingly, a considerable increase in health care services in geriatrics in the State of Ohio has been achieved with a modest appropriation of $500,000 initially in 1977, followed by minimal increases each year to a total of $1.13 million in the 1984 fiscal year. The impact of public funding on geriatrics care was enhanced by its timeliness and genuine public need.

### REFERENCES

*Annual Reports,* Offices of Geriatrics of Ohio Medical Schools, on file at the Office of the Ohio Board of Regents.

R. L. Clark and J. A. Menefee, "Federal Expenditures for the Elderly: Past and Future," *The Gerontologist,* 21(2), 1981, pp. 132-37.

D. L. Klemmack and L. L. Roff, "Predicting General and Comparative Support for Government's Providing Benefits to Older Persons," *The Gerontologist,* 21(6), 1981, pp. 592-99.

R. H. Lee and J. Hadley, "Physicians' Fees and Public Medical Care Programs," *Health Services Research,* 16:2, Summer 1981.

I. J. Lewis, "Evolution of Federal Policy on Access to Health Care 1965 to 1980," *Bulletin of New York Academy of Medicine,* 59(1), January-February 1983, pp. 9-20.

Medical College of Ohio, "Report of the Office of Geriatric Medicine/Gerontology as of June 30, 1983," Office of the Ohio Board of Regents.

"Medicare Program; Prospective Payments for Medicare Inpatient Hospital Services; Interim Final Rule With Comment Period," *Federal Register,* 48(171), September 1, 1983, pp. 39752-890.

D. O. Parsons, "Demographic Effects on Public Charity to the Aged," *The Journal of Human Resources,* XVIII(1), 1982, pp. 144-52.

R. Stevens, " 'A Poor Sort of Memory:' Voluntary Hospitals and Government Before the Depression," *Milbank Memorial Fund Quarterly,* 60(4), 1982.

## Primary Care Delivery System for Pregnant Adolescents

# Chapter Thirty

MARTA SILVERBERG,
ALBERT R. TAMA,
SUSAN WALLNER,
LEONARD E. BRAITMAN

### Introduction

For the period January 1, 1981 through December 31, 1981, maternal and newborn outcome data were examined for all adolescents who delivered at Cooper Hospital in Camden, New Jersey. The hypothesis of the study was that adolescents who received primary nursing care, as offered by Women's Care Center, fared better than those who did not receive such care. The groups were identified as those adolescents 19 years of age and younger who received prenatal care in private physician offices located near Cooper Hospital and those who received their prenatal care at the Women's Care Center.

The purpose of this study is to evaluate the short–term effectiveness of primary nursing in the care of the pregnant adolescent. Short–term effectiveness will be measured in terms of pregnancy outcomes. It is hypothesized that by improving pregnancy outcome, the cost to society will be minimized in terms of its impact on the consumption of health resources. This study:

1. Compares two similar groups of pregnant teenagers, one receiving primary nursing care and the other receiving traditional care in a private setting;

2. Examines maternal and fetal outcomes to determine if there are any significant differences between these two groups; and

3. Analyzes admission rate and length of stay in neonatal intensive care units for the infants in both groups, and obstetrical length of stay to determine differences, if any, in patterns of consumption of hospital resources.

### Adolescent Pregnancy Program

The Adolescent Pregnancy Program, instituted at the Women's Care Center in 1980, was made possible through Title VI which established the Office of Adolescent Pregnancy Programs within the U.S. Department of Health and Human Services.

The Women's Care Center, as a subcontractor of the Camden Adolescent Pregnancy Program, was charged with the responsibility of delivering prenatal care and an array of other services to pregnant adolescents in the

311

City of Camden. It has an average of 1,000 patients a year, 300 of whom are adolescents.

In order to meet the goals of the Adolescent Pregnancy Program, an interdisciplinary team composed of professionals in medicine, nursing, social work, nutrition, and health education was formed. This team functioned under the co-direction of an administrative director and a medical director.

Services provided to adolescents included comprehensive medical care, nutritional and social service evaluations and follow-up, and health education with emphasis on selection and utilization of birth control methods. These services continue to be offered throughout the pregnancy as well as during the first 12 months post-partum. The social worker offered psychosocial counseling to both teen parents as well as to other members of their families. Great emphasis was placed on assisting the young woman to explore every option open to her following the birth of her baby. To this end, referrals were made to vocational training and counseling services and to a variety of educational programs. Day care referrals were made in order to help the young mother remain in school, or to return to employment. The young father was also eligible for, and referred to, these programs, and all referrals were meticulously tracked.

Case management is provided by four registered nurses who practice primary nursing care and work exclusively within the adolescent pregnancy program. In addition, primary nurses are also responsible for the patient education program; family members and prospective fathers are encouraged to participate in the educational program as well. During clinic visits, classes are offered by the Primary Care Nurse in the following areas: (1) labor and delivery; (2) fetal growth and development; (3) immediate post-partum period, and introduction to available social services; and (4) emotional and physiological changes of pregnancy. Patients participate in the classes appropriate to their stage of gestation. In addition, other classes such as food preparation and an introduction to the General Educational Development program are offered on an occasional basis.

The topic of contraception is introduced by the Primary Care Nurse late in the third trimester, and this teaching is reinforced during the hospital stay and again at the time of the post-partum examination. A parenting class is also offered immediately prior to the post-partum examination.

The first post-partum home visit is scheduled during the second post-partum week, and subsequent visits are made at three, six, and 12 months post-partum. Additional visits are made as needed. The nurse does whatever teaching is appropriate regarding maternal and infant care and ensures that both mother and infant are receiving appropriate medical services. She is also trained to refer the patient, and her family members as well, to a wide variety of additional services which may be required.

Following the 12 month post-partum follow-up period, patients are terminated from the program, with encouragement to return for regular care for both mother and baby.

## Characteristics of Camden, New Jersey

*Demographic Characteristics*

Camden is located along the western border of Camden County, one mile from Philadelphia. It is the fourth largest city in the State of New Jersey and the largest city in South Jersey. The city contains the majority of the indigent people of the larger metropolitan area of close to a million residents living east of the Delaware River. In 1980 its population was 86,000, with a density of 9,212 per square mile. Among the population 19 years of age and younger, 56 percent are black, 26 percent Hispanic, and 18 percent white.

*Socio-Economic Characteristics*

The Brookings Institute has ranked Camden as the ninth most distressed city in the nation on the basis of the percentage of citizens living in poverty, the percentage of pre-1940 housing and the rate of population decline. The most severe poverty exists in the Hispanic community which comprises approximately 25 percent of the city's population. The per capita income of Hispanics was 57 percent less than whites and 18 percent less than blacks.

*Educational Characteristics*

The educational picture of Camden is consistent with the other socio-economic data. Only 20 percent of the population has graduated from high school and the public school system is predominately black and Hispanic with over a 50 percent dropout rate. Only 45 percent of 1,420 students entering Camden's high schools in 1973 graduated in 1977.

*Health Status Characteristics*

In 1981, there were 94,502 births in the State of New Jersey. Camden had one of the highest birth rates in the state with 22.9 per 1,000 population. This rate exceeds Camden County and the State of New Jersey by 8.2 and 10.1, respectively. Statewide, the percentage of all births to mothers 19 years of age and younger was 11.6; within Camden County it was 15, and within the city of Camden it was 25. In contrast to state and county figures, in Camden there are more non-married mothers than married mothers. In fact, the rate of births to unwed mothers in the city is three times the state average and 2.4 times the county average. Of the non-married mothers, 72.1 percent are either black or Hispanic.

## The Experimental Group

In 1981, there were a total of 228 adolescents ranging in ages from 14 to 19 who participated in the Adolescent Pregnancy Program. Their mean age was 17.3 with a 1.4 standard deviation. Within this group, whites tended to be a little older with a mean age of 17.7 with a 1.1 standard deviation. More than half of these adolescents were black or 56.1 percent, 24.1 percent were Hispanic, and 19.7 percent were white.

Of this group, 80 percent were applying for, or receiving public assistance at the time of registration for prenatal care, 13.3 percent had other third party coverage, and the rest had no insurance. At the time of registration, 57 percent were attending school. This percentage increased to 70 percent by the third prenatal visit. Twenty-five percent began prenatal care during the first trimester, 61.1 percent during the second trimester, and the rest during the third trimester. The percentage of prenatal appointments kept was 78 percent.

Among the experimental group, 63.8 percent were primiparous. This is a low figure compared with the 83 percent reported for all adolescents who participated in Adolescent Pregnancy Programs throughout the nation. For the 228 young women who delivered, there were a total of 229 live births. There were two neonatal deaths and no stillborns or maternal deaths were reported. Of the group, 19.2 percent had maternal or fetal complications. This figure compared well with the national figure of 17 percent.[1]

### The Control Group

In 1981, there were a total of 182 adolescents, ranging in ages from 13 to 19, who delivered at Cooper Hospital but received prenatal care in private physicians' offices. This group had a mean age of 17.4 with a 1.6 standard deviation. For this group, the Hispanic population tended to be a little older with a mean age of 17.7 and a 1.1 standard deviation. Blacks accounted for 70.3 percent, whites for 20.3 percent, and Hispanics for 9.3 percent. Of this group, 61.5 percent were primiparous. This rate is slightly lower than that of the experimental group. Unfortunately, for this group, the following data are unavailable: (1) which trimester prenatal care began; (2) kept prenatal appointment rate; (3) school attendance; and (4) type of third party insurance coverage. For the 182 young women who delivered, there were a total of 184 live births, one neonatal death, two stillborns, and no maternal deaths. The maternal–fetal complication rate was 19.2 percent.

### Program Goals

One of the original goals of the Adolescent Pregnancy Program was the promotion of improved outcomes for young mothers and their infants. This analysis defines improved outcome in the following areas:

---

[1] Information on nationwide adolescent pregnancy programs was obtained through telephone communication with Mary Burt from the Urban Institute on October 17, 1983. At the time this paper was being written, the Urban Institute was completing the final draft of the *Report on Evaluation of Adolescent Pregnancy Programs.*

1. *APGAR Scores.* This is the composite measure to evaluate the newborn's general condition. APGAR scores are given at one and five minutes after birth. A score of 10 is optimum and less than 7 is undesirable. An APGAR score was defined as low when either the one or five minute score is less than 7.

2. *Birthweight.* The birthweight is the weight of the infant at time of delivery. Low birthweight was defined as equal or less than 2,500 grams, or 5 pounds, 8 ounces.

3. *Maternal–Fetal Complications.* These are complications before and during labor for both the mother and the fetus. These were defined as: (a) premature rupture of membranes; (b) membranes ruptured 24 hours; (c) maternal death; (d) pregnancy-induced hypertension, anemia, abruptio placenta, placenta previa, uterine atony, heart disease, and diabetes; (e) cetal distress; (f) arrested progress; and (g) fetopelvic disproportion.

4. *Caesarean Section.* This only included primary Caesarean section.

5. *Pre–Term Pregnancies.* These are pregnancies of 36 weeks or less.

The economic impact of the above outcomes was measured in terms of: (1) admission rate to the neonatal intensive care unit with its corresponding number of hospital days and the antepartum admissions; and (2) the average number of hospital obstetrical days consumed by the participant.

Annual cost of neonatal intensive care in 1981 has been estimated at more than $1.5 billion [Budetti, 1980]. Low birthweight alone represents a good indicator of larger consumption of resources in neonatal intensive care units. An extensive study done at the H. C. Moffitt Hospital, in San Francisco, showed that while 42 percent of infants admitted to the hospital's neonatal intensive care unit had low birthweight, they were responsible for 60 percent of total costs [Phibbs, *et al,* 1981, p. 315].

Maternal–fetal complications, low APGAR scores, and morbidity after Caesarean section also contribute to the high cost of hospital care.

## Data Collection

Maternal and child outcome was obtained by examining both the Cooper Hospital 1981 maternity service records and the newborn record log book. Information collected in these two books is used by the New Jersey State Department of Health to gather data on the state maternal and child health status.

Six adolescents who first appeared at Cooper Hospital for delivery and did not receive prenatal care were excluded from this study.

The newborn record log book was examined to obtain data on special care nursery admissions of infants born to adolescents. The number of days were computed to determine the difference, if any, in the consumption of resources.

Data on the number of obstetrical days and antepartum admissions were obtained through patient identification cards in the medical records department.

Through examination of patients' cards, the place of residence was determined, along with the length of stay for the 1981 delivery and any obstetrical admission nine months prior to the delivery, which was then defined as an antepartum admission.

Other information on the experimental group was obtained through program evaluation reports submitted to the Office of Adolescent Pregnancy Program in Washington, D.C., and preliminary data on the Adolescent Pregnancy Program prepared by two of the authors.

### Data Analysis

There were a total of 29 admissions to the neonatal intensive care unit out of 229 live births in the experimental group, or a rate of 12.7 percent. Within the control group, there was a total of 19 admissions out of 184 live births, or a rate of 10.3.

The average length of stay of infants in the neonatal intensive care unit, for both intensive and intermediate days, in the experimental and control groups was 18.4 and 21.0 days, respectively. Of interest was to find that the average length of intensive care days for infants in the control group was more than twice as high (5.5 days as compared to 2.0 days) as infants in the experimental group. This finding leads one to believe (although not empirically proven) that infants in the control group tend to be sicker than their counterparts in the experimental group.

Unfortunately, since the hospital does not separate cost between the intensive care and the intermediate care unit, the authors were unable to calculate the difference in total costs associated with the findings. However, since the ratio of nurse to patient required for intensive and intermediate care is known, the authors were able to calculate the difference in nursing cost associated with the care of newborns from both groups admitted to the neonatal intensive care unit.

It was found that nursing care cost for the control group was $2,231 per admission, while that of the experimental group was $1,665. Even though the results indicate that the control group consumed more nursing resources than the experimental group, one cannot conclude that this is the case in the overall cost of caring for these patients, unless it can be empirically demonstrated.

Data on antepartum admissions and length of stay in the obstetrical unit was obtained for both groups. The antepartum admission rate per participant was found to be slightly lower in the control group than in the experimental group, 7.8 and 8.8 percent, respectively. The overall maternal length of stay for both antepartum admissions and admissions for delivery was 3.9 for the experimental group and 3.6 for the control group, or a difference of 0.3 of a day. It is obvious that the difference in hospital resources consumed for obstetrical care is minimal and, therefore, financial analysis is not necessary.

The proportions with undesired outcomes were compared in the experimental and control groups. Undesired outcomes include:

1. *Low Birth Weight.* The number of low birth weight babies was calculated for both groups. A rate per group was obtained by dividing the number of low birth weight babies by the total number of live births within the group. The rate of low birth weight babies in the experimental group was slightly lower (12.6 percent) than that of the control group (13.0 percent).

2. *Pregnancies of 36 Weeks or Less.* The rate of pregnancies in this category for the experimental and control groups were 7.9 and 8.8 percent, respectively. The rate for the experimental group was slightly lower than the reported 8.0 percent for adolescents participating in adolescent pregnancy programs nationwide.

3. *Maternal–Fetal Complications.* Both groups were found to have the same rate of complications, 19.2 percent.

4. *Caesarean Section Rate.* The experimental group was found to have a higher primary Caesarean section rate (16.2 percent) than the control group (13.2 percent).

5. *APGAR Scores.* Low APGAR scores among babies of mothers in the experimental and control groups were found to be 9.6 and 7.0 percent, respectively. Further analysis was made by comparing both groups at the five minute score. The experimental group experienced a 3.9 percent rate and the control group a 3.3 percent rate.

$P$-values for the Chi–square test of the difference of proportions were calculated. For each of the five outcomes listed above, $P < 0.10$, so that none of the differences were found to be statistically significant.

The experimental and control groups were found to share maternal characteristics which have been documented in the literature as contributory to poor pregnancy outcome [Battaglia, *et al,* 1963; Davidson, 1979, p. 12; Grazi, *et al,* 1982, p. 89; McCormick, *et al,* 1984; McLean, *et al,* February 1979; Menken, 1975; Shah, *et al,* 1975]. These characteristics are: (1) Maternal age; (2) Socio–economic status; and (3) Parity status.

The authors carefully examined all variables documented in the literature which could have biased the results and determined that both groups shared equally in the risk factors associated with poor outcome.

## Conclusions

The goal of this study was to determine the effectiveness of the Adolescent Pregnancy Program in terms of short–term maternal and newborn outcomes. Cost of the program is approximately $438 per adolescent to provide primary nursing, nutritional, and social services.

Although some differences were noted when calculating the rates of low birth weight, pregnancies equal or less than 36 weeks, maternal–fetal complications, Caesarean section rate, and APGAR scores, none of them turned out to be statistically significant.

In comparing admission rates and length of stay in the neonatal intensive care unit the authors found a longer length of stay among infants in the control group than their counterparts in the experimental group. Antepartum admissions and obstetrical length of stay were found to be similar among both groups.

Based on these findings, it is concluded that these two groups fared equally in their outcomes, at least in the short run.

However, the results found in this study cannot be used to draw overall conclusions as to the long-term effectiveness of the Cooper Hospital Adolescent Pregnancy Program. Because data were obtained at the time of delivery, the long-term impact on the lives of the adolescent parent and her infant could not be measured. Consequently, it becomes necessary to conduct a study on this group to evaluate such long-term factors.

Such a study requires the establishment of a sophisticated management information system to enable one to locate and assess the status of both project participants and mothers within the control population along these parameters. Although this is an ambitious task requiring substantial resources, the authors believe that it must be undertaken to complete the evaluation of the Adolescent Pregnancy Program so that those services can be provided which significantly and positively impact upon the lives of young mothers and their families.

## REFERENCES

F. C. Battaglia, T. M. Frazier, and A. Helleghers, "Obstetrics and Pediatric Complications of Juvenile Pregnancy," *Pediatrics,* 32:902, 1963.

P. Budetti, P. McManus, and N. Barrand, *et al,* "The Cost Effectiveness of Neonatal Intensive Care," Washington D.C. Office of Technology Assessment Contract No. 933-22.60.0, 1980.

Susan M. Coupey, "Pregnancy in Teenage Girls: More than a Medical Problem," *Montefiore Medicine,* p. 36.

Ezra Davidson, "Adolescent Perinatal Health, A Guidebook for Services," *The American College of Obstetricians and Gynecologists,* 1979.

Richard V. Grazi, Ramakreshnan Redheendran, Nirmala Mudaliar, and Robin M. Bannerman, "Offspring of Teenage Mothers, Congenital Malformations, Low Birth Weight, and Other Findings," *The Journal of Reproductive Medicine,* 27, No. 2, February 1982.

Marie C. McCormick, Sam Shapiro, and Barbara Starfield, "High Risk Mothers: Infant Mortality and Morbidity in Four Areas in the United States, 1973-1978," *American Journal of Public Health,* 74, No. 1, January 1984.

Roderick McLean, Ernest Mattison, Nancy Cochrance, and Karen Fall, "Teenage Pregnancy and Maternal Mortality in New York State," *New York State Journal of Medicine,* February 1979.

Jane Menken, "The Health and Demographic Consequences of Adolescent Pregnancy and Childbearing," presented at the Conference on Research on the Consequences of Adolescent Pregnancy and Childbearing, Center for Population Research, National Institute of Health, Bethesda, Maryland, October 29-30, 1975.

Ciaran S. Phibbs, Ronald L. Williams, and Roderic H. Phibbs, "Newborn Risk Factors and Cost of Neonatal Intensive Care," *Pediatrics,* 68, No. 3, September 1981.

Farida Shah, Melvin Zelnik, and John F. Kantner, "Unprotected Intercourse Among Unwed Teenagers," *Family Planning Perspectives,* 7, No. 1, January/February 1975.

# Chapter Thirty-One

## A Self-Supporting Hospital Dental Service

### STEPHEN M. PATZ

### Introduction

The dental service at Sinai Hospital of Detroit originally treated only the dental indigent population. As dental care was provided by dental general practice residents, and one of the major reasons for having a dental service was to teach residents, the staff of the dental and oral surgery department thought that the dental service should be limited to dental indigent patients. This would ensure the support of the entire dental staff because the staff members would not be in competition with each other.

However, limiting care to the dental indigent of the community created a deficit of $110,000 in 1975 and jeopardized the future of the dental service. A decision had to be reached: either changes had to be made to eliminate or significantly reduce the deficit, or the program would be eliminated.

Through a close working relationship, the administration and the dental and oral surgery department were able to transform the deficit program into a self-supporting service. This was accomplished by the development of a plan of action that altered the concept of the original dental service by changing the financial mix of patients from 100 percent indigent to a 75 percent private patient and 25 percent indigent patient mix.

### Pressures on Dental Care in the United States

During the 1970's, the dental profession was faced with a dichotomy of pressures. As inflation surpassed wage increases, less and less disposable income was available for dental services. Thus, many families were priced out of the dental care market, even though dental fees have risen only at the same rate as the cost of living.

This trend towards reduced accessibility to dental care has been replicated in other countries with advanced economies outside the U.S. Even in nations with nationalized health delivery systems, there has been a tendency towards higher deductibles and co-payments.

One mitigating factor in the United States' situation is the increase in the number of people covered by dental insurance and an increase in competition among dentists. Approximately 18-20 percent (60 million people) of the population is covered by dental insurance [Wotman and

319

Goldman, 1982, p. 685]. Even with the federal government's support for oral health care as part of the national health policy and the efforts for prevention and treatment of oral disease for the poor and indigent population, the dental needs of the poor are not being met. In 1964, 65 percent of the poor and 40 percent of the non-poor had not visited a dentist in two years, a difference of 25 percent. In 1977, 53 percent of the poor and 33 percent of the non-poor had not visited a dentist for two years, a difference of 20 percent [Wotman and Goldman, 1982, p. 687]. This comparison indicates that low income still presents a major barrier to dental care and that significant groups of the population are not served by dentists.

This problem of dental care for the poor and indigent exists in different forms in most of the developing countries. Although this paper focuses on an urban, U.S. experience, its lesson for the role which hospitals can play in this area is, in general terms, potentially applicable elsewhere. In many depressed urban environments, inadequately staffed with private physicians and dentists, the local hospital is inevitably a focal point for all forms of health delivery. People will seek ways to get dental care at an affordable price. Dental schools have provided this opportunity for patients. Hospitals can also fill this void but, due to limited resources, must be in a position to provide these services without draining resources from other programs.

## History

The department of dental and oral surgery has existed since Sinai Hospital of Detroit's inception in January 1953. Community service, teaching, education, and self-improvement were the desired goals of the department.

An outpatient dental facility was established that included four operatories, a small dental laboratory, a darkroom, and a waiting room. The initial service to the community began with the dental staff providing free care to indigent dental patients. Later, a modest fee schedule was developed to help defray some of the costs of operation. This fee schedule was far below the prevailing fee schedules of the dental community.

In 1954, the Council on Dental Education of the American Dental Association approved a general rotating dental internship, which began that year. This was the second step in meeting the goals of the dental staff—teaching and education. In 1960, the rotating dental internship was expanded to two dental interns. The facility was originally staffed by the members of the dental department but, after the establishment of the internship, the facility was staffed by the interns with the dental staff supervising and teaching. To ensure high quality dental education, the dental service was divided into specialty care areas—operative dentistry, oral surgery, pedodontics, orthodontics, endodontics, periodontics, prosthodontics, and restorative dentistry.

Each specialty was directed by a section chief who was responsible to the chairman of the department. A dental advisory committee directed the professional affairs, established policies, and enhanced the growth of the program. This committee was comprised of the dental section chiefs, the department chairman, the ambulatory care manager, and the administration's liaison to the dental department.

In addition to the general practice residence dental program (the internship name was changed in the early 1970's) as described above, Sinai Hospital has had an oral surgery residency program since 1959. The program originated in 1949 at Mount Carmel Mercy Hospital, a neighboring hospital, and was transferred to Sinai Hospital. The oral surgery program began with one resident, and expanded to two residents. In 1965, the hospital developed a four-year residency program in oral surgery affiliated with the Wayne State University School of Medicine. This was the first four-year oral surgery training program offered in the United States, and led to a master of science degree from Wayne State University for the oral surgery residents, in addition to a certificate of an approved oral surgery residency from the hospital.

The oral surgery training program eventually expanded to six residents, and also became formally affiliated with Mount Carmel Mercy Hospital. Sinai Hospital provides oral surgery coverage for Mount Carmel Mercy Hospital's emergency room and responds to its consultative needs for the inpatient service. Mount Carmel Mercy Hospital reimburses Sinai Hospital for the salary and fringe benefits for one third-year oral surgery resident. (The affiliation was approved by the American Dental Association.)

In addition to the general dental and oral surgery services, Sinai Hospital has a large and sophisticated prosthetic service. In 1964, the chief of the prosthetic section joined the hospital on a full-time salaried basis as the outpatient department (OPD) dental clinic coordinator. He established a maxillofacial prosthetic service.

In July 1973, the hospital initiated a geographic, full-time department chairmanship. This provided the department of dental and oral surgery with full-time leadership for its growing programs, which now included a general practice residency, a maxillofacial prosthetic service, an oral surgery teaching program, and cleft palate and head and neck teams.

**Financial Analysis**

By the early 1960's, the volume of outpatient visits in the dental facility expanded from the initial 1,200 to almost 6,000. The clinic, however, operated with a substantial deficit. Much of this deficit was paid by Blue Cross when it covered the cost of the hospital operation on the basis of the percent of patients belonging to its programs. However, when accounting methods changed, and all departments were separated into cost centers for both revenue and expenses, Blue Cross no longer funded the outpatient deficits previously integrated into total hospital operations.

The OPD deficit in the late 1960's and early 1970's, therefore, became a significant fiscal problem. Dental materials and laboratory costs were increasing rapidly. With a reduced fee schedule for indigent patients, laboratory services for full and partial dentures cost more than the fee schedule rates. Because of fee schedule restrictions by Medicaid, the hospital was not able to increase its fee schedule to compensate for the laboratory cost increases. By 1975, the deficit reached $110,000.

The major hurdle in eliminating or significantly reducing the deficit was that the clinic, as a revenue-producing department, was allocated costs from the nonrevenue-producing departments based on the Medicare Step-Down Report. This burdened the cost center with an excessive amount of indirect costs, such as costs allocated for personnel services, administration, maintenance, and so forth, far in excess of what the department used or what a private dental office would have for indirect expenses.

For example, a general dentist figures that 50 percent of his gross revenue is overhead, both direct and indirect. The other 50 percent would be his net income. An oral surgeon works on a percentage of 40 percent overhead and 60 percent profit, as he does not have the high laboratory fees of a general dentist. In fiscal year 1974-1975, the indirect costs alone for the clinic were 114 percent of revenue. The total costs, both direct and indirect, in that fiscal year were 225 percent of revenue.

Another major problem that had to be addressed was the attitude and acceptance of change by the dental staff. Some felt that it was the hospital's responsibility to treat the indigent community, regardless of the deficit; others felt that a deficit was the price the hospital had to pay for a dental teaching program. In 1975, a discussion of the fiscal deficit received considerable attention from the dental staff, as it raised concern regarding the future role of dental care in a voluntary hospital. Compounding the problem, the majority of the dentists did not understand the new and complex methods of cost accounting, which allocated large indirect costs to the outpatient department.

Before 1974, the department was physically separated into three facilities—oral surgery, general dentistry, and maxillofacial prosthetics. In 1974, the oral surgery section moved into a new 2,500 square foot facility in the hospital's medical office building. The maxillofacial prosthetic section was relocated to the medical office building opposite the oral surgery section the following year.

In 1975, the administration was faced with the decision of whether effective changes could be made to eliminate or reduce the deficit or whether it would be necessary to close the clinic and, thus, eliminate the general practice residency. The overriding issues were the need to preserve the integrity of the teaching program and to provide dental service to the patient population that had been receiving care at the hospital for 25 years, while keeping a check on inflation and cost containment. The fact that the general dental facility was located in an area that was to be part of an expansion to the emergency service area forced an early decision.

## Finding a Solution

A task force was created to study the problem of the fiscal feasibility of maintaining a dental program. The task force included the chairman of the department of dental and oral surgery, the associate department chairman, the director of fiscal affairs, the ambulatory care manager, and an associate administrator who was the administrative liaison to the dental program.

After numerous meetings, the task force reached several conclusions. Because of the excessive amount of indirect cost allocated to the clinic on the basis of the Medicare Step-Down Report, it was not feasible to think that the program could run without a deficit.

The administration's goal, if the elimination of the deficit was not feasible, was to reduce the deficit to an acceptable level that would permit the hospital to continue its care of the indigent. By changing the patient mix from all indigent patients to a majority of private patients, it was anticipated that the deficit could be significantly reduced. It was estimated that a 75 percent private and 25 percent indigent patient mix would produce adequate revenue for the dental department to reach an acceptable economic level.

The facility needed a dynamic, full-time general practice dentist to create a private practice in conjunction with the teaching program and to supervise the productivity of the general practice residents and hygienist.

The following recommendations were made: It was suggested that the OPD facility consolidate with the other clinical dental programs in the outpatient medical office building and be located adjacent to the maxillofacial unit and across from the oral surgery suite. This would centralize the dental services and improve efficiency in supervision and function. This relocation would necessitate some capital expenditures but would immediately improve the cost report, since the cost of space in the office building was less than the cost per square foot in the hospital. The relocation was projected to save $9,000 per year of indirect cost.

A geographic, full-time general practice dentist should be recruited to both manage and coordinate the general practice clinic and the residency program. This dentist would also develop a private practice, in conjunction with the clinic, that would bring in private patients to change the patient mix and offset much of the dental clinic write-offs.

As a dentist would need a start-up period to develop a practice, the dental department was given two years to implement these two recommendations and thus reduce the deficit, which had reached $110,679 in fiscal year 1974-1975, to a deficit no greater than $50,000 per year. Even if an established dentist with an ongoing practice joined the staff as the general practice dentist, it was anticipated that only a small segment of his practice would follow him. Therefore, two years seemed realistic.

In the spring of 1977, the general practice clinic relocated to space immediately adjacent to the maxillofacial section. That summer, in response to the dental department recruitment endeavors, 18 dentists applied for the position of geographic, full-time general practitioner. The dental department's reputation for professional excellence and high quality service attracted dentists who wanted to have stronger academic orientation in their professional life. The selected candidate began working on campus in January 1978.

## Administrative Decision

An administrative-dental task force was established to explore the dental needs of the community surrounding the hospital and the marketability of the proposed dental program aimed at the insured and self-paying consumer. Information was gathered from the Comprehensive Health Planning Council of Southeastern Michigan, meetings were held with members of the dental staff, and a meeting was held with the general manager of the largest dental supply company in the area. Information from the Comprehensive Health Planning Council and dental supply company manager confirmed the assumption that many of the dentists who previously practiced in Wayne County had moved their practices to the growing suburbs of Oakland County. As the hospital was located in Wayne County, an attempt to market a dental service to private patients in the local community could be successful.

The majority of the staff dentists interviewed felt that there were more patients in need of dental care than dentists available, and that the hospital's venture into the private sector of dental care would not create competition for them. Many also believed that the addition of private patients to the dental teaching program would benefit the residents and the program, as this would give the residents a more representative patient population to prepare them for their future practices. The indigent patient population is a difficult one to manage, from the dental care point-of-view, because many patients do not have routine dental care and frequently do not return for scheduled visits.

The director of fiscal affairs was asked to prepare a cost analysis of relocating the OPD clinic to the medical office building and to compare the relocation plus the relocating of the clinic, including the addition of a full-time dentist, with the present operation. The report showed that the hospital could reduce the deficit from an anticipated $119,061 to $55,641 by relocating the clinic and to $51,072 by relocating and having a full-time, general practice dentist.

By this time, in 1977, the hospital had experience with the oral surgery and maxillofacial prosthetics services operating in the medical office building. The fiscal analysis plus the success the hospital had with the maxillofacial service during the previous two years, with an approximate $13,000 profit in fiscal year 1975-1976 and an anticipated $52,000 profit for fiscal year 1976-1977, led to the following conclusions:

1. The relocation of the clinic to the medical office building and the change in patient mix would significantly reduce the deficit.

2. The entire dental service could be viewed as a whole department and the excess revenue in one area could offset a deficit in another.

The oral surgery clinic was experiencing a deficit owing to the high indirect cost and the fact that all of the educational costs, such as the department secretary, conference room space, and so forth, were charged to the oral surgery clinic instead of an oral surgery education account. A fiscal study was also prepared in 1978 that projected that the addition of a second oral surgeon to the oral surgery clinic would generate enough income to offset the indirect costs.

**Results**

The hospital proceeded with its plan and the results were:

1. The newly appointed geographic, full-time general practice dentist increased the revenue of the general dental clinic during his first full year (fiscal year 1978-1979) to $248,446. The operating deficit was reduced to $64,694. This was an excellent beginning. The revenue of the dental clinic continued to grow for the next three fiscal years (FY). The revenue increased 38 percent from FY 1978-1979 to FY 1981-1982. The deficit increased from $64,694 to $79,547; however, this was due to a 46 percent increase in the indirect costs allocated by the hospital to the clinic. The direct dental expense increased only 34 percent.

2. The maxillofacial prosthetic section continued to grow and be successful. The maxillofacial prosthodontist generated $601,642 revenue in 1978-1979, and had an excess income over expenses of $156,474. The profits for the maxillofacial section continued over the next three years. Not only did this provide an additional operating profit for the hospital, but the service created an additional referral source for the hospital's oral surgery program.

3. In oral surgery, a second oral surgeon joined the hospital for fiscal year 1978-1979. With a minimum of additional expenses, the oral surgery clinic increased its utilization of facilities and revenue. The revenue increased by more than $120,000, from $191,842 to $312,197, whereas the expenses rose only approximately $107,000. The operating surplus was $29,000. The operating surplus for oral surgery continued over the next three years to a high of $111,900 in FY 1981-1982.

The oral surgery suite had originally been developed for two oral surgeons. Although one oral surgeon could generate adequate income, he would not utilize the personnel and office space adequately. Because the suite was geographically based and a developing referral center for oral carcinoma treatment, a significant portion of the oral surgeon's work week was spent in the operating room, as well as attending meetings and performing other administrative duties. The addition of a second oral surgeon increased the use of the personnel and operatories. In fiscal year 1980-1981, the oral surgery section operated with only one oral surgeon.

4. In addition, to maximize reimbursement, an oral surgery administrative account was developed. Some of the costs allocated to the oral surgery account were expenses that related to the departmental administration and teaching activities, such as a department secretary, a percentage of the department chairman's time allotted for teaching and administration, and office space. Therefore, these expenses were allocated to the oral surgery administrative account—an inpatient account, the expenses of which are covered by third party payers. This increased the profitability of the oral surgery office by approximately $50,000 in 1977-1978 and by $22,500 in 1978-1979. The profitability of the total department of dental and oral surgery changed from the deficit of approximately $148,000 in 1975-1976 to a profit of $120,759 in 1978-1979 and $156,162 in 1981-1982.

The results have been gratifying. The goal of maintaining a strong, high-quality dental department, while significantly reducing the deficit in the general dental service, has been accomplished. The patient mix has reached an approximate 75 percent private and 25 percent indigent mix. Both the administration and department of dental and oral surgery are satisfied with the results.

### Dental Care in Hospitals in the 1980's

The solution discussed in this paper to permit hospitals to maintain dental programs either for education or service were relative for the 1970's. Currently, in the United States, adding a dental ambulatory program in a hospital may fall on deaf ears because the United States hospitals are living through a tide of economic changes in their reimbursement systems. However, the changing reimbursement systems (DRG's) and changes to the corporate structure of hospitals (diversification) makes it all the more necessary for hospitals to evaluate their ambulatory programs and provide even greater opportunity for ambulatory and dental programs to be successful in a hospital setting.

One of the major problems that hospitals have had to overcome in their ambulatory care programs, as previously discussed in this paper, was the allocation of indirect costs from 24 hours per day, seven days per week departments to the ambulatory departments which are only open 40 hours per week. Hospitals that have diversified, i.e., set up a corporate structure that has both profit and non-profit subsidiaries, can use this mechanism to create a dental subsidiary—either profit or non-profit, depending on state laws.

The dental subsidiary, being a separate corporation, would not have the hospital's indirect costs. Therefore, this subsidiary can be profitable as direct expenses can be controlled. The indirect expenses allocated to the dental department, as discussed in this paper, were beyond the control of a dental department.

Since the hospital would have to apply for dental residency approval, the hospital could, for example, contract the residents' services to the dental corporation. The dental corporation would provide the education to the residents and use the residents to provide service to the patient population. Having control, the parent corporation can assure itself that the residents are receiving education and the target community is being served. A dental subsidiary would provide services at a relatively low labor cost and thus be able to exist with a patient mix that includes a substantial Medicaid population.

It is the author's opinion that a dental subsidiary is the best financial mechanism for the ambulatory dental program in a hospital.

The DRG reimbursement system, as established in New Jersey and potentially other parts of the country, will not change the problem of allocation of indirect costs to ambulatory departments and will limit hospitals' ability to cost shift, which will limit the potential profitability of hospitals. Cost shifting is charging commercial paid patients significantly higher charges than cost, which provides hospitals a slight margin to offset free care and patients paying less than cost. Controlled charges also limit profitability from ambulatory services. Again, the separate dental corporation, outside of the direct hospital controls, will permit hospital dentistry to survive.

## Conclusion

This article focuses on the business aspects of dentistry in a hospital. However, there is another aspect of hospital dentistry that needs to be written. That aspect deals with the relationship of dentistry to medicine in a hospital and the tertiary dental services that can be developed with a strong dental program.

A strong dental sevice has benefits for a hospital in addition to its service to an indigent dental community and the teaching of general practice dental residents. A strong dental service will attract oral surgeons and, potentially, an oral surgery residency program. Oral surgeons fill beds, use the operating room, and interact with other medical disciplines.

Having oral surgery residents will attract the more difficult oral surgery patients, i.e., oral carcinoma, maxillofacial surgery, and the like. Having residents available for 24 hour coverage will encourage these major cases to be admitted to the hospital. Oral surgeons will also refer dental emergencies to the emergency room, which will also be a potential source of admissions.

The relationship of medicine and dentistry can also be found in the following programs: (1) cleft palate teams; (2) head and neck surgery; (3) temporal-mandibular joint (TMJ) problems; (4) maxillofacial surgery; and (5) mandibular fractures. These programs will encourage physicians to admit patients with these health care needs to the hospital, since the full range of services are available.

This facet of hospital dentistry should be written by the dental professionals and would be an excellent corollary to this article.

In closing, there are many reasons for a hospital to evaluate all possible alternatives for survival of hospital ambulatory dentistry or to evaluate the start of a program.

### REFERENCES

Stephen Wotman and Harriet Goldman, "Pressures on the Dental Care System in the United States," *American Journal of Public Health*, 72, July 1982.

# Contributors

# Contributors

**John M. Virgo,** editor of this book, is a specialist in manpower, labor, and economic theory, as well as personnel, business law, and social responsibility. He is the author of six books and over 35 articles and has served as consultant to the U.S. Department of Labor, State of California, State of Virginia, and numerous regional private and public groups. Dr. Virgo founded the Atlantic Economic Society and the *Atlantic Economic Journal* in 1973, where he serves as Executive Vice President and Managing Editor, respectively. In addition, he founded the International Health Economics and Management Institute, where he serves as Chief Executive Officer. He currently teaches at Southern Illinois University at Edwardsville.

**Martha S. Albert** is a health systems consultant specializing in strategic management of health care, business, and educational structure. Dr. Albert was previously adjunct Associate Professor at the Robert O. Anderson Schools of Management at the University of New Mexico and consultant to the Michigan Department of Public Health. She has recently been appointed to the Masters of Business Administration Division of the Chinese University of Hong Kong. She is the author of numerous published articles and chapters of books in the health field.

**Roger M. Battistella** has been Coordinator of the Sloan Program in Hospital and Health Services Administration at Cornell University since 1968. His particular fields of interest encompass health services policy, medical sociology, international health, and social and economic development planning. Professor Battistella holds a B.S. degree in Public Health, University of Massachusetts; a M.P.H. in Public Health Administration, University of Michigan; and a Ph. D. in Medical Care Organization, University of Michigan. He has authored 40 articles in his field and is also the author of a book, *Health Care Policy in a Changing Environment.* He serves on the New York State Health Research Council, and is a consultant to the U.S. Government and the World Bank.

**Ronald E. Beller** has been the president of East Tennessee State University since September 1980. His previous experience includes senior administrative and teaching responsibilities at Virginia Commonwealth University, the University of South Alabama, and the University of Florida. He has authored several articles appearing in both business and medical publications and has conducted sponsored studies and projects for the U.S. Department of Health, Education, and Welfare; the Association of American Medical Colleges; and the Department of Housing and Urban Development. Dr. Beller is active in community affairs including service as an officer and director on the local boards of the United Way, Salvation Army, and Chamber of Commerce.

**Otis R. Bowen** is a former governor of the State of Indiana. He was elected to the Indiana House of Representatives where he served in the 1957 and 1958 sessions. He was re-elected to the House in 1960. In 1965, he was selected by his Republican colleagues as Minority Leader for the 1965 and 1966 sessions and then was elevated to the position of Speaker where he served three terms until his election as Governor. He currently serves as Chairman of the Advisory Council on Social Security to President Reagan. He is also a member of the Advisory Council of the United Student Aid Fund. In addition, he is a member of the Two-Year Study of Nursing and Nursing Education, Institute of Medicine of the National Academy of Sciences. He has received 19 honorary doctorates from Indiana colleges and universities.

**Leonard E. Braitman** is the Associate Editor of *Annuals of Internal Medicine*. He received his M.A. in Mathematics from Temple University and his Ph.D. in Medical Sociology from the University of Chicago. Dr. Braitman has served as Instructor of Sociology at Rush College of Nursing and Rush College of Medicine in Chicago. He has also taught statistics and research methods at Temple University. He has done consulting work for Campbell Soup Company and for the Temple University Department of Medicine and has co-authored several publications on nutrition.

**Thomas R. Burke** is Special Assistant to the Administrator of the Health Care Financing Administration, Department of Health and Human Services. He has also served as Executive Director of the Advisory Council on Social Security for the Department of Health and Human Services. Previously he served in numerous different health positions in the Office of the Assistant Secretary of Defense, including Deputy Director for Health Planning and Director for Policy Analysis. In 1978, Mr. Burke was a member of the White House Staff that prepared the President's Report on International Health. Prior to his service with the Department of Defense, Mr. Burke was Senior Health Economist on the Health Services Industry Committee and the Health Industry Advisory Committee of the Cost of Living Council during the Economic Stabilization Program.

**Carolyne K. Davis** is the Administrator of the Health Care Financing Administration (HCFA), Department of Health and Human Services. Dr. Davis oversees the functions of the Medicare and Medicaid programs, which help to finance health care services for nearly 50 million poor, elderly and disabled Americans. Prior to coming to HCFA, Dr. Davis was Associate Vice-President for the Academic Affairs at the University of Michigan. As such, she was responsible for coordinating the activities of Michigan's five health science schools. In addition, she chaired the university's hospital cost containment committee. During this time, Dr. Davis also served on the Board of Trustees of the Johns Hopkins University. Previously, she was Dean of the School of Nursing at Michigan while holding professorships in both nursing and education. Earlier, she chaired the Baccalaureate Nursing Program at Syracuse University.

**Paul F. Detrick** has been the President of Christian Health Services Development Corporation in St. Louis, Missouri since 1981. Christian Health Services Development Corporation is the first hospital in the St. Louis area to undergo corporate reorganization. The parent company has six subsidiaries, one of which is the hospital. Mr. Detrick is also the President of three of the corporate subsidiaries. Prior to his current position, Mr. Detrick was Chief Executive Officer of Christian Hospitals since 1960. He has also served as a hospital consultant with Hewitt & Royer, Inc., hospital architects in Kansas City, Missouri and Arkansas City Memorial Hospital. Mr. Detrick was recently honored by the Missouri Hospital Association with the awarding of their Distinguished Service Award for 1983.

**Jaime Rivera Dueno** is the former Secretary of Health of the Commonwealth of Puerto Rico. He graduated as a physician from the School of Medicine of Puerto Rico and became a pediatrician at the University Hospital in Puerto Rico. Since 1966, he has devoted his professional life to the public service in different capacities. Among other roles he has been Assistant Professor in Pediatrics at the Puerto Rico School of Medicine, assistant Secretary for Maternal and Child Health Services, under Secretary of Health, Regional Health Administrator of the Public Health Service, Region II, in New York, and Director of the Department of Health of San Juan, Puerto Rico. He has also served on different committees at the state and federal levels, on various governor's committees, on the Children's Commission and on the Child Development Committee of the National Academy of Sciences in Washington, D.C.

**Reinaldo A. Ferrer** is a health care consultant based in Puerto Rico. He has held positions in health care research and administration in Puerto Rico, including Deputy Secretary of Health. Dr. Ferrer has also served as Associate Director for Medical Care, Department of Health, Washington, Associate Director for Professional and Academic Affairs, Beth Israel Medical Center and Commissioner of Health of the City of New York. Dr. Ferrer is a founding member of Puerto Rico's Society of Hospitals and Health Services Administrators, former Rockefeller Foundation Travel Fellow and has teaching appointments from Mount Sinai School of Medicine and School of Public Health, Columbia University, New York. He served as consultant to the Pan American Health Organization, Ministry of Health, Jamaica, West Indies and is consultant to the Job Corps Program, U.S. Department of Labor.

**Frank W. Fournier** is currently Executive Director, Seguros de Servicio de Salud de Puerto Rico, Inc. He received his training from the University of Puerto Rico, Inter American University of Puerto Rico, and the Wharton School of Finance. Mr. Fournier is a member of the Puerto Rico Bar Association and the Puerto Rico Medical Association. He is the Director of the Puerto Rico Chamber of Commerce, Director of the Spanish Chamber of Commerce, President of the State Health Coordinating Committee, and on the Board of Directors, Puerto Rico Life Guaranty Association. He was selected as Outstanding Citizen of 1983 by the Puerto Rico Products Association and was selected among the 20 most outstanding citizens of the last 20 years by the Jaycees of Puerto Rico. Mr. Fournier has also served as President for the Fund Raising Campaign for the Crippled Children's Association, Easter Seals.

**Lewis Freiberg** is an Associate Professor of Economics at Northeastern Illinois University in Chicago. Dr. Freiberg held faculty positions at Morehead State University and Kentucky State University until 1976 when he joined the National Association of Blue Shield Plans as Research Economist. From 1978 to 1982 he served as Director of Economic Research for the merged Blue Cross and Blue Shield Associations. He currently serves as a Director of the Arlington Heights Federal Savings and Loan Association. In addition, he is an adjunct Professor at the Lake Forest School of Management and heads his own consulting firm. He has published in the areas of medical economics, regional economics, public finance, and the economics of financial institutions. Dr. Freiberg's current research interests include the allocative functioning of medical markets-agency relationships, direct regulation, and the achievement of efficiency.

**Helmuth Jung** is a consultant for Health Care Services and Welfare Institutions. He serves hospitals, welfare institutions, and political and labor organizations. Dr. Jung is a specialist in organizational development. He has previously taught at the Freie Universitat Berlin, the Verwaltungsakademie Berlin, and the Ev. Fachhochschule fur Sozialarbeit und Sozialpadagogik giving lectures in economics, social politics, and hospital administrations. Dr. Jung was Wissenschaftlicher Assistent at the Osteuropa-Institut at the Freie Universitat Berlin. His research focused on social affairs and health economic analysis of east European countries, especially of the German Democratic Republic.

**John P. Kemph** is Vice President for Academic Affairs and Dean of the School of Medicine at the Medical College of Ohio in Toledo. He has previously served on the faculty of Ohio State University, the University of Michigan, the State University of New York Downstate Medical Center, and the Medical College of Ohio in Toledo. His professional orientation is eclectic in Psychiatry and Child Psychiatry with a major emphasis on physiological aspects of the central nervous system function. While serving as a faculty member in four institutions, Dr. Kemph has held administrative positions and directed laboratories and programs throughout his professional career.

**R. Kenneth McGeorge** is currently the Chief Executive Officer of the Queen's University Faculty of Medicine. He has, in the past 15 years, held a number of administrative positions in the health field with increasing responsibilities. He has worked in community hospitals as well as teaching hospitals. Mr. McGeorge has spent five years on the Board of Directors of the Canadian College of Health Service Executives. He has held lectureship positions at Dalhousie University and Queen's University Faculties of Medicine. He is the author of many articles ranging from metric conversion to case mix management. In addition to his current position he is a member of the Executive Committees of the Ontario Hospital Association and the Ontario Council of Administrators of Teaching Hospitals.

**Richard C. McKibbin** is the Director of Policy Analysis for the American Nurses' Association where he is responsible for economic and manpower policy analysis, projects, reports, and programs, analysis of federal legislation and policies which affect health care and nursing, and economic consultation services to association executives, staff and officials. He has published and appeared extensively on programs dealing with the economics of health, and is on the editorial board of a major health journal. He has been listed in *Who's Who in Health Care*, *Who's Who in Wichita*, and *American Men and Women of Science*.

**P. Donald Muhlenthaler** is presently the Administrator of Marion General Hospital in Ohio. He has previously served as Executive Director of Dearborn County Hospital; Administrator, Walters Hospital; and Assistant Administrator, Mercer Medical Center. Mr. Muhlenthaler is a Fellow in the American College of Hospital Administrators. He is a past member of the Cincinnati Hospital Council Board of Trustees; the Indiana Hospital Association Government Relations Committee; and the Southern Indiana Health Systems Agency Board of Trustees. He is also a past member of the Lawrenceburg/Greendale Chamber of Commerce.

**Stephen M. Patz** is Executive Vice President and Chief Operating Officer for Cooper Hospital/University Medical Center in Camden, New Jersey. Past positions include Associate Administrator of Sinai Hospital in Detroit and Vice President of Lancaster General Hospital. Mr. Patz is a fellow in the American College of Hospital Administrators and has authored four articles.

**Pamela Paul-Shaheen** is Division Chief of Policy and Planning at the Michigan Department of Public Health. She was previously Division Chief, Office of Local Health Services, Michigan Department of Public Health; Health Policy Analyst, Michigan House of Representatives, Democratic Research Staff; Director, ECHO Program, Flint/Genesee County Health Department, Flint, Michigan; and Social Research Analyst, Michigan Center for Health Statistics, Michigan Department of Public Health. She is a specialist in health care cost containment, including the drafting of related legislation. Her experience includes extensive liaison work between the legislature and public health agencies. She has been involved in public health strategic planning for eight years.

**Richard W. Rahn** joined the Chamber of Commerce of the United States on February 1, 1980, as Vice President and Chief Economist. He also holds the positions of Director and Vice President of the National Chamber Foundation. Prior to joining the Chamber staff, Dr. Rahn served as Executive Director of the American Council for Capital Formation, and Chief Executive Officer of the American Council for Capital Formation: Center for Policy Research. Specializing in economic and tax policy issues, Dr. Rahn has addressed many professional, business, academic and civic groups. He is a frequent guest commentator on tax and economic issues on national radio and television, and has frequently testified before various Congressional committees.

**Edward P. Robinson** is the first and only Administrator and the Executive Director of the Community Hospital in Munster, Indiana, where he has been since 1966. Previously, Mr. Robinson was the Administrator for Gottlieb Memorial Hospital, the Assistant Administrator for Louis A. Weiss Memorial Hospital, and the Assistant Administrator for Western Pennsylvania Hospital. He has served as a member of the Board of Trustees for the State of Indiana Medical and Nursing Distribution Loan Fund and as a member of the Board of Directors for Hospice of Northwest Indiana.

**Jesus M. Rodriguez** has, over the last 30 years, held administrative posts in Puerto Rico's Health Delivery System. He is presently Executive Director of the Industrial Hospital of the Puerto Rico Medical Center Complex. A graduate of Columbia University's Master's Degree Program in Hospital Administration Science, Mr. Rodriguez was a founder and past president of the Puerto Rico Hospital Administrators Association and a member of the Council of Regents of the American College of Hospital Administrators. He is a member of the Faculty of the Health and Administrative Medicine Program of the University of Puerto Rico.

**Carlos Romero-Barceló** is the former governor of Puerto Rico. He was elected in 1977 and was re-elected in 1980; the first governor of Puerto Rico to be re-elected since 1960. Mr. Romero-Barceló served as Mayor of San Juan for eight years. He was co-founder of the New Progressive Party of Puerto Rico and was elected Party Vice-President in 1971 and President in 1974. He has also served on the Board of Directors of the United States Conference of Mayors, and was 1975 President of the National League of Cities, the first Hispanic ever elected to the NLC presidency. His memberships include the National Governors' Association, Southern Governors' Association, of which he was chairman 1980-1981, and the Council on Foreign Relations.

**Michael D. Rosko** is an Associate Professor in the Graduate Program in Health and Medical Services Administration of Widener University. He has been a faculty member at Widener University since 1975. His previous teaching position was at Stockton State College. He is a specialist in health economics, prospective payment systems, program evaluation, and health care marketing. He is the author of over 20 papers, including empirical analysis of the New Jersey prospective payment system and qualitative analysis of the Medicare prospective payment system.

**Marta C. Silverberg** is Assistant Vice President of Cooper Hospital/University Medical Center in Camden, New Jersey. Ms. Silverberg has taught at Temple University and Glassboro State College. She was instrumental in increasing the number of deliveries at Cooper Hospital which at the time was declining. She has successfully obtained state and federal grants for maternal and child health care and implemented a management by objectives program within her areas of responsibilities. Ms. Silverberg also wrote a major Certificate of Need to establish the Southern New Jersey Regional Perinatal Center.

338

**Gloria R. Smith** is the Director of the Michigan Department of Public Health. Dr. Smith has been Dean and Professor at the University of Oklahoma College of Nursing, a Medicare nurse consultant, a district nurse supervisor and a senior public health nurse. She is a member of the Board of Directors of the National League for Nursing and the Midwest Alliance for Nursing. Dr. Smith has been a consultant to the U.S. Department of Health, Education, and Welfare, the Veterans Administration Hospital, the University of Michigan School of Nursing and Federal Government of Nigeria. She is the author of numerous articles presented at a wide variety of universities, national professional organizations and symposiums, principally in the areas of public health, health care policy and strategy, ethnicity, and affirmative action. She has received many awards for leadership in education and in nursing.

**Lyndsey Stone** is Vice President of Operations and Nursing Administration at Presbyterian Hospital and adjunct Professor of Nursing at the University of Oklahoma College of Nursing. He has a total of 40 years experience working in clinical nursing and nursing administration, including 22 years of duty with the U.S. Army Nurse Corp attaining the rank of colonel. His former positions include Chief, Department of Nursing, Hawley Army Hospital, Indianapolis; Assistant Chief Nurse, U.S. Army Hospital, Fort Carson, Colorado Springs; Chief Nurse, 24th Evacuation Hospital, Republic of Viet Nam; and Chief Nurse, 7th Army and 7th Medical Brigade, Europe.

**Albert R. Tama** is the Executive Vice President for Medical Affairs at Cooper Hospital/University Medical Center in Camden, New Jersey. Dr. Tama received his M.D. from Hahnemann Medical College in Philadelphia where he completed his residency in Obstetrics and Gynecology. He served as an Assistant Professor at Hahnemann, and at Jefferson Medical College with responsibilities in the education of residents as well as outpatient service administration. Dr. Tama served as Acting Chief, Department of Obstetrics and Gynecology and Medical Director of the Women's Care Center at Cooper Hospital/University Medical Center from 1981 to 1983 and provided the clinical direction for the Adolescent Pregnancy Program.

339

**Malcolm Gordon Taylor** is Professor of Administrative Studies at York University in Toronto, Canada. He has also been the Hannah Lecturer of the Hannah Institute for the History of Medicine; First President, University of Victoria; First Principal, University of Alberta; and Professor, University of Toronto. Professor Taylor has served as advisor to the Ontario Education Communications Authority; Research Consultant, Health Services Review; President, Canadian Society for Higher Education; Chairman, National Manpower Council; Chairman, National Committee on Education and Manpower for the Social Services. His books on Canadian health insurance and public policy are considered by many to be the best in the field.

**Kytja K.S. Voeller** is the Division Chief of Pediatric Neurology at the Medical College of Ohio in Toledo. She received her M.D. degree from Columbia University, College of Physicians and Surgeons. She is board certified in both Pediatrics and Neurology, with special competence in Child Neurology. Faculty appointments have been held at the State University of New York, Downstate Medical Center, and Columbia University. Since 1975, she has been on the faculty of the Medical College of Ohio and established the Division of Pediatric Neurology. Dr. Voeller has a special interest in the application of modern management techniques to the delivery of health care, particularly within the context of medical education.

**Susan Weiss Wallner** is the Administrative Director for Medical Affairs at Cooper Hospital/University Medical Center in Camden, New Jersey. She received her M.A. in Psychology from Pacific Lutheran University in Washington. Mrs. Wallner has developed an innovative, hospital-based adolescent pregnancy program providing high quality, comprehensive care to the pregnant adolescent as well as to her family members, while emphasizing continuity of care through the pregnancy and first postpartum year. In addition, she has practiced as a psychologist in both outpatient and residential settings and has taught psychology at the college level.

**William J. Winston** is currently Dean, School of Health Services Management and Assistant Professor of Management, Golden Gate University, San Francisco. He is the Editor of *Health Marketing Quarterly*, The Haworth Press, New York, and Managing Associate, Professional Services Marketing Group, Health Marketing Consulting Firm, San Francisco. Formerly, Mr. Winston was Principal at Business Economics Development Institute. Graduate education was completed at the Johns Hopkins University, Baltimore, Maryland, in Health Administration and Planning. His major instructional areas are economic analysis and marketing strategy development for health services organizations.

**Charles Wood** is the President of the Foundation of the Massachusetts Eye and Ear Infirmary in Boston. His hospital management career began at Roanoke Memorial Hospital where he was an Administrative Resident and then Assistant Administrator. His 30-year career with the Massachusetts Eye and Ear Infirmary began in 1955 when he assumed the position of Assistant Director. In 1963 he was promoted to Associate Director and in 1966 was named General Director of the Infirmary. In 1964, Mr. Wood became a Fellow of the American College of Hospital Administrators. He has served as President of the New England Hospital Assembly, chairman of the Massachusetts Hospital Association and was on the Regional Advisory Board of the American Hospital Association. Mr. Wood lectures on the benefits of cost containment and reimbursement methods for health care facilities.